Nutritional Epidemiology of Breast Cancer

Alvaro Luis Ronco • Eduardo De Stéfani

Nutritional Epidemiology of Breast Cancer

Springer

Alvaro Luis Ronco
IUCLAEH School of Medicine
Department of Epidemiology
and Scientific Methods
Convención 1490 dep. 202
11100 Montevideo
Uruguay
alronco@gmail.com

Eduardo De Stéfani
School of Medicine
Department of Pathology
Epidemiology Group
Universidad de la República
Av. Brasil 3080 dep. 402
11300 Montevideo
Uruguay
edestefani@gmail.com

ISBN 978-94-007-2396-2 e-ISBN 978-94-007-2397-9
DOI 10.1007/978-94-007-2397-9
Springer Dordrecht Heidelberg London New York

Library of Congress Control Number: 2011939191

Printed on acid-free paper

Springer is part of Springer Science+Business Media (www.springer.com)

Preface

Since several decades ago, breast cancer has been recognized as the most frequent malignant tumour among women in the world. Although it is an extremely known and frequent health problem in developed societies it has been recently emerging as a new situation in developing countries. These latter have witnessed a sustained translocation of cervical cancer moving downward from the first place in their cancer rankings while breast cancer aroused firmly to the top. Such changes have usually taken place together with the positive evolution of certain indicators of human development. Breast cancer is a polygenic and multifactorial disease for which estrogens have been recognized as the main risk factor, and for which lifestyle plays a key role.

From the beginning of our epidemiologic research on breast cancer next to two decades ago up to now, we still believe like then that the disease constitutes a major intellectual challenge of oncology. It is so in all its features, from the molecular and biological ones, through the clinical ones such as its diagnosis and therapy up to the prevention. Why? Because breast cancer, which is a complex hormonal, metabolic and immune problem, does not offer the possibility of a simple diagnosis like a cancer of the cervix uteri, nor a preventive strategy can be so efficient as smoking ceasing is for prevention of lung cancer. Breast cancer is much more complex than that. Perhaps we only are in the way towards better solutions to the problem.

Breast cancer is an essentially preventable tumour, through the different ways that prevention can be developed. Although secondary prevention or screening is currently the accepted way to impact on mortality due to diagnosis of early and even non-palpable tumours, primary prevention has begun lately to emerge as a useful tool to face the problem. Primary prevention attempts to reduce the incidence of the disease through a reduction in the exposure to risk factors, through an increase in exposure to protective factors, or both combined. The risk reduction through influencing on dietary factors could reach a base of 30–35%, which is non-negligible and could overcome a 60% when including body composition, physical activity, metabolic diseases such as insulin resistance, hypovitaminosis D, diabetes and also psychosocial stress. What we are proposing to do in primary prevention is mainly a quantitative and qualitative change in the bioavailability and exposure to estrogens.

Epidemiologic case-control studies on nutrition and breast cancer carried out in Uruguay since 1994 to the present time, allowed us to explore and identify the main risk and protective factors for the disease in this country. Research has been performed at institutions within the frame of public hospitals as well as of the pre-paid healthcare system, something that enabled us to be highly comprehensive regarding the local population at risk. Albeit in a small scale but mostly original, the papers generated by our research group have seen the light mainly through international specialized journals. Furthermore, a few years ago the National Academy of Medicine of Uruguay awarded our monography entitled "Epidemiología Nutricional del Cáncer de Mama" with a national Prize – which derived in the publication of a limited edition of a book in Spanish –. This was a new step given by our team. The logic satisfaction that it has meant for us is now followed by the publication of the present updated, expanded and improved international edition by Springer Publishers, due to which we feel highly encouraged and it probably represents a hallmark in our personal and collective research careers.

We believe that this technical material, supported by several hundreds of updated bibliographic references, will be certainly useful for all those who are interested in the area. Whether the book somehow contributes in expanding the knowledge and view of the disease among health professionals – from the prevention to the treatment fields –, our effort will have been worthwhile.

The editors

Contents

Chapter 1
General Epidemiology of Breast Cancer

Breast cancer (BC) in women is a major health burden worldwide. It is the most frequent cause of cancer among women in both developed and undeveloped societies (Fig. 1.1), and is responsible for more than one million of the estimated 10 million of cancers diagnosed worldwide each year in both sexes [1]. It is also the primary cause of cancer death among women globally, responsible for 23% of the total new cancer cases and 14% (458.400) of the total cancer deaths in 2008 [2].

Figure 1.2 shows the geographical variation in BC incidence worldwide, as estimated for the year 2008. The highest incidence rates occur in Northern and Western Europe, North America, Australia and New Zealand, Israel and in Southern Latin American are two exceptions: Uruguay and Argentina. According to GLOBOCAN [2], the incidence age-adjusted rate in the more developed areas is currently 66.4/100.000 women compared to 27.3/100.000 in the less developed areas. Also mortality is higher in the developed societies, when it is compared to the one in the less developed countries: 15.3/100.000 vs. 10.8/100.000 respectively. Cancer survival tends to be poorer in developing countries, most likely because of a combination of a late stage at diagnosis and limited access to timely and standard treatment [3].

Although BC is still a major public health issue in developed societies, its incidence has been rising in several developing countries over the past few years. International data [1] indicate that Uruguay is among those with the highest rates in the world. Furthermore, its capital city, Montevideo, displays the highest incidence rate for a city until new data are published. Albeit Uruguay is a South American developing country, it shares some features of developed societies, i.e. a very high level of red meat consumption [4], a high human development index (50° in the world ranking according to United Nations, by factors as birth rate, infant mortality, life expectancy, literacy among others) [5] and an aged population [6]. In other words, a developing country has displayed a high occurrence of a disease typical of developed countries. The fact that the above quoted countries are cattle producers and high meat consumers might not be a coincidence: Uruguay is the country with the highest beef per capita intake in the world [7].

Being a developed country is not mandatory for having high incidence rates: Japan, for example, has lower rates than the quoted countries from Northern hemisphere.

A.L. Ronco and E. De Stéfani, *Nutritional Epidemiology of Breast Cancer*,
DOI 10.1007/978-94-007-2397-9_1, © Springer Science+Business Media B.V. 2012

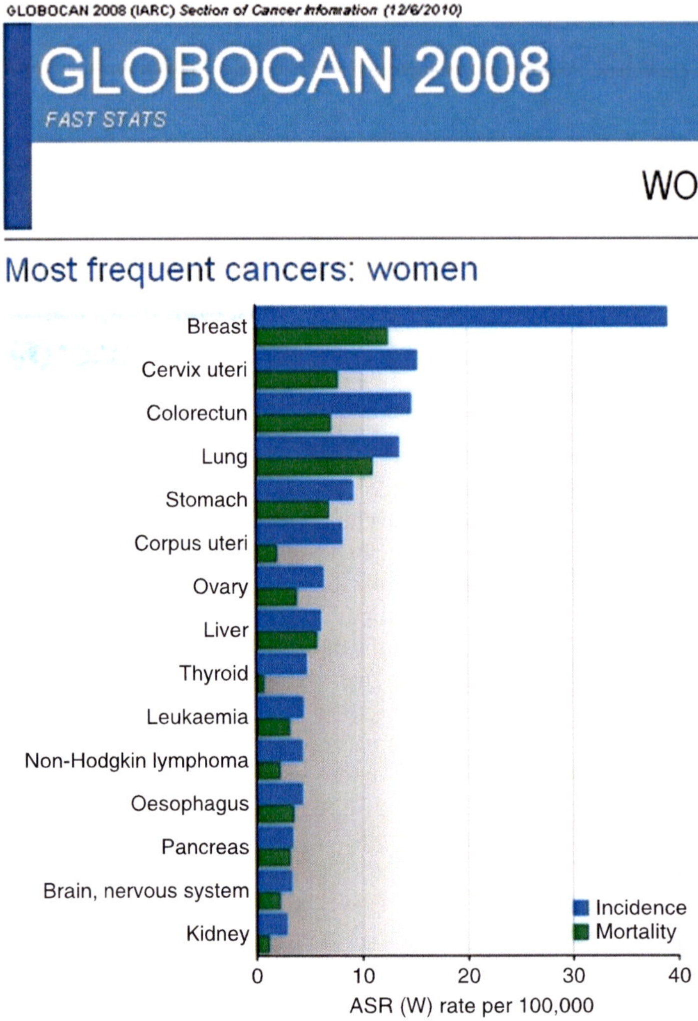

Fig. 1.1 Bar graphics showing the incidence of female cancers in the world

Conversely, countries as Uruguay and Argentina have shown higher rates in the region than in the rest of the Latin American developing countries.

As a result of the 'westernisation' of lifestyles (change of habits, stronger urbanization, increase of educational levels) the occurrence of BC increases. The incidence ranking of the last years has notably changed, due to the rise. The most rapid rises have been seen in developing countries, including some of them which belonged to the former Soviet Union and some other underdeveloped ones, where BC risk has historically been low relative to industrialised societies [8]. Urbanization implies an

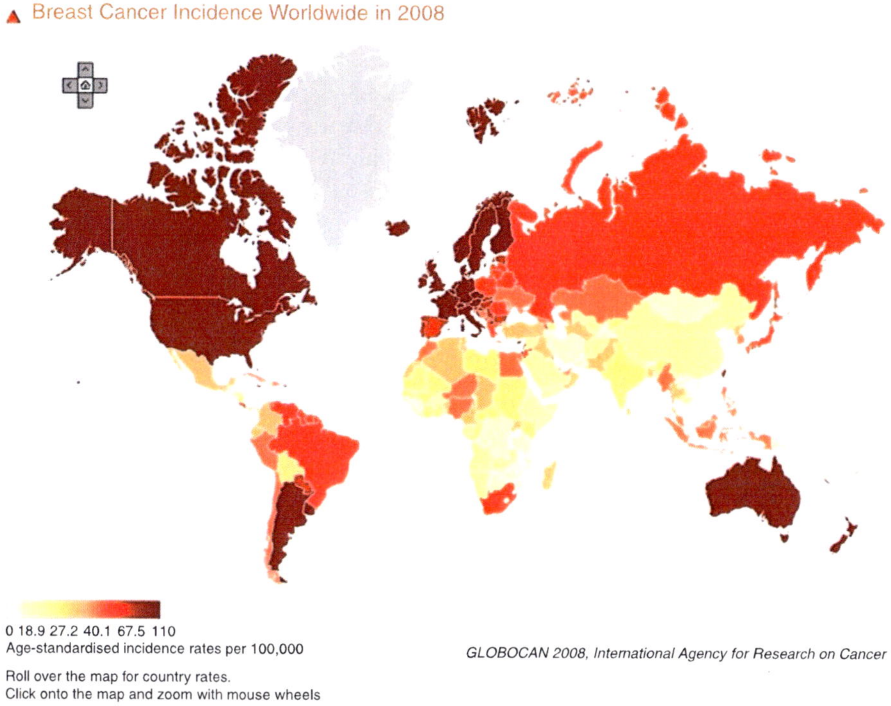

Fig. 1.2 Breast cancer incidence worldwide: age-standardised rates (world population) (Source: Ref. [2])

increase in job types that are less active than rural ones: outdoor jobs performed by women, regardless of their conditions, are associated with high caloric- and fast-foods and this is favourable for the development of health problems such as excess weight and obesity. Also psychosocial stress might play a role [9], albeit it can be difficult to quantify. Higher educational levels correspond to a reduction in the average number of pregnancies and births, an increase of age at the first birth, as well as reduced times of breastfeeding.

Therefore, as a consequence of changing exposures to reproductive and nutrition-related determinants over time, it should be recognized that women are at increasingly high risk of BC in most regions of the world during the past few decades [8]. The most severely affected women from developing countries, at least within the Latin America region, are those who belong to the mid-to-high socioeconomic and cultural classes and who accumulate menstrual and reproductive risk factors with some environmental ones. Due to such socio-economic and environmental factors, we have recognized that these women belong to a "first world" within the third world [10], in other words, women have been acquiring a profile which is closer to that of women in industrialized countries. Additionally, an increased screening intensity can explain partially the quoted rise in incidence [11].

Risk Factors

Estrogens were recognized five decades ago as the main risk factor for developing BC [12]. Currently, the importance of other risk factors different from the classic ones (menstrual and reproductive factors and family history of cancer) has been somehow underestimated until few years ago, in our opinion. In general, the high rates of BC in developed societies are a consequence of a higher prevalence of the known "classic" risk factors for the disease, many of which – early age at menarche, nulliparity, late age at first birth, late age at any birth, low parity, and late menopause – relate to the hormonal (specially estrogen) milieu to which the breast is exposed from menarche to the cessation of ovulation at menopause [13].

Previous knowledge on classic risk factors (menstrual-reproductive history and family history) has led to the idea that women who have been exposed for a longer time period or more intensely to endogenous estrogens will have an increased risk of BC. However, scientific research has demonstrated that diet, fat excess and a low level of physical activity can also strongly affect the hormonal production and availability, independently from having or not any of the quoted "classic" risk factors [14, 15]. The higher parity and earlier age at first pregnancy of women seen in many developing countries might account for part of the lower incidence of BC in these regions relative to developed countries. The greater risk for women from affluent (developed) backgrounds is, however, outweighed by their lower mortality. On the other hand, women from deprived backgrounds often present more advanced stages of the disease, and this applies not only to BC but cancers in general [3].

Exposure to exogenous hormones as oral contraceptives [16] and hormone replacement therapy [17] result in an increase in the risk of BC. Incidence rates in some of the developed countries, including the United States, United Kingdom, France, and Australia, sharply decreased from the beginning of the current century, in part due to a lower use of combined postmenopausal hormone therapy [18–22]. On the contrary, BC mortality rates have been decreasing in North America and several European countries over the past 25 years, largely as a result of early detection through mammography and improved treatment [11, 23, 24].

Excessive alcohol intake also seems to increase risk, with a recent re-analysis of 53 studies indicating that about 4% of BCs in developed countries might be attributable to its consumption [25]. The accompanying evidence on exposure to endogenous and exogenous oestrogen indicates that the lifetime length of exposure to endogenous oestrogen has been increasing, which is consistent with upward trends in incidence of BC, particularly in developed countries.

The changing patterns of childbearing and breastfeeding, of exogenous hormonal intake and of dietary factors including obesity and reduced physical activity have certainly contributed to trends in incidence and mortality. Currently, the experts suggest that maintaining a healthy body weight, increasing physical activity, and minimizing alcohol intake are the best available strategies to reduce the risk of developing BC [26]. Early detection through mammography has been shown to increase treatment options and at the same time to save lives, although this approach is not feasible in most economically developing countries due to its costs [27]. Recommended early detection strategies in these countries include the promotion of awareness of early signs and symptoms and screening by clinical breast examination [28]. The recognition that several particular factors have contributed to the incidence of BC in different populations worldwide has meant a major challenge. The underlying reasons are multiple and interactive. The analysis of the possible role of nutrition as an indicator of the major factor, lifestyle, and its relationships with BC is the main purpose of this book, since this information has potential impact on public health.

References

1. Parkin DM, Whelan SL, Ferlay J, Teppo L et al (eds) (2002) Cancer incidence in five continents, vol VIII, IARC Scientific Publications No. 155. IARC, Lyon
2. Ferlay J, Shin HR, Bray F, et al (2010) GLOBOCAN 2008, Cancer incidence and mortality worldwide: IARC CancerBase no 10. International Agency for Research on Cancer, Lyon. Available at: http://globocan.iarc.fr. Accessed 17 Aug 2010
3. Jemal A, Bray F, Center MM et al (2011) Global cancer statistics. Ca Cancer J Clin. doi:10.3322/caac.20107
4. Food and Agricultural Organization (2010) http://faostat.fao.org/site/610/DesktopDefault.aspx? PageID=610#ancor. Accessed 30 April 2010
5. United Nations Organization, Program of Human Development (2010) Human development index rankings. Available at: http://hdr.undp.org/en/statistics/;2009. Accessed 27 April 2010
6. U.S. Census Bureau (2010) International data base, http://www.census.gov/ipc/www/idb/country.php. Accessed 30 April 2010
7. Matos E, Brandani A (2002) Review on meat consumption and cancer in South America. Mutat Res 506–507:243–249
8. Bray F, Mc Carron P, Parkin DM (2004) The changing global patterns of female breast cancer incidence and mortality. Breast Cancer Res 6:229–239
9. Ronco AL, Silveira S, De Stéfani E et al (2007) Factores socioculturales y psicológicos y cáncer de mama: un estudio caso-control en Montevideo, Uruguay. Biomedicina 3(1):6–17
10. Ronco AL, De Stéfani E, Stoll M (2010) Hormonal and metabolic modulation through nutrition: towards a primary prevention of breast cancer. Breast 19:322–332
11. Althuis MD, Dozier JD, Anderson WF et al (2005) Global trends in breast cancer incidence and mortality 1973–1997. Int J Epidemiol 34:405–412
12. MacMahon B, Feinleib M (1960) Breast cancer in relation to nursing and menopausal history. J Natl Cancer Inst 24:733–753
13. Pike MC, Krailo MD, Henderson BE et al (1983) 'Hormonal' risk factors, 'breast tissue age' and the age-incidence of breast cancer. Nature 303:767–770
14. Hanf V, Gonder U (2005) Nutrition and primary prevention of breast cancer: foods, nutrients and breast cancer risk. Eur J Obstet Gynecol Reprod Biol 123:139–149
15. Duncan AM (2004) The role of nutrition in the prevention of breast cancer. AACN Clin Issues 15:119–135
16. Collaborative Group on Hormonal Factors in Breast Cancer (1996) Breast cancer and hormonal contraceptives: collaborative reanalysis of individual data on 53 297 women with breast cancer and 100 239 women without breast cancer from 54 epidemiological studies. Lancet 347:1713–1727
17. Beral V (2003) Breast cancer and hormone-replacement therapy in the million women study. Lancet 362:419–427

18. Ravdin PM, Cronin KA, Howlader N et al (2007) The decrease in breast-cancer incidence in 2003 in the United States. N Engl J Med 356:1670–1674
19. Cronin KA, Ravdin PM, Edwards BK (2009) Sustained lower rates of breast cancer in the United States. Breast Cancer Res Treat 117:223–224
20. Parkin DM (2009) Is the recent fall in incidence of post-menopausal breast cancer in UK related to changes in use of hormone replacement therapy? Eur J Cancer 45:1649–1653
21. Seradour B, Allemand H, Weill A et al (2009) Changes by age in breast cancer incidence, mammography screening and hormone therapy use in France from 2000 to 2006. Bull Cancer 96:E1–E6
22. Canfell K, Banks E, Moa AM et al (2008) Decrease in breast cancer incidence following a rapid fall in use of hormone replacement therapy in Australia. Med J Aust 188:641–644
23. Jemal A, Center MM, Desantis C et al (2010) Global patterns of cancer incidence and mortality rates and trends. Cancer Epidemiol Biomarkers Prev 19:1893–1907
24. Autier P, Boniol M, La Vecchia C et al (2010) Disparities in breast cancer mortality trends between 30 European countries: retrospective trend analysis of WHO mortality database. BMJ 341:c3620
25. Hamajima N, Hirose K, Tajima K et al (2002) Alcohol, tobacco and breast cancer – collaborative reanalysis of individual data from 53 epidemiological studies, including 58,515 women with breast cancer and 95,067 women without the disease. Br J Cancer 87:1234–1245
26. Kushi LH, Byers T, Doyle C et al (2006) American Cancer Society Guidelines on Nutrition and Physical Activity for cancer prevention: reducing the risk of cancer with healthy food choices and physical activity. Ca Cancer J Clin 56:254–281, quiz 313–4
27. Anderson BO, Yip CH, Ramsey SD et al (2006) Breast cancer in limited-resource countries: health care systems and public policy. Breast J 12(Suppl 1):S54–S69
28. Anderson BO, Yip CH, Smith RA et al (2008) Guideline implementation for breast healthcare in low-income and middle-income countries: overview of the Breast Health Global Initiative Global Summit 2007. Cancer 113(8 Suppl):2221–2243

Part I
Current Knowledge

Chapter 2
Energy and Related Factors

In the preface of this book, BC was recognized as a complex hormonal, metabolic and immune problem. These areas combine themselves through "bridges" given by lifestyle. At the same time, we can simplify the concept of lifestyle, remarking what is the most important: nutrition (diet and anthropometry) and physical activity. These elements interact among themselves and the endocrine activity of ovaries and adipose tissue is modified by the influence of the former ones.

Anthropometric measures are considered to be linked with risk of BC. There is a parallelism among BC incidence, dietary caloric excesses and obesity. These latter are enhancers of endocrine and metabolic phenomena associated to the development of the disease. Whichever the factors were the conditioning ones, the resultant fact is **a frame of high levels of bioavailable estrogens all along the reproductive life and even after it**, in the case of postmenopausal women.

Growth and Menarche

The rates of growth and early development in women are partially determined by nutritional factors, within a range of genetic potential. Fast growth speeds lead to earlier ages of puberty, which is an accepted risk factor for BC. Fast growth and development are evidenced by higher heights in childhood as well as in adulthood.

Prospective studies examined nutritional factors in girls as potential predictors of age at menarche [1–3]. Items such as energy intake, total fat, saturated fat, proteins and other nutrients, and also some food groups like dairy, meats, legumes, vegetables among others were analyzed. No associations between among dietary factors previous to onset of menarche and its age were observed. One of the studies found a significant association of high fat intakes with an earlier menarche, taking into account body fat and physical activity levels. Results also described a later age for menarche in girls with higher sport activity.

A previous study had found that high meat intakes were associated with an earlier age at menarche [4]. An association between menarche with high level of energy

A.L. Ronco and E. De Stéfani, *Nutritional Epidemiology of Breast Cancer*,

DOI 10.1007/978-94-007-2397-9_2,

intake was found, when adjusting for body weight [5]. Besides, ecologic studies showed that a high-protein or a low-fibre diet was correlated with an earlier menarche [6]. Additionally, vegetarian girls experienced their menarche later [7]. Besides, whereas fat intake has increased, the average age of menarche has decreased along the last century [1]. Based on an analysis of several studies, Kelsey et al. [8] concluded that the earlier menarche is, is higher the risk of BC for a woman.

The thesis of a protective effect based on nutritional restrictions is based on a study about mortality of BC in Norwegian women, in particular in the cohort exposed to starve during the 2nd world war [9]. Those women who were exposed under such conditions during age of menarche had a lesser risk (−13%) for dying due to BC.

Although findings led to a possible role of diet in sexual maturation, the study could not discriminate on the possible roles of fat, meats, energy or other dietary features. Following a similar orientation, studies performed in the Netherlands and Scandinavian countries are consistent in supporting a modest association between height and risk of BC [10–12].

THERE IS CONVINCING EVIDENCE THAT A FAST GROWTH INCREASES THE RISK OF BREAST CANCER.

Caloric Restriction

Human and animal studies have given support for possible protective effects in the risk of BC of dietary energy restriction, through favourable changes in circulating levels of insulin, leptin, sex hormone binding globulin, insulin-like growth factor-1, estradiol, testosterone, reactive oxygen species, and the production and secretion of adipokines and inflammatory cytokines, that is, increased adiponectin and decreased interleukin-6 [13].

More than 70 years ago experimental observations on caloric restrictions in the diet of mice reported an increase of their life expectancy and a reduction of degenerative diseases and cancer, especially in the breast [14]. Through wide varieties of tumour models, the reduction of energy intake has substantially and consistently reduced the occurrence of mammary tumours [15], independently from the fat intake. Other study [16] showed a reduction of incidence of breast tumours through caloric restriction, also keeping constant the fat composition of diet, suggesting that reduction of BC probably involves other factors as a delay in the onset of menarche, since the incidence reduction included other tumour types. Nevertheless, an increase of risk (+ 48%) was also found in Dutch women who were severely exposed to the famine during the World War II compared to those who were not exposed [17].

Some benefits were achieved in primates through caloric reduction: increased insulin sensitivity, lower serum insulin levels and of some cytokines produced by adipose tissue, lower serum levels of total cholesterol and triglycerides, lower blood pressure and arterial stiffness, and a higher serum level of HDL cholesterol [18].

Investigations confirmed an improvement of maximal survival and of average life expectancy in similar proportions to the caloric reduction, also reporting a delay in the aging process followed by lesser number of cancer cases.

Restriction of calories by 10–40% has been shown to decrease cell proliferation, increasing apoptosis through anti-angiogenic processes [19]. In addition, reduced expressions of genes in the lipid metabolism and glycolytic pathways were recently reported as detectable in breast tissue following dietary energy restriction [20]. Mechanistic studies have shown that dietary energy restriction inhibits cell proliferation, creates a proapoptotic environment, and reduces blood vessel density adjacent to premalignant and malignant mammary pathologies [21].

Animal and human data suggest that intermittent energy restriction may have cancer preventative effects beyond that of chronic energy restriction and weight loss. It seemed that an intermittent caloric restriction (i.e. one day weekly) could be more efficient in the prevention of BC than the chronic caloric restriction, something which could have potential implications at the human level [13], for example on metabolic disease risk markers [22].

THE EVIDENCE SUGGESTS THAT INTERMITTENT ENERGY RESTRICTION HAS A PREVENTIVE EFFECT AGAINST THE RISK OF BREAST CANCER.

The Body Mass Index

The Body Mass Index (BMI) is a measure of relationship between height and weight, usually expressed by the formula: weight/height^2, in terms of kg/m^2. There is an internationally known range, which is the following:

< 18.5 kg/m^2 = malnourished
18.5–24.9 kg/m^2 = normal weight
25–29.9 kg/m^2 = overweight
>=30 kg/m^2 = obesity, which could be a morbid type (BMI>=40)

In the last years, the association between BMI and BC has been systematically examined in expert evaluations [23, 24]. The available data have shown a contrast: Heavier women have been found to be at increased risk of postmenopausal BC in most studies, whereas BMI is inversely associated with the risk of cancer among premenopausal [25–27] women. Recently, high weight and body fat in elder women were reported as an independent risk factor [28]. Also, fat-free mass has been found positively associated with the risk of BC in postmenopausal women [29]. Absence of association in premenopausal women has been also described for certain anthropometric measures (body size, BMI, fat distribution) in some populations such as Chinese [30, 31], Japanese [32], or African American women [33], different from what has been consistently described in the Western and Caucasian societies. Recently, waist-to-hip ratio was also associated with an increase of risk in premenopausal Nigerian [34] and Asian American women [35].

The BMI is highly correlated with body fat level, but it is very unspecific: even a highly muscled woman can have a BMI that is within overweight and that constitutes a mistake in itself. Furthermore, if an overweight person begins with an exercise plan with which he/she gains muscle mass and at the same time loses adiposity, it is likely that the weight increases and lead this person to think that he/she is not doing adequately the plan. Since muscle is more dense than fat (similar volumes of the former are heavier than the latter), the inner changes might not be expressed adequately by the weighing scale.

In spite of these limitations, BMI has been very popular and accepted in the epidemiologic research because it is known that it is strongly associated with the amount of body fat and at the same time is extremely practical to be done and easy to calculate. When we faced the study on the fat/muscle ratio [36] we realized that in fact, BMI was highly correlated with the calculated fat weight ($r=.67$) but we also found a strong correlation with muscle weight ($r=.57$), in both cases very significantly ($p<0.0001$). Hence, BMI does not discriminate well between both components, suggesting that muscle and fat effects might cancel each other out. Then we thought that perhaps the observations made in large populations indicating an inverse behaviour of BMI among pre- and postmenopausal women could reveal something: probably an elevated BMI reflects a high correlation with fat in older women (in whom fat mass occupies a higher fraction) and a high correlation with muscle mass in younger women (in whom muscle mass is a higher fraction). The same measure seems to indicate a risk effect among ones and a protective effect among others, but it could be that indirectly reflecting a different body composition.

A HIGH BODY MASS INDEX COULD INCREASE THE RISK OF BREAST CANCER, BUT THE EVIDENCE IS STILL NOT ENOUGH TO STATE IT CATEGORICALLY.

Body Mass and Menopausal Status

The associations between body mass and BC have been widely investigated. On one hand, as it was quoted above, some prospective studies have shown that the BMI was significantly and inversely associated with the risk of BC among premenopausal women [37], although with weak risks. On the other side, other studies showed that the current body weight and the weight gain were strong predictors of BC in postmenopausal women [38]. Lahmann et al. reported that in postmenopausal women not taking exogenous hormones, general obesity was a significant predictor of BC, while abdominal fat assessed as waist-hip ratio or waist circumference was not related to excess risk when adjusted for BMI [26]. In the same study, weight and BMI showed nonsignificant inverse associations with BC among premenopausal women. In this sense, the risk increases in women with low BMI at the end of adolescence and who had overweight during adulthood. The inverse situation is also valid, that is, a reduction of risk when in a 30 year period women moved from over to under median BMI [39].

Besides, other case-control studies have also found an association between obesity and increased risk of BC among postmenopausal women [40–42]. Few studies have found an increased risk association in both pre- and postmenopausal women [23, 43]. The available data suggest some type of interaction between BMI and menstrual status.

A review of some years ago recognized that some of these epidemiologic studies in postmenopausal women indicate a relatively higher risk for obese women than in other studies [44], but it is also evident that a clear cutpoint of BMI still does not appear and this latter cannot be managed as a fix international reference, since there is so much variability among populations as currently exist. It is obvious that morphologic differences between Anglo-Saxon and Hispanic women could turn inaccurate the same cutpoints of BMI: for example, "overweight" can be a very clear strip among the former ones and not so much in the latter.

Concerning the inverse relationship between body weight and risk of BC in premenopausal women (the higher BMI, the lesser risk and viceversa), the specialized literature hypothesized that it could be due to an effect of obesity on the anovulatory cycles. Less ovulatory cycles could be associated with a reduced risk of BC [45, 46] and obesity could derive into a state of frequent anovulation [47].

Regarding postmenopausal women, we will repeat again further in the present book that obesity can increase the risk of BC by changing the endogen estrogenic levels through a higher androgen aromatization. Adipose tissue does not have the capability of synthesizing hormones de novo, but in compensation it accounts for the appropriate biochemical machinery to transform circulating steroid hormones, particularly those produced at adrenal glands. More than 20 years ago, it was reported that premenopausal women from countries with caloric excesses (North America, some Western European countries) had higher hormonal levels compared to those of women from countries without caloric excesses, as rural Chinese women [48]. These differences were also observed in postmenopausal women: the more advanced was the age, the higher were such differences.

Particularly in the postmenopausal woman, from the moment of the permanent cessation of ovarian function, the estrogen synthesis will be produced mostly by adrenal glands and the adipose tissue. In the last two decades, it has been recognized that the adipose tissue, far from being only a compartment of fat reserves, is a functionally active organ. When it is exceeded in its fat content, the adipocytes produce pro-inflammatory cytokines, which stimulate the insulin resistance and promote the development of new vessels (pro-angiogenic), among other capabilities. The environment around the adipose tissue is unique in the sense that it offers a growth development for transformed cells, such as BC cells. In addition, adipose tissue is the only organ with an unlimited growth potential at any stage of human life. In order to accomodate the fat depots (mostly triglycerides) the adipocyte can increase its diameter up to 20 times, equivalent to a possible volume increase in hundreds of times.

A LARGER BODY MASS PROBABLY INCREASES THE RISK OF BREAST CANCER, BUT RESTRICTED TO THE POSTMENOPAUSE.

Weight Gain

Along the past decade, several studies have remarked that weight gain between adolescence and adult age is linked to BC. Having as base age 18 years old – the age in which the body development of a woman has the basic adult build-weight gain is generally associated with an increased risk of BC [38]. A double risk has been reported for a gain of 25 kg compared to those women that increased only 2 kg [49], although this was observed only among women who had not received hormones in the climacteric. An increase of 77% was observed in Uruguayan women of mid-to-high social classes who gained more than 12 kg between age 18 and adulthood, when compared to the lowest tertile (from weight loss up to 3 kg of weight gain) The studied subpopulations differ notably, since in around 2,000 patients recruited at public hospitals (where low social strata are admitted), weight gain does not keep association with the risk of BC [50].

Body fatness at young ages has a strong and independent inverse relation to BC risk throughout life [51]. We can state that in general there is an agreement about the fact that an important weight gain through adulthood is associated to a risk increase [52], apparently also the same among BRCA 1/2 mutation carriers [53, 54] and that the maintenance of a normal weight as well as the reduction of an overweight are associated to a reduction of BC risk. Talking about body weight, we are taking into account mainly the weight of body fat, which has been the major body component associated to the disease.

AN EXCESSIVE WEIGHT GAIN FROM THE ADOLESCENCE TO ADULTHOOD INCREASES THE RISK OF BREAST CANCER.

Central Obesity

There have been studies which examined regional adiposity (localized) and the risk of BC [55–59]. In these works – except for the Dutch study [58] – a positive association of central adiposity (abdominal, android type) with the risk of BC was found: the more adiposity, the higher the risk. Among premenopausal women the association was weaker although positive too. Several studies have shown an increased risk associated with fat distribution in the upper body parts [33, 55–57, 60–65]. Besides, more than three decades ago Levshin [66] had reported the usefulness of 14 anthropometric measurements and certain selected indexes in the study of BC. This author remarked then a positive association between obesity and BC in both extreme age groups (young women and elder women).

An upper or central distribution of body fat is associated to multiple metabolic and hormonal changes, including insulin resistance, hyperinsulinism, a reduction in SHBG (sexual hormone binding globulins) levels, increase in the androgens and increase of aromatization [67, 68]. Hence, international scientific literature – proceeding mostly from developed societies – recognizes that women having this body pattern which is associated to an increased risk of type II diabetes [69], blood hypertension and cardiovascular disease [70], can have a higher risk of BC and also a higher risk of endometrial cancer [71] than those women whose fat is mainly distributed in hips, buttocks and lower limbs. The global evidence seems to be in favour of this hypothesis, although the studied Uruguayan population does not fit entirely these patterns, according to a recent study on somatotype and risk of BC [72]. Anyway, since BC is a multifactorial disease, it is admissible that Western lifestyle may act on the incidence of the disease through an influence on body fat distribution and the resulting changes in sex hormones availability [73].

ABDOMINAL (CENTRAL) FAT ACCUMULATION HAS BEEN ASSOCIATED TO AN INCREASE OF RISK OF BREAST CANCER PREFERENTLY IN DEVELOPED SOCIETIES.

Physical Exercise

Analytic studies have investigated some aspects of the relationship physical activity – BC. The cohort studies have shown increased risks in non-athlete subjects compared with athletes [74], increased risk in women with low-physical activity occupations [75], and also the absence of association [76]. Case-control studies agreed with previous findings, in the sense of a reduction of BC risk associated to more physical activity [77], also taking into account the occupation mentioned in the death certificates and classified according to occupational physical activity [78]. Among women with a diagnosed and treated BC, it has been described as associated to a reduction of the recurrence risk and of mortality risk [79].

The plausible biologic mechanisms that account for the inhibitory effects of physical activity on the carcinogenic process are reduction in fat stores, activity related changes in sex-hormone levels [80], altered immune function i.e. in T lymphocytes and Natural Killers [81, 82], effects in insulin and insulin-like growth factors, reduced free radical generation, and direct effect on the tumour [19].

In response to muscle contraction, some cytokines called "myokines" [83, 84] such as Interleukin-6 [IL-6], IL-8, and IL-15 are produced. They can modulate the metabolic and immunological response to exercise in several tissues. After the release of IL-6 into the circulation, it works in a hormone-like fashion inducing lipolysis and fat oxidation. It mediates anti-inflammatory effects by stimulating the production of anti-inflammatory cytokines and by suppressing TNF-alpha production [85]. Some differences observed between normal and obese animals suggest that IL-15 may play an important role in the control of fat deposition in adipose tissue [86]. It is involved in the reciprocal metabolic regulation between adipose tissue and skeletal muscle. It stimulates muscle fibers to accumulate increased amounts of proteins [87], induces T-cell proliferation [82], enhances NK cell cytotoxicity [88], and protects these immune cells and neutrophils from apoptosis [89, 90]. Since two decades ago, animal experimentation has agreed with the facts observed in humans [91, 92], in the sense of a protective effect of exercise against BC.

Because physical activity, body size, and metabolic efficiency are highly related to total energy intake and expenditure, it is difficult to assess the independent effect of energy intake on cancer risk [93]. Caloric restriction and physical exercise seem to exert their effects on mammary carcinogenesis through distinct pathways [94].

IT IS ACCEPTED THAT PHYSICAL ACTIVITY PROBABLY REDUCES THE RISK OF BREAST CANCER, ESPECIALLY IN THE POSTMENOPAUSE.

References

1. Maclure M, Travis LB, Willett WC et al (1991) A prospective cohort study of nutrient intake and age at menarche. Am J Clin Nutr 54:649–656
2. Moisan J, Meyer F, Gingras S (1990) Diet and age at menarche. Cancer Causes Control 1:149–154
3. Merzenich H, Boeing H, Wahrendorf J (1993) Dietary fat and sports activity as determinants for age at menarche. Am J Epidemiol 138:217–224
4. Kissinger DG, Sanchez A (1987) The association of dietary factors and age at menarche. Nutr Res 7:471–479
5. Meyer F, Verreault R (1987) Erythrocite selenium and breast cancer risk. Am J Epidemiol 125:917–919
6. Hughes RE, Jones E (1985) Intake of dietary fibre and age of menarche. Ann Hum Biol 12: 325–332
7. Sanchez A, Kissinger DG, Phillips RI (1981) A hypothesis on the etiological role of diet on age of menarche. Med Hypotheses 7(11):1339–1345
8. Kelsey JL, Gammon MD, Esther MJ (1993) Reproductive factors and breast cancer. Epidemiol Rev 15:36–47

9. Tretli S, Gaard M (1996) Lifestyle changes during adolescence and risk of breast cancer: an ecologic study of the effect of World War II in Norway. Cancer Causes Control 7(5):507–512
10. Tornberg SA, Holm LE, Carstensen JM (1988) Breast cancer risk in relation to serum cholesterol, serum beta-lipoprotein, height, weight, and blood pressure. Acta Oncolog 27:31–37
11. Vatten LJ, Kvinnsland S (1990) Body mass index and risk of breast cancer. A prospective study of 23.826 Norwegian women. Int J Cancer 45:440–444
12. Vatten LJ, Kvinnsland S (1992) Prospective study of height, body mass index and risk of breast cancer. Acta Oncolog 31:195–200
13. Harvie M, Howell A (2006) Energy balance adiposity and breast cancer – energy restriction strategies for breast cancer prevention. Obes Rev 7(1):33–47
14. McCay CM, Crowell MF (1934) Prolonging the life span. Sci Mon 39:405
15. Welsch CW (1994) Interrelationship between dietary lipids and calories and experimental mammary gland tumorigenesis. Cancer 74(Suppl):1055–1062
16. Boissoneault GA, Elson CE, Pariza MW (1986) Net energy effects of dietary fat on chemically induced mammary carcinogenesis in F344 rats. J Natl Cancer Inst 76:335–338
17. Elias SG, Peeters PH, Grobbee DE et al (2004) Breast cancer risk after caloric restriction during the 1944–1945 Dutch famine. J Natl Cancer Inst 96(7):539–546
18. Roth GS, Ingram DK, Lane MA (2001) Caloric restriction in primates and relevance to humans. Ann NY Acad Sci 928:305
19. Fair AM, Montgomery K (2009) Energy balance, physical activity, and cancer risk. Methods Mol Biol 472:57–88
20. Ong KR, Sims AH, Harvie M et al (2009) Biomarkers of dietary energy restriction in women at increased risk of breast cancer. Cancer Prev Res (Phila) 2(8):720–731
21. Thompson HJ, Zhu Z, Jiang W (2004) Weight control and breast cancer prevention: are the effects of reduced energy intake equivalent to those of increased energy expenditure? J Nutr 134(12 Suppl):3407S–3411S
22. Harvie MN, Pegington M, Mattson MP et al (2010) The effects of intermittent or continuous energy restriction on weight loss and metabolic disease risk markers: a randomized trial in young overweight women. Int J Obes (Lond). doi:10.1038/ijo.2010.171
23. World Cancer Research Fund/American Institute for Cancer Research (2007) Food, nutrition, physical activity, and the prevention of cancer: a global perspective. American Institute for Cancer Research, Washington, DC
24. International Agency for Research on Cancer (2002) IARC handbooks of cancer prevention, vol 6, Weight control and physical activity. IARC Press, Lyon
25. Macinnis RJ, English DR, Gertig DM et al (2004) Body size and composition and risk of postmenopausal breast cancer. Cancer Epidemiol Biomarkers Prev 13:2117–2125
26. Lahmann PH, Hoffmann K, Allen N et al (2004) Body size and breast cancer risk: findings from the European Prospective Investigation into Cancer and Nutrition (EPIC). Int J Cancer 111:762–771
27. Lahmann PH, Schulz M, Hoffmann K et al (2005) Long-term weight change and breast cancer risk: the European prospective investigation into cancer and nutrition (EPIC). Br J Cancer 93:582–589
28. Krebs EE, Taylor BC, Cauley JA et al (2006) Measures of adiposity and risk of breast cancer in older postmenopausal women. J Am Geriatr Soc 54:63–69
29. Mellemkjaer L, Bigaard J, Tjonneland A et al (2006) Body composition and breast cancer in postmenopausal women: a Danish prospective cohort study. Obesity (Silver Spring) 14: 1854–1862
30. Shu XO, Jin F, Dai Q et al (2001) Association of body size and fat distribution with risk of breast cancer among Chinese women. Int J Cancer 94:449–455
31. Chow LW, Lui KL, Chan JC et al (2005) Association between body mass index and risk of formation of breast cancer in Chinese women. Asian J Surg 28:179–184
32. Hirose K, Tajima K, Hamajima N et al (2001) Association of family history and other risk factors with breast cancer risk among Japanese premenopausal and postmenopausal women. Cancer Causes Control 12:349–358

33. Hall IJ, Newman B, Millikan RC et al (2000) Body size and breast cancer risk in black women and white women: the Carolina Breast Cancer Study. Am J Epidemiol 151:754–764
34. Okobia MN, Bunker CH, Zmuda JM et al (2006) Anthropometry and breast cancer risk in Nigerian women. Breast J 12:462–466
35. Wu AH, Yu MC, Tseng CC et al (2007) Body size, hormone therapy and risk of breast cancer in Asian-American women. Int J Cancer 120:844–852
36. Ronco AL, Boeing H, De Stéfani E et al (2009) A case-control study on fat to muscle ratio and risk of breast cancer. Nutr Cancer 61(4):466–474
37. Tretli S (1989) Height and weight in relation to breast cancer morbidity and mortality. A prospective study of 570,000 women in Norway. Int J Cancer 44:23–30
38. Barnes-Josiah D, Potter JD, Sellers TA et al (1995) Early body size and subsequent weight gain as predictors of breast cancer incidence. Cancer Causes Control 6:112–118
39. Le Marchand L, Kolonel LN, Earle ME et al (1988) Body size at different periods of life and breast cancer risk. Am J Epidemiol 128:137–152
40. Kato I, Miura S, Kasumi F et al (1992) A case-control study of breast cancer among Japanese women: with special reference to family history and reproductive and dietary factors. Breast Cancer Res Treat 24:51–59
41. La Vecchia C, Decarli A, Parazzini F et al (1987) General epidemiology of breast cancer in Northern Italy. Int J Epidemiol 16:347–355
42. Toti A, Agugiaro S, Amadori D et al (1986) Breast cancer risk factors in Italian women: a multicentric case-control study. Tumori 72:241–249
43. Van den Brandt PA, Spiegelman D, Yaun S-S et al (2000) Pooled analysis of prospective cohort studies on height, weight, and breast cancer risk. Am J Epidemiol 152:514–527
44. Friedenreich CM (2001) Review of anthropometric factors and breast cancer risk. Eur J Cancer Prev 10:15–32
45. Henderson BE, Ross RK, Judd HL et al (1985) Do regular ovulatory cycles increase breast cancer risk? Cancer 56:1206–1208
46. Pike MC (1990) Reducing cancer risk in women through lifestyle-mediated changes in hormone levels. Cancer Detect Prev 14:595–607
47. Sherman B, Wallace R, Bean J et al (1981) Relationship of body weight to menarcheal and menopausal age: implications for breast cancer risk. Clin Endocrinol Metab 52:488–493
48. Key TJ, Chen J, Wang DI et al (1990) Sex hormones in women in rural China and in Britain. Br J Cancer 62:631
49. Huang Z, Hankinson SE, Colditz GA et al (1997) Dual effects of weight and weight gain on breast cancer risk. JAMA 278:1407–1411
50. Ronco AL, De Stéfani E, Deneo-Pellegrini H et al (2008) Epidemiología nutricional del cáncer de mama. Ediciones de la Plaza, Montevideo
51. Baer HJ, Tworoger SS, Hankinson SE et al (2010) Body fatness at young ages and risk of breast cancer throughout life. Am J Epidemiol 171(11):1183–1194
52. Shi J, Zhang M, Li L et al (2010) Body mass index and its change in adulthood and breast cancer risk in china. Asian Pac J Cancer Prev 11(5):1213–1218
53. Suzuki R, Iwasaki M, Inoue M et al (2011) Body weight at age 20 years, subsequent weight change and breast cancer risk defined by estrogen and progesterone receptor status-the Japan public health center-based prospective study. Int J Cancer 129:1214–1224
54. Kotsopoulos J, Olopado OI, Ghadirian P et al (2005) Changes in body weight and the risk of breast cancer in BRCA1 and BRCA2 mutation carriers. Breast Cancer Res 7(5):R833–R843
55. Ballard-Barbash R, Schatzkin A, Carter CL et al (1990) Body fat distribution and breast cancer in the Framingham Study. J Natl Cancer Inst 82:286–290
56. Folsom AR, Kaye SA, Prineas RJ et al (1990) Increased incidence of carcinoma of the breast associated with abdominal adiposity in postmenopausal women. Am J Epidemiol 131:794–803
57. Sellers TA, Kushi LH, Potter JD et al (1992) Effect of family history, body-fat distribution, and reproductive factors on the risk of post-menopausal breast cancer. N Engl J Med 326: 1323–1329

58. Den Tonkelaar I, Seidell JC, Collette JH et al (1994) A prospective study on obesity and subcutaneous fat patterning in relation to breast cancer in post-menopausal women participating in the DOM project. Br J Cancer 69:352–357
59. Kaaks R, van Noord PAH, Den Tonkelaar I et al (1998) Breast cancer incidence in relation to height, weight and body-fat distribution in the Dutch "Dom" cohort. Int J Cancer 76:647–651
60. Schapira DV, Kumar NB, Lyman GH et al (1990) Abdominal obesity and breast cancer risk. Ann Intern Med 112:182–186
61. Kumar NB, Lyman GH, Allen K et al (1995) Timing of weight gain and breast cancer risk. Cancer 76:243–249
62. Männistö S, Pietinen P, Pyy M et al (1996) Body size indicators and risk of breast cancer according to menopause and estrogen-receptor status. Int J Cancer 68:8–13
63. Ng E-H, Gao F, Ji C-H et al (1997) Risk factors for breast carcinoma in Singaporean Chinese women. Cancer 80:725–731
64. Magnusson C, Baron J, Persson I et al (1998) Body size in different periods of life and breast cancer risk in postmenopausal women. Int J Cancer 76:29–34
65. Sonnenschein E, Toniolo P, Terry MB et al (1999) Body fat distribution and obesity in pre- and postmenopausal breast cancer. Int J Epidemiol 28:1026–1031
66. Levshin VF (1980) Importance of anthropometric parameters in breast cancer. Vopr Onkol 26:69–73
67. Bruning PF, Bonfrer JMG, van Noord PAH et al (1992) Insulin resistance and breast cancer risk. Int J Cancer 52:511–516
68. Ballard-Barbash R (1994) Anthropometry and breast cancer: body size – a moving target. Cancer 74:1090–1100
69. Moller R, Tafeit TE, Sudi TK et al (2000) Quantifying the 'appleness' or 'pearness' of the human body by subcutaneous adipose tissue distribution. Ann Hum Biol 27:47–55
70. Folsom AR, Kushi LH, Anderson KE (2000) Associations of general and abdominal obesity with multiple health outcomes in older women: the Iowa Women's Health Study. Arch Intern Med 160:2117–2128
71. Schapira DV, Kumar NB, Lyman GH et al (1991) Upper-body fat distribution and endometrial cancer risk. JAMA 266:1808–1811
72. Ronco AL, Mendoza B, Varas X et al (2008) Somatotype and risk of breast cancer: a case-control study in Uruguay. Braz J Epidemiol 11(2):215–227
73. Bruning PF (1987) Endogenous estrogens and breast cancer a possible relationship between body fat distribution and estrogen availability. J Steroid Biochem 27:487–492
74. Frisch RE, Wyshak G, Albright NL et al (1985) Lower prevalence of breast cancer and cancers of the reproductive system among former college athletes compared to nonathletes. Br J Cancer 52:885–891
75. Albanes D, Blair A, Taylor PR (1989) Physical activity and risk of cancer in the NHANES I population. Am J Public Health 79:744–750
76. Paffenbarger RSJ, Hyde RT, Wing AL (1987) Physical activity and incidence of cancer in diverse populations: a preliminary report. Am J Clin Nutr 45(Suppl):312–317
77. Bernstein L, Henderson BE, Hanisch R et al (1994) Physical exercise and reduced risk of breast cancer in young women. J Natl Cancer Inst 86:1403–1408
78. Vena JE, Graham S, Zielezny M et al (1987) Occupational exercise and risk of cancer. Am J Clin Nutr 45:318–327
79. Demark-Wahnefried W, Kenyon AJ, Eberle P et al (2002) Preventing sarcopenic obesity among breast cancer patients who receive adjuvant chemotherapy: results of a feasibility study. Clin Exerc Physiol 4(1):44–49
80. Bernstein L, Ross RK, Lobo RA et al (1987) The effects of moderate physical activity on menstrual cycle patterns in adolescence: implications for breast cancer prevention. Br J Cancer 55:681–685
81. Hutnick NA, Williams NI, Kraemer WJ et al (2005) Exercise and lymphocyte activation following chemotherapy for breast cancer. Med Sci Sports Exerc 37(11):1827–1835

82. Burton JD, Bamford RN, Peters C et al (1994) A lymphokine, provisionally designated interleukin T and produced by a human adult T cell leukemia line, stimulates T cell proliferation and the induction of lymphokine-activated killer cells. Proc Natl Acad Sci USA 91:4935–4939
83. Pedersen BK, Akerström TC, Nielsen AR et al (2007) Role of myokines in exercise and metabolism. J Appl Physiol 103:1093–1098
84. Pedersen BK, Fischer CP (2007) Physiological roles of muscle-derived interleukin-6 in response to exercise. Curr Opin Clin Nutr Metab Care 10:265–271
85. Pedersen BK (2007) IL-6 signalling in exercise and disease. Biochem Soc Trans 35(Pt 5): 1295–1297
86. Alvarez B, Carbó N, López-Soriano J et al (2002) Effects of interleukin-15 (IL-15) on adipose tissue mass in rodent obesity models: evidence for direct IL-15 action on adipose tissue. Biochim Biophys Acta 1570:33–37
87. Quinn LS, Anderson BG, Drivdahl RH et al (2002) Overexpression of interleukin-15 induces skeletal muscle hypertrophy in vitro: implications for treatment of muscle wasting disorders. Exp Cell Res 280:55–63
88. Carson WE, Giri JG, Lindemann MJ et al (1994) Interleukin (IL)15 is a novel cytokine that activates human natural killer cells via components of the IL-2 receptor. J Exp Med 180: 1395–1403
89. Akbar AN, Borthwick NJ, Wickremasinghe RG et al (1996) IL-2 receptor common gamma-chain signaling cytokines regulate activated T-cell apoptosis in response to growth factor withdrawal: Selective induction of anti-apoptotic (bcl-2, bcl-xL) but not proapoptotic (bax, bcl-xS) gene expression. Eur J Immunol 26:294–299
90. Girard D, Paquet ME, Paquin R et al (1996) Differential effects of interleukin-15 (IL-15) and IL-2 on human neutrophils: Modulation of phagocytosis, cytoskeleton rearrangement, gene expression and apoptosis by IL-15. Blood 88:3176–3184
91. Cohen LA, Boylan E, Epstein M et al (1992) Voluntary exercise and experimental mammary cancer. Adv Exp Med Biol 322:61
92. Thompson HJ (1992) Effect of treadmill exercise intensity on hepatic glutathione content and its relevance to mammary tumorigenesis. J Sports Med Phys Fitness 32(1):59–63
93. Pan SY, Des Meules M (2009) Energy intake, physical activity, energy balance, and cancer: epidemiologic evidence. Methods Mol Biol 472:191–215
94. Padovani M, Lavigne JA, Chandramouli GV et al (2009) Distinct effects of calorie restriction and exercise on mammary gland gene expression in C57BL/6 mice. Cancer Prev Res (Phila Pa) 2(12):1076–1087

Chapter 3
Foods

Vegetables and Fruits

The associations between intake of fruits and vegetables and the risk of breast cancer (BC) have been examined in several papers. The studies have reported conflicting evidence on the role of fruit and vegetables in BC prevention. A study in California reported essentially null associations for total vegetables, total fruits, dark leaf and yellow leaf vegetables [1]. Other study in Canada communicated a non significant risk reduction for the high intakes of vegetables and fruits rich in carotenoids and vitamins [2]. In other studies, on the contrary, most researchers have found significant associations in a protective sense for one or more categories of vegetables and/or fruits [3–6]. Such studies were performed in the United States, Switzerland, Japan, Argentina, Canada, Italy, Poland and Greece. Similar associations were also observed in the study performed in Uruguay [7].

More recently, a multisite study carried out in this population [8] showed that a high intake of fruits and vegetables combined was associated with a decreased risk of BC (OR=0.47, 95% CI: 0.31–0.71). Estimates were slightly more protective for total vegetables (OR=0.53, 95% CI 0.35–0.81) than for total fruits (OR=0.60, 95% CI 0.42–0.87).

The global consideration of more than 20 epidemiologic studies [9] determined 70 associations: these are related with different types of vegetables and fruits, as well as also in some studies there were results derived from the analysis of diet according to age groups, age at diagnosis, country of origin of the studied women and even with the comparison of pre- and postmenopausal women. Of the 70 associations found, 37 risk estimations suggested a protective association and 30 were labelled as "without association". Only 3 results displayed an increase of risk, higher than 1.5.

Considering total vegetables as a general category, most studies which analyzed them found RR from 0.3 to 0.8 for the highest intakes [9–11]. A minor fraction of those studies did not communicate risk associations between BC and total vegetables [12, 13]. Besides, most studies which analyzed the intake of green leaf vegetables observed statistically significant protective associations, with RR from 0.2 to

A.L. Ronco and E. De Stéfani, *Nutritional Epidemiology of Breast Cancer*,
DOI 10.1007/978-94-007-2397-9_3,

0.5 for the high intakes [14, 15]. Also here few studies reported absence of association [13, 16].

Some studies examined specially the intakes of cruciferous vegetables – which are of particular interest in BC due to the presence of indole compounds, as indol-3-carbinol – which exert some effect on the estrogen metabolism, and therefore on the risk of BC. Except one of them, the rest observed risk reduction (RR = 0.6) for the highest consumptions of cruciferous. The intake of carrot has suggested risk reduction for the highest levels, although they were not significant [6, 17]. The intake of onion was reported by a study as reducing the risk to the half, among high consumers [17]. Finally, the preparation condition of vegetables does not enable to be conclusive about the association degree: a study revealed a risk reduction for the intake of raw vegetables and absence of association in cooked ones [18], but other study showed also a risk reduction even for the intake of cooked vegetables [19].

Of those studies which examined the intake of fruit or raw fruit in general, around half have reported a null association [12, 17, 20]. One part observed risk reduction among the highest intake levels [10, 21]. There were also studies which found a risk reduction among pre-menopausal and risk increase among postmenopausal women [22]. Most studies have not reported an association with the intake of oranges or citrus fruits.

A study of around two decades ago studied the relationship between the intake of vegetables and fruits and vegetables with the prognosis and survival in women who were surgically operated in small BC cases. Those who had previously eaten more vegetables and fruits had tumours with more favourable prognostic features, including among others, more normal cell differentiation, less vascular invasion, a smaller size and positive estrogen receptors [23].

Experimental studies have demonstrated that the inclusion of different vegetables in the diet of rats resulted in a lesser incidence of experimentally induced mammary tumours [24, 25]. These studies involved a feeding based on cabbage, cauliflower, Brussels sprouts or broccoli, generally in levels around 5–20% of total diet. The inclusion of orange oil in a proportion of 1–5% of diet produced a lesser incidence of tumours and a lesser number of tumours per animal [24].

A meta-analysis found evidence that fruit intake was negatively associated with the risk of BC in cohort studies, but not in case-control studies [26]. Conversely, in the case of vegetables this analysis described that there was an inverse association among case-control studies, but not cohort studies. In a pooled analysis of eight cohort studies there was evidence only of a possible weak effect of fruit and vegetable intake [27]. In a large American cohort there was a slight positive association with vegetables, but a slight inverse association with fruit intake [28].

The contribution of vegetables in general, albeit it has been favourable, has not been so much remarkable as the other large group proceeding from plants, which are the fruits. Several substances contained in vegetables have potential actions as anti-tumour, antioxidant and bioactive. There have been long and comprehensive epidemiologic studies whose analyses have not shed so good results as it could be expected, just as the EPIC study where was little evidence of an association [29], although they have given evidence of risk reduction [30]. The AICR/WCRF report [31] stated that the data on fruits and vegetables and BC were limited or inconsistent for any conclusion, something that clearly indicates that the issue is far from being defined.

A dietary pattern based on "salad" type vegetables (raw vegetables with olive oil) has been recognized as protective among Italian women [32], although the protection was restricted to those ones who had normal weight (BMI <25 kg/m2). A study carried out in German women under age 50 found a risk reduction for the intake of total vegetables intake [33]. Other study performed in Chinese women [34] found a protective effect for vegetables as a group, however no effect was described for individual foods. A protective association was also described for the plant foods only in postmenopausal but not in pre-menopausal ones [35]. Also a protective effect was seen for raw vegetables but not for cooked ones [36]. According a more recent study [37], there could be differences in risk reduction depending on the receptor status of tumours, that is, if they are ER+(positive for estrogen receptors) or ER- (negative for estrogen receptors).

A DIET RICH IN VEGETABLES AND FRUITS PROBABLY REDUCES THE RISK OF BREAST CANCER.

Legumes

Most case–control [7, 34, 38–40] studies and a cohort study [41] suggested significant or nonsignificant 20–30% reductions in BC risk with high legume intake. A Japanese cohort study revealed a risk reduction of BC associated with a high intake of a soup made with soybean paste [2]. Other study performed in Singapore showed a RR=0.4, that is, a risk reduction of 60% of BC in pre-menopausal women who had the highest intake of soy products, although it did not show association among postmenopausal ones [42].

Some previous case–control studies [43, 44] found no association between legume intake and BC risk. In China, case-control studies did not showed association for the intake of soy protein, neither for soymilk or tofu [45].

A recent multisite study performed in Uruguay [46] reported absence of association with the risk of BC for legumes (OR=0.89, 95% CI 0.65–1.20) neither for beans or lentils separately (OR=1.06, 95% 0.77–1.46 and OR=0.86, 95% CI 0.66–1.21 respectively).

At an experimental level, a reduction in the incidence of BC in rats fed with 50% of soybeans compared with the control group was observed after being irradiated [47]. Also a reduction of chemically induced tumours in rats was observed when soy was administered in the diet [48].

As it will be mentioned in the chapter *Vitamins and bioactive substances*, soybeans have large amounts of isoflavones, so it is reasonable to think that its consumption could inhibit cancers in whose promotion participate estrogens. Menstrual cycles in young women were described as correlated with their intakes of polyunsaturated fats, soy and dietary fibre [49], something that gives plausible bases for the protective action of soy-derived products. A recent meta-analysis recognized that even though a general trend towards a risk reduction with soy intake has been found, it is still premature recommend the supplementation of high doses of isoflavones to reduce the risk of developing a BC or for preventing its recurrence [50]. There is some evidence that the intake of soy is not dangerous for BC survival [51].

ALTHOUGH THE EVIDENCE BETWEEN LEGUMES AND THE RISK OF BREAST CANCER IS LIMITED, THEY COULD BE PROTECTIVE.

Meats, Poultry, Fish

Meat

Along the decade of the 90s the most conclusive studies on meat consumption and who investigated its eventual association with the risk of BC were carried out. A study in New York revealed a moderately high risk associated with the intake of red meat and adjusted for calories (RR = 1.9) for the group with highest intake, although no significant statistical relationship with total fat or some particular fat was seen [52].

Some cohort studies reported also a risk increase [2, 53]. Two previous meta-analyses of several case-control studies and cohort studies on meat consumption and BC risk found evidence of increased risk. The former one reported a significant RR = 1.54 for the highest intake of red meat [54] and the more recent one, based on 22 case-control studies and 9 cohort studies, found a summary RR of 1.17 (95% CI: 1.06–1.29) for high vs. low total meat intake [55].

Nevertheless, other cohort studies did not reveal any association between BC risk and red meat consumption [56, 57]. In addition, a pooled analysis of seven cohort studies reported no association [58]. More recent studies have also found conflicting results, with some case-control [38, 59, 60] and cohort [61–63] studies reporting positive associations while others found no association [64–66].

One of the Uruguayan studies [67] indicated a fourfold RR among the highest consumers of red meat, after adjusting for calories. The risk increase was even higher with fried and barbecued meats, something that led the authors to propose a possible effect of the cooking method using high temperatures. This hypothesis was emphasized in our following case-control study, through the estimation of the production of Heterocyclic Amines (HAs) in the cooking process [68].

Other study assessed the exposure to HAs by interrogating individuals with questions supported with photographs which showed different cooking levels for the meats [69]. This study displayed a fourfold risk of BC among those consumers of well-done meats compared to the consumers of intermediate or less cooked meat.

Recently, a multisite study on meat and the risk of cancer [70] reported moderate to strong increases in the risk of BC with high intakes of total meat (OR=2.05 [1.23–3.42]), red meat (OR=1.97 [1.04–3.75]), beef (OR=1.58 [1.11–2.24]), lamb (OR=1.88 [1.12–3.15]) and processed meat [OR=1.53 [1.01–2.30]). Besides, another multisite study in Uruguay [71] has not reported an increased risk of BC for high intake of salted meat (OR=1.16 0.87–1.53). On the other hand, other studies have reported an increased risk for processed meats (sausage, saucisson, etc.) [72], as well as with the intake of salami [73].

An old ecologic study reported strong correlations (r=0.7–0.8) between meat consumption and BC [74]. Other ecologic study communicated that among the members of the Adventist Church in the United States – who have a low meat intake – the BC mortality was slightly lower (around 10%) compared with the mortality occurring in North American white women with similar socio-economic status [75].

The evaluation of meat as a risk factor for BC was initially focused on its role as a source of dietary fat or animal protein. But the study of Toniolo et al. from 1994 [52] found that the intake of meat (but not of total fat or protein) increased significantly the risk of BC. Then it is possible, that if meat consumption plays some role in the etiology of BC, the risk cannot be related with meat as a source of fats and proteins, but mainly as a source of mutagens and/or carcinogens, specifically HAs, N-Nitroso compounds and Polycyclic Aromatic Hydrocarbons. Some HAs are powerful breast carcinogens in rodents and could be risk factors in humans. In addition, some HAs distribute themselves in the mammary gland, they provoke alterations and cause cancer in rats [76].

DIETS RICH IN MEAT, IN PARTICULAR RED MEAT COOKED WITH DIRECT HEAT, INCREASE THE RISK OF BREAST CANCER.

Poultry

A meta-analysis done on a basis of case-control and cohort studies reported that the intake of poultry did not keep relationship with the risk of BC, having found a non significant RR=0.94 [54]. Two cohort studies done after that meta-analysis did not find an association between poultry intake and BC either [52, 77]. A case-control study in Chinese women did not show significant associations between poultry intake and the risk of BC [78]. No associations were observed either with consumption of chicken regarding circulating concentrations of Steroid Hormon Binding Globulins (SHBG) and estradiol [79]. Nevertheless, also a positive and significant association has been reported [80]. A recent review poses that a high intake of poultry (among other items) may play a causative role in this disease [81].

In the last decade we studied in Uruguay the intake of chicken at a medical institution belonging to the pre-paid healthcare system [82]. It was possible to observe important differences in the consumption style of white meat: chicken with skin prevailed in the BC cases ($p<0.001$), while women with normal mammograms had preference for skinless chicken ($p=0.0000$). In the chapter corresponding to the research performed in Uruguay are detailed the estimated risks for each one of the consumption modalities.

The preparation and/or consumption modality is a possible factor for the absence of association evidence in several studies, even in the own Uruguayan studies performed in population admitted at public hospitals, perhaps based on the presence of saturated, monounsaturated and Ω-6 polyunsaturated fats (PUFA) in the chicken skin, as well as on the production of HAs in the surface of the skin due to the frying or to the barbecue process. It is not unlikely that the studies which asked about poultry consumption without discriminating the preparation method could have covered an eventual protective effect of the skinless poultry or even an eventual risk increase of such meat with skin.

THERE IS NO CERTAINTY THAT POULTRY INTAKE IS RELATED TO BREAST CANCER. THE PREPARATION METHOD CAN BE ASSOCIATED WITH THE DISEASE.

Fish

Few epidemiologic studies have investigated the associations between fish (or oil fish) intake and BC. The prospective studies have reported lack of association [52] or a weak protective effect [83]. A Japanese case-control study has also communicated a weak protective effect [5]. Our study in Uruguayan women affiliated to the prepaid health system [82] showed a significant increase of risk for the highest intake of fried fish ($OR=2.0$) whereas there was a significant negative association for the high intake of not fried fish ($OR=0.50$).

The ecologic studies have reported findings in the same sense of the other epidemiologic studies: absence of association [84] or a protective effect [85]. At an experimental level, results support a possible protective effect for the oil fish in the mammary tumorigenesis [86]. The contribution of PUFA Ω-3 type, just as it is described in the corresponding chapter, can be an important reason for the observed protective effect.

Again, in the same sense that we observed for chicken consumption, we have the opinion that similar considerations can be done regarding the preparation forms and intake of fish. When this item is queried as an only variable, several studies could have possible not shown the differences which actually exist, due to reciprocal cancellation of effects. It should not be forgotten that fried forms of cooking imply the association of PUFA Ω-6 type to the fish, with which the balance Ω-6/Ω-3 would direct towards values which are potentially harmful.

DIETS RICH IN FISH COULD REDUCE THE RISK OF BREAST CANCER, BUT THE EVIDENCE SEEMS TO BE STILL INSUFFICIENT.

Dairy Foods

Several epidemiologic analytic studies analyzed the relationship between dairy products and the risk of BC. In the case of milk, a relative majority of studies reported an elevation of risk with large intakes [15, 53, 87], in similar proportions to those studies which have not found a relationship [88, 89]. Only some of them found a risk reduction [72, 90]. Among the cohort studies, most of them communicated an absence of association and only a few of them found an increase of risk or a risk reduction [77, 90, 91].

Respect of the cheese intake, the proportion of findings is rather similar to the one of milk: reasonably similar proportions have described an increase of risk [12, 17] and absence of association [88, 90] and on the other hand, some isolated study found a risk reduction [92].

A meta-analysis of cohort and case-control studies communicated that a high milk and cheese intake was associated with very weak increases of BC risk (RR = 1.20) [54]. Besides, ecologic studies have usually found positive correlations between milk or dairy consumption and the incidence of BC [74, 93]. Dairy foods together were examined by a cohort study like a general category of foods, and from there was reported a moderately protective association, with a RR = 0.6 after adjusting for energy, considering the quintile of higher consumption.

Fats, which are usually present in milk and dairy foods, possibly increase the risk of BC, although on the other hand, these foods are good sources of calcium and conjugated linoleic acid, a fatty acid which has showed its partially protective capability against chemically induced mammary tumours in animals [94].

In the corresponding chapter, the results obtained in a case-control study carried in Uruguay in the last decade about the role of dairy foods and the risk of BC [95]. Summarily, whole milk, chocolate milk and Gruyere cheese were associated with significant risk increases of BC, whereas the intake of ricotta cheese and skimmed yoghurt were associated with significant reduced risk. Low-fat and fermented dairy foods seemed to be the most protective ones. Concerning this point, our results suggested us the convenience for the future to continue making separate queries and analyses for milk, yoghurt and cheese types, since the combined inclusion could lead results to the null.

THE EVIDENCE OF DAIRY CONSUMPTION AND BREAST CANCER IS INCONSISTENT. SKIMMED AND FERMENTED PRODUCTS COULD REDUCE THE RISK OF BREAST CANCER.

Sweet Foods

The possible role of sweet foods and sugar on the risk of BC has been analyzed in several types of scientific studies, but results are inconsistent. Some of the ecologic studies found a positive correlation between sugar or sweet intakes and incidence or mortality from BC [96]. Also case-control and cohort studies reported positive associations between sweet foods and the risk of BC [53, 90, 97–101], but there were also papers reporting absence of or no consistent associations [12, 16–18, 72, 73, 102–105].

The positive risks found were usually modest (up to OR = 1.5), with the exception of the Spanish study [98], with an OR = 2.3 for the highest intake of sweets. Apparently, none of the studies found a protective effect of these foods suggested by results. As in other epidemiological studies, some inconsistencies might rely on different approaches to data analysis and interpretation, also on possible biases, but we emphasize the actual differences in the recipes among populations all over the world as well as in the composition of sweet foods. Even mono- or disaccarides did not show either consistent associations with BC risk [22, 106].

It is difficult to analyze completely separated the sweets due to high collinearity among several foods and nutrients playing different possible roles [107]. Some of the sweet foods like desserts are also rich in saturated fats, which have been associated with BC risk [27] as well as in trans-fats, which are considered unhealthy [108]. In addition, the effect of high-energy dietary patterns cannot be excluded from the considerations about the sweet foods.

A simultaneous reduction in the intake of favourable foods substituted by sweets may lead directly (through the intake of sugar) or indirectly (through the increase of Insulin-like Growth Factors) to an increase of insulin, promoting carcinogenesis and chronic inflammation, which is also linked to the cancer origin and a critical component of tumour progression [109–113].

THE INTAKE OF SWEET FOODS MIGHT INCREASE THE RISK OF BREAST CANCER BUT THE EVIDENCE IS STILL INCONSISTENT.

References

1. Hirayama T (1978) Epidemiology of breast cancer with special reference to the role of diet. Prev Med 7:173–195
2. Hirayama T et al (1986) A large-scale study on cancer risks by diet – with special reference to the risk reducing effects of green-yellow vegetable consumption. In: Hayashi Y, Magao M, Sugimura T (eds) Diet, nutrition and cancer. Japan Scientific Societies Press, Bunkyo-ku, pp 41–53
3. Cohen LA, Kendall ME, Zang E et al (1991) Modulation of N-nitrosomethylurea-induced mammary tumor promotion by dietary fiber and fat. J Natl Cancer Inst 83:496–501
4. Hirohata T, Nomura AMY, Hankin JH et al (1987) An epidemiological study on the association between diet and breast cancer. J Natl Cancer Inst 78:595–600
5. Hirose K, Tajima K, Hamajima N et al (1995) A large-scale, hospital based case-control study of risk factors of breast cancer according to menopausal status. Jpn J Cancer Res 86:146–154
6. Hislop TG, Coldman AJ, Elwood JM et al (1986) Childhood and recent eating patterns and risk of breast cancer. Cancer Detect Prev 9:47–58
7. Ronco AL, De Stéfani E, Boffetta P et al (1999) Vegetables, fruits, and related nutrients and risk of breast cancer: a case control study in Uruguay. Nutr Cancer 35(2):111–119
8. Aune D, De Stéfani E, Ronco AL et al (2009) Fruits, vegetables and the risk of cancer: a multisite case-control study in Uruguay. Asian Pac J Cancer Prev 20:419–428
9. Holmberg L, Ohlander EM, Byers T et al (1994) Diet and breast cancer risk: results from a population-based, case-control study in Sweden. Arch Int Med 154:1805–1811
10. Freudenheim JL, Marshall JR, Vena JE et al (1996) Premenopausal breast cancer risk and intake of vegetables, fruits, and related nutrients. J Natl Cancer Inst 88:340–348
11. Katsouyanni K, Trichopoulous D, Boyle P et al (1986) Diet and breast cancer: a case-control study in Greece. Int J Cancer 38:815–820
12. Toniolo P, Riboli E, Protta F et al (1989) Calorie-providing nutrients and risk of breast cancer. J Natl Cancer Inst 81:278–286
13. Shibata A, Paganini-Hill A, Ross RK et al (1992) Intake of vegetables, fruits, beta-carotene, vitamin C and vitamin supplements and cancer incidence among the elderly: a prospective study. Br J Cancer 66:673–679
14. La Vecchia C, Decarli A, Parazzini F et al (1987) General epidemiology of breast cancer in Northern Italy. Int J Epidemiol 16:347–355
15. Kato I, Miura S, Kasumi F et al (1992) A case-control study of breast cancer among Japanese women: with special reference to family history and reproductive and dietary factors. Breast Cancer Res Treat 24:51–59
16. Ewertz M, Gill C (1990) Dietary factors and breast cancer risk in Denmark. Int J Cancer 46:779–784
17. Levi F, La Vecchia C, Gulie C et al (1993) Dietary factors and breast cancer risk in Vaud. Switzerland Nutr Cancer 19:327–335
18. Simard A, Vobecky J, Vobecky JS (1990) Nutrition and life-style factors in fibrocystic disease and cancer of the breast. Cancer Detect Prev 14:567–572
19. Pawlega J (1992) Breast cancer and smoking, vodka drinking and dietary habits. Acta Oncol 31:387–392
20. Rohan TE, Howe GR, Friedenreich CM et al (1993) Dietary fiber, vitamins A, C, and E, and risk of breast cancer: a cohort study. Cancer Causes Control 4:29–37
21. Van't Veer P, Kalb CM, Verhoef P et al (1990) Dietary fiber, beta-carotene and breast cancer: results from a case-control study. Int J Cancer 45:825–828
22. Zaridze D, Lifanova Y, Maximovitch D et al (1991) Diet, alcohol consumption and reproductive factors in a case-control study of breast cancer in Moscow. Int J Cancer 48:493–501
23. Ingram DM, Roberts A, Nottage EM (1992) Host factors and breast cancer growth characteristics. Eur J Cancer 28 A(6–7):1153–1161

24. Wattenberg LW (1983) Inhibition of neoplasia by minor dietary constituents. Cancer Res 43(Suppl):2448S–2453S
25. Wattenberg LW, Schafer HW, Waters L Jr et al (1989) Inhibition of mammary tumor formation by broccoli and cabbage. Proc Am Assoc Cancer Res 30:181
26. Vainio H, Weiderpass E (2006) Fruit and vegetables in cancer prevention. Nutr Cancer 54:111–142
27. Smith-Warner S, Spiegelman D, Adami H-O et al (2001) Types of dietary fat and breast cancer: a pooled analysis of cohort studies. Int J Cancer 92:767–774
28. George SM, Park Y, Leitzmann MF et al (2009) Fruit and vegetable intake and risk of cancer: a prospective cohort study. Am J Clin Nutr 89:347–353
29. van Gils CH, Peeters PH, Bueno-de-Mesquita HB et al (2005) Consumption of vegetables and fruits and risk of breast cancer. JAMA 293(2):183–193
30. Malin AS, Qi D, Shu XO et al (2003) Intake of fruits, vegetables and selected micronutrients in relation to the risk of breast cancer. Int J Cancer 105(3):413–418
31. World Cancer Research Fund/American Institute for Cancer Research (2007) Food, nutrition, physical activity and the prevention of cancer: a global perspective. AICR, Washington DC
32. Sieri S, Krogh V, Pala V et al (2004) Dietary patterns and risk of breast cancer in the ORDET cohort. Cancer Epidemiol Biomarkers Prev 13(4):567–572
33. Hermann S, Linseisen J, Chang-Claude J (2002) Nutrition and breast cancer risk by age 50: a population-based case-control study in Germany. Nutr Cancer 44(1):23–34
34. Shannon J, Ray R, Wu C et al (2005) Food and botanical groupings and risk of breast cancer: a case-control study in Shanghai, China. Cancer Epidemiol Biomarkers Prev 14(1):81–90
35. Gaudet MM, Britton JA, Kabat GC et al (2004) Fruits, vegetables, and micronutrients in relation to breast cancer modified by menopause and hormone receptor status. Cancer Epidemiol Biomarkers Prev 13(9):1485–1494
36. Adzersen KH, Jess P, Freivogel KW et al (2003) Raw and cooked vegetables, fruits, selected micronutrients, and breast cancer risk: a case-control study in Germany. Nutr Cancer 46(2): 131–137
37. Olsen A, Tjonneland A, Thomsen BL et al (2003) Fruits and vegetables intake differentially affects estrogen receptor negative and positive breast cancer incidence rates. J Nutr 133(7): 2342–2347
38. Bessaoud F, Daures JP, Gerber M (2008) Dietary factors and breast cancer risk: a case control study among a population in southern France. Nutr Cancer 60:177–187
39. Shu XO, Jin F, Dai Q et al (2001) Soyfood intake during adolescence and subsequent risk of breast cancer among Chinese women. Cancer Epidemiol Biomarkers Prev 10:483–488
40. Dos Santos SI, Mangtani P, McCormack V et al (2002) Lifelong vegetarianism and risk of breast cancer: a population-based case-control study among South Asian migrant women living in England. Int J Cancer 99:238–244
41. Adebamowo CA, Cho E, Sampson L et al (2005) Dietary flavonols and flavonol-rich foods intake and the risk of breast cancer. Int J Cancer 114:628–633
42. Lee HP, Gourley L, Duffy SW et al (1991) Dietary effects on breast cancer risk in Singapore. Lancet 337:1197–1200
43. Franceschi S, Parpinel M, La Vecchia C et al (1998) Role of different types of vegetables and fruit in the prevention of cancer of the colon, rectum, and breast. Epidemiology 9:338–341
44. Morales Suarez-Varela M, Jimenez Lopez MC, Almenar CD et al (1998) Effect of the ingestion of food and gynecologic risk factors on breast cancer risk in Valencia. Nutr Hosp 13:325–329
45. Yuan JM, Wang Q, Ross RK et al (1995) Diet and breast cancer in Shanghai and Tianjin, China. Br J Cancer 71:1353–1358
46. Aune D, De Stéfani E, Ronco AL et al (2009) Legume intake and the risk of cancer: a multisite case–control study in Uruguay. Cancer Causes Control 20(9):1605–1615
47. Troll W (1991) Prevention of cancer by agents that suppress oxygen radical formation. Free Radic Res Commun 12–13(Pt 2):751–757
48. Barnes S, Grubbs C, Setchell KD et al (1990) Soybeans inhibit mammary tumors in models of breast cancer. Prog Clin Biol Res 347:239–253

49. Nagata C, Oba S, Shimizu H (2006) Associations of menstrual cycle length with intake of soy, fat, and dietary fiber in Japanese women. Nutr Cancer 54(2):166–170
50. Trock BJ, Hilakivi-Clarke L, Clarke R (2006) Meta-analysis of soy intake and breast cancer risk. J Natl Cancer Inst 98(7):459–471, Comment in: J Natl Cancer Inst 2006; 98(7): 430–1
51. Boyapati SM, Shu XO, Ruan ZX et al (2005) Soyfood intake and breast cancer survival: a followup of the Shanghai breast cancer study. Breast Cancer Res Treat 92(1):11–17
52. Toniolo P, Riboli E, Shore RE et al (1994) Consumption of meat, animal products protein, and fat and risk of breast cancer – a prospective cohort study in New York. Epidemiology 5: 391–397
53. Gaard M, Tretli S, Loken EB (1995) Dietary fat and the risk of breast cancer: a prospective study of 25.982 Norwegian women. Int J Cancer 63:13–17
54. Boyd NF, Martin L, Noffel M et al (1993) A metaanalysis of studies of dietary-fat and breast-cancer risk. Br J Cancer 68:267–275
55. Boyd NF, Stone J, Vogt KN et al (2003) Dietary fat and breast cancer risk revisited: a meta-analysis of the published literature. Br J Cancer 89:1672–1685
56. Willett WC, Hunter DJ, Stampfer MJ et al (1992) Dietary fat and fiber to relation to risk of breast cancer: an eight year follow-up. JAMA 268:2037–2044
57. Kinlen LJ (1982) Meat and fat consumption and cancer mortality: a study of strict religious orders in Britain. Lancet 1(8278):946–949
58. Missmer SA, Smith-Warner SA, Spiegelman D et al (2002) Meat and dairy food consumption and breast cancer: a pooled analysis of cohort studies. Int J Epidemiol 31:78–85
59. Kruk J (2007) Association of lifestyle and other risk factors with breast cancer according to menopausal status: a casecontrol study in the region of Western Pomerania (Poland). Asian Pac J Cancer Prev 8:513–524
60. Aune D, Ronco A, Boffetta P et al (2009) Meat consumption and cancer risk: a multisite case-control study in Uruguay. Cancer Ther 7:174–187
61. Cho E, Chen WY, Hunter DJ et al (2006) Red meat intake and risk of breast cancer among premenopausal women. Arch Intern Med 166:2253–2259
62. Egeberg R, Olsen A, Autrup H et al (2008) Meat consumption, N-acetyl transferase 1 and 2 polymorphism and risk of breast cancer in Danish postmenopausal women. Eur J Cancer Prev 17:39–47
63. Taylor EF, Burley VJ, Greenwood DC et al (2007) Meat consumption and risk of breast cancer in the UK Women's Cohort Study. Br J Cancer 96:1139–1146
64. Cross AJ, Leitzmann MF, Gail MH et al (2007) A prospective study of red and processed meat intake in relation to cancer risk. PLoS Med 4:e325
65. Holmes MD, Colditz GA, Hunter DJ et al (2003) Meat, fish and egg intake and risk of breast cancer. Int J Cancer 104:221–227
66. Kabat GC, Miller AB, Jain M et al (2007) Dietary iron and heme iron intake and risk of breast cancer: a prospective cohort study. Cancer Epidemiol Biomarkers Prev 16:1306–1308
67. Ronco AL, De Stéfani E, Mendilaharsu M et al (1996) Meat, fat and the risk of breast cancer: a case-control study from Uruguay. Int J Cancer 65:328–331
68. De Stéfani E, Ronco AL, Mendilaharsu M et al (1997) Meat intake, heterocyclic amines, and risk of breast cancer: a case-control study in Uruguay. Cancer Epidemiol Biomarkers Prev 6: 573–581
69. Zheng W, Gustafson DR, Sinha R et al (1998) Well-done meat intake and the risk of breast cancer. J Natl Cancer Inst 90:1724–1729
70. Aune D, De Stéfani E, Ronco AL et al (2009) Meat consumption and cancer risk: a case-control study in Uruguay. Asian Pac J Cancer Prev 10:1–10
71. De Stéfani E, Aune D, Boffetta P et al (2009) Salted meat consumption and the risk of cancer: a multisite case-control study in Uruguay. Asian Pac J Cancer Prev 10(5):853–857
72. Iscovich J, Iscovich R, Howe J et al (1989) A case-control study of diet and breast cancer in Argentina. Int J Cancer 44:770–777
73. Goodman MT, Nomura AMY, Wilkens LR et al (1992) The association of diet, obesity and breast cancer in Hawaii. Cancer Epidemiol Biomark Prev 1:269–275

74. Armstrong B, Doll R (1975) Environmental factors and cancer incidence and mortality in different countries, with special reference to dietary practices. Int J Cancer 15:617–631
75. Phillips RL, Garfinkel L, Kuzma JW et al (1980) Mortality among California Seventh-day Adventists for selected cancer sites. J Natl Cancer Inst 65:1095–1107
76. Snyderwine EG (1994) Some perspectives on the nutritional aspects of breast cancer research: food-derived heterocyclic amines as etiologic agents in human mammary cancer. Cancer 74: 1070–1077
77. Tavani A, La Vecchia C (1995) Fruit and vegetable consumption and cancer risk in a Mediterranean population. Am J Clin Nutr 61:1374S–1377S
78. Zhang CX, Ho SC, Chen YM et al (2009) Meat and egg consumption and risk of breast cancer among Chinese women. Cancer Causes Control 20(10):1845–1853
79. Brinkman MT, Baglietto L, Krishnan K et al (2010) Consumption of animal products, their nutrient components and postmenopausal circulating steroid hormone concentrations. Eur J Clin Nutr 64(2):176–183
80. Bissonauth V, Shatenstein B, Ghadirian P (2008) Nutrition and breast cancer among sporadic cases and gene mutation carriers: an overview. Cancer Detect Prev 32(1):52–64
81. Jayalekshmi P, Varughese SC, Kalavathi S et al (2009) A nested case-control study of female breast cancer in Karunagappally cohort in Kerala, India. Asian Pac J Cancer Prev 10(2): 241–246
82. Ronco AL, De Stéfani E, Fabra A (2003) White meat intake and the risk of breast cancer: a case-control study in Montevideo, Uruguay. Nutr Res 23(2):151–162
83. Vatten LJ, Kvinnsland S (1990) Body mass index and risk of breast cancer. A prospective study of 23.826 Norwegian women. Int J Cancer 45:440–444
84. Caygill CP, Hill MJ (1995) Fish, n-3 fatty acids and human colorectal and breast cancer mortality. Eur J Cancer Prev 4(4):329–332
85. Kaizer L, Boyd NF, Kriukov V et al (1989) Fish consumption and breast cancer risk: an ecological study. Nutr Cancer 12:61–68
86. Rose DP, Rayburn J, Hatala MA et al (1994) Effects of dietary fish oil on fatty acids and eicosanoids in metastasizing human breast cancer cells. Nutr Cancer 22:131–141
87. Talamini R, La Vecchia C, Decarli A et al (1984) Social factors, diet and breast in a northern Italian population. Br J Cancer 49:723–729
88. Lubin JH, Burns PE, Blot WJ et al (1981) Dietary factors and breast cancer risk. Int J Cancer 28:685–689
89. Ursin G, Bjelke E, Heuch I et al (1990) Milk consumption and cancer incidence. A Norwegian prospective study. Br J Cancer 61:454–459
90. Knekt P, Jarvinen R, Seppanen R et al (1996) Intake of dairy products and risk of breast cancer. Br J Cancer 73:687–691
91. Mills PK, Annegers JF, Phillips Rl (1988) Animal product consumption and subsequent fatal breast cancer risk among Seventh-day Adventists. Am J Epidemiol 127(3):440–453
92. Van't Veer P, Kok FJ, Hermus RJ et al (1989) Alcohol dose, frequency and age at first exposure in relation to the risk of breast cancer. Int J Epidemiol 18(3):511–517
93. Rose DP, Boyar AP, Wynder EL (1986) International comparisons of mortality rates for cancer of the breast, ovary, prostate, and colon, and per capita food consumption. Cancer 58: 2263–2271
94. Ip C, Scimeca JA, Thompson H (1995) Effect of timing and duration of dietary conjugated linoleic acid on mammary cancer prevention. Nutr Cancer 24(3):241–247
95. Ronco AL, De Stéfani E, Dáttoli R (2002) Dairy foods and risk of breast cancer: a case-control study in Montevideo, Uruguay. Eur J Cancer Prev 11(5):457–463
96. Burley VJ (1998) Sugar consumption and human cancer in sites other than the digestive tract. Eur J Cancer Prev 7:253–277
97. Richardson S, Gerber M, Cenee S (1991) The role of fat, animal protein and some vitamin consumption in breast cancer: a case control study in southern France. Int J Cancer 48:1–9

98. Landa MC, Frago N, Tres A (1994) Diet and the risk of breast cancer in Spain. Eur J Cancer Prev 3:313–320
99. Bala DV, Patel DD, Duffy SW et al (2001) Role of dietary intake and biomarkers in risk of breast cancer: a case control study. Asian Pac J Cancer Prev 2:123–130
100. Potischman N, Coates RJ, Swanson CA et al (2002) Increased risk of early-stage breast cancer related to consumption of sweet foods among women less than age 45 in the United States. Cancer Causes Control 13:937–946
101. Tavani A, Giordano L, Gallus S et al (2006) Consumption of sweet foods and breast cancer risk in Italy. Ann Oncol 17:341–345
102. Nomura A, Henderson BE, Lee J (1978) Breast cancer and diet among the Japanese in Hawaii. Am J Clin Nutr 31:2020–2025
103. Ingram DM, Nottage E, Roberts T (1991) The role of diet in the development of breast cancer: a case–control study of patients with breast cancer, benign epithelial hyperplasia and fibrocystic disease of the breast. Br J Cancer 64:187–191
104. Mannisto S, Pietinen P, Virtanen M et al (1999) Diet and the risk of breast cancer in a case–control study: does the threat of disease have an influence on recall bias? J Clin Epidemiol 52:429–439
105. Katsouyanni K, Willett W, Trichopoulos D et al (1988) Risk of breast cancer among Greek women in relation to nutrient intake. Cancer 61:181–185
106. Rohan TE, McMichael AJ, Baghurst PA (1988) A population-based case–control study of diet and breast cancer in Australia. Am J Epidemiol 128:478–489
107. Negri E, La Vecchia C, Franceschi S (2002) Relations between vegetable, fruit and micronutrient intake. Implications for odds ratios in a case–control study. Eur J Clin Nutr 56:166–170
108. Ascherio A, Willett WC (1997) Health effects of trans fatty acids. Am J Clin Nutr 66: 1006S–1010S
109. Kaaks R (1996) Nutrition, hormones, and breast cancer: is insulin the missing link? Cancer Causes Control 7:605–625
110. Yu H, Rohan T (2000) Role of the insulin-like growth factor family in cancer development and progression. J Natl Cancer Inst 92:1472–1489
111. Renehan AG, Zwahlen M, Minder C et al (2004) Insulin like growth factor (IGF)-I, IGF binding protein-3, and cancer risk: systematic review and meta-regression analysis. Lancet 363: 1346–1353
112. Shi R, Yu H, McLarty J et al (2004) IGF-I and breast cancer: a meta-analysis. Int J Cancer 111:418–423
113. Coussens LM, Werb Z (2002) Inflammation and cancer. Nature 420:860–867

Chapter 4
Nutrients

Carbohydrates

Carbohydrates have not been intensively investigated in epidemiological studies of diet and cancer. According to a recent review, the available data on carbohydrates and other cancers than colorectal cancer are too sparse to draw even tentative conclusions [1]. The issue deserves a separate analysis in relation to breast cancer (BC) and that is the reason of this next part of the present chapter.

Starch

In a previous stage of research, ecologic studies had shown negative correlations between mortality rates of BC and per capita intake of starch [2]. Afterwards, some analytic studies have investigated the association between the intake of starch and the risk of BC. On one hand, two studies have communicated small variations in the risk [3, 4] although an Italian study [5] found a significant but small (40%) increase in risk for the group with highest consumption (more than 191 grams per day), having controlled for confusion factors. In Italy white bread and pasta are recognized as the most important sources of starch. Although initially was not possible to find a plausible explanation for the finding, the metabolic link with high-glycemic foods, insulin peaks, inflammation and the development of cancers should be taken into account. Besides, starchy foods have been associated with an increase of risk of BC [6, 7] and with reduced risk in other study [8]. The results of a study on dietary patterns suggested that a diet characterized by a low intake of starches and a high intake of legumes is associated with a reduced risk of BC in Asian Americans [9]. Lack of association for starch intake among postmenopausal women, including by hormonal status, was reported by a Danish study [10].

A.L. Ronco and E. De Stéfani, *Nutritional Epidemiology of Breast Cancer*,
DOI 10.1007/978-94-007-2397-9_4,

THE EVIDENCE RELATING STARCH CONSUMPTION AND THE RISK OF BREAST CANCER IS STILL INCONSISTENT.

Dietary Fibre

The hypothesis that fibre-rich diets could be protective against BC has been postulated, but not many epidemiologic studies have analyzed the association. Cohort studies have shown absence of association or borderline situations [11, 12], as well as a 30% risk reduction for the group of highest consumption [7]. A meta-analysis on ten case-control studies reported a weak although significant protective association, given by a 15% reduction for consumers of 20 or more grams per day [13].

Other studies have also communicated protective associations for components of diet which are rich in fibre, for example, in the case of cellulose [14], raw fibre [15], and the fibre proceeding from vegetables and fruits but not from cereals [16]. High-fibre bread was significantly associated with a decreased BC incidence (OR=0.75, 95% CI 0.57–0.98, for highest compared with lowest quintile) in Swedish women [17]. A British study reported in pre-menopausal, but not post-menopausal women a statistically significant inverse relationship between total fibre intake and risk of BC (OR=0.48, 95% CI 0.24–0.96) compared with the lowest quintile [18]. On the other hand, an Italian study did not show relationship with total dietary fibre [5].

When we compare the levels of fibre consumption in some parts of the World, just as rural Chinese population (70–80 g/day) with the observed intake in Western countries (5–20 g/day), such intake is very low in the latter, therefore, the probability of finding an association is also reduced from a statistical viewpoint. The Uruguayan study on fibre and BC [19] found a protective for the highest consumption (between 23 and 44% of protection depending on the source foods). Nevertheless, in the interviewed population a very low intake of fibre-rich foods was found, thus, we experienced a similar risk of other studies, in the sense that possible differences between cases and controls tended to the null. Animal research supports also the epidemiologic findings, since a fibre-rich diet was seen as associated to a reduced incidence of chemically induced BC [20].

Several biologic mechanisms were proposed, through which fibre could prevent BC [21]. There are non-soluble components of fibre which are excreted relatively unchanged, and on the other hand, several soluble fractions have varied biologic effects. Fibre can reduce the intestinal reabsortion of estrogens which are excreted through the bile [22]. Also, fibre could act more indirectly through beneficial effects as the reduction of body weight or improving the sensibility to insulin [23], each one of them could be playing a certain role in the etiology of BC. In addition, it has been recognized that other bioactive components of fibre-rich foods, such as carotenoids, isoflavones or lignans, could explain at least partially the epidemiologic associations between the fibre and the risk of BC.

THE AVAILABLE EPIDEMIOLOGIC EVIDENCE AND THE BIOLOGIC PLAUSIBILITY SUGGEST THAT DIETARY FIBRE POSSIBLY REDUCES THE RISK OF BREAST CANCER.

Sugar

Sugar is part of foods with high glycemic index (together with ice cream, potatoes, bread, bakery, etc.), the products whose ingestion cause the major increase of blood sugar. Therefore, they finally imply high glucose loadings. The results of several case-control studies which have included in their analysis the relationship between sugar consumption and BC are inconsistent. The intake of sugar and confitures were reported as associated to a risk increase [24], non significant risk increase [25], absence of association [4, 5, 26] and even protective effects [14].

Mortality rates due to BC and the per capita intakes of glucose and sucrose displayed direct correlations, which were reported in international ecologic studies [27].

Insulin could be involved in the development of BC [28, 29], as an expression of insulin resistance syndrome, in which high insulin levels are associated with an increased risk of BC [30]. The point is developed in the chapter on Metabolism and Breast Cancer.

THE EVIDENCE OF ASSOCIATION BETWEEN SUGAR AND BREAST CANCER IS CURRENTLY STILL INCONSISTENT. IT CANNOT BE CONCLUSIVE.

The Glycemic Index

The Glycemic Index (GI) has proven to be a useful nutritional concept since it contributes to have a new view of the relationships between foods and chronic diseases like cancer. The GI is the measure of entrance of different carbohydrates sources into the bloodstream. The faster the Index is the higher is the effect on the insulin secretion. Examples of high GI are white bread, white rice, potatoes, soft drinks, dry fruits. Examples of median GI are: orange juice, banana, sweet potato, chocolate, fruit cocktail, spagetti. Finally, some foods with low GI include: skimmed yoghurt, plums, apples, beans, lentils and tomatoes.

Also the concept of Glycemic Load (GL) exists, which is the product of multiplying the GI of a given food by its carbohydrates contents. A diet with a high GL can contribute to a metabolic environment prone to carcinogenesis, beginning with the stimulation on the insulin and the insulin-like growth factors (IGF-1, i.e.).

The results of studies on foods with high GI or high GL are not conclusive. There is evidence of risk increase for foods which are rich in carbohydrates having high GI [31–33], as well as absence of association [34–36]. Some effects were observed only in pre-menopausal [37] or only in postmenopausal women [38], and even showing opposite effects according BMI [39].

FOODS WITH HIGH GLYCEMIC INDEX OR WITH HIGH GLYCEMIC LOAD CAN INCREASE THE RISK, ALTHOUGH THE EVIDENCE IS STILL NOT CONCLUSIVE.

Fats and Cholesterol

Total Fat

The main dietary hypothesis related with BC has been by far that fat-rich diets increase the risk of the disease. Although such hypothesis had its experimental support almost seven decades [40] where fat-rich diets increased the occurrence of mammary tumours in rodents, it was reinforced on a basis of strong statistical correlations (r=0.7–0.9) which were shown in international ecologic studies, based on food disappearance from market [41, 42]. This hypothesis, in addition, has been subject of large controversies along the last two decades.

A large series of prospective and case-control type studies examined the relationship between the intake of fats, cholesterol and the risk of BC. Most of prospective studies, performed in cohorts of Western developed countries (where is usual 30% or higher of dietary energy coming from fats) showed elevated risks but not statistically significant, for the group of highest intake respect the one of least intake in each studied population sample. We mention herewith some of them [12, 43, 44]. The results implied previously adjustments by variables of reproductive history and family predisposition to cancer, as well as by alcohol intake or other factors such as body mass and education. When a part of these studies were analyzed in a meta-analysis [45], no increase of risk was observed with the highest intake of fat or a risk reduction with intakes lesser than 20% of total energy coming from fat. More recent prospective cohort studies [46–49] have shown no association either.

Besides, the case-control studies have shown inconsistent results. The fraction of highest intake was associated with an increase of risk [8] or absence of significant association [50–52], having controlled for the main confounding variables. A meta-analysis of 12 case-control studies [13] displayed elevated risks for high intakes of total fat (>100 g/day), with a stronger association among postmenopausal than among pre-menopausal women (RR=1.5 vs. RR=1.1 respectively). Based on such numbers, the authors proposed that (at least in North America) a reduction of average consumption of total fat around 25–30% could lead to a reduction of the BC incidence of 24% and 16% among post- and pre-menopausal women respectively, assuming that those observed association were causal.

Other meta-analysis including 23 studies on dietary fat and BC [53] did not use the data of the original studies but averaged the relative risks of the groups with highest intake. With this methodology, the authors obtained a weak but significant risk increase (RR = 1.12, CI 1.04–1.21) for total fat. A further meta-analysis of 45 epidemiologic studies (14 cohort studies and 31 case-control studies) by the same principal investigator [54] found again a weak but statistically significant relation between high fat intake and greater BC risk. A Recent study [55] found no significant association of BC with total, monounsaturated, or polyunsaturated fat. Finally, another recent meta-analysis and review of epidemiological cohort studies [56] reported no significant association comparing the highest category of animal fat intake with the lowest, and no significant association between a 5% increment of energy from animal fat intake and BC either.

The discrepancies observed between the findings obtained from cohort and from case-control studies, have been matter of controversy, based on the possibility that the information in some cases could have been biased to null due to methodological errors or due to factors which are not easily assessed. The persistency of such controversies was confirmed in a review on diet and BC [57].

Even after adjusting by per capita gross product and by mean age at menarche, the intake of total fat in international indexes keeps a close correlation with BC rates [58]. Nevertheless, other heavy known risk factors for BC such as late age at first delivery, low number of births, high body mass index and high stature are also more common in developed societies and they could confound the ecologic association between dietary fat and BC. This viewpoint should be taken into account when analyzing what happened in Japan along the XXth century, in which the fat consumption has increased parallel to BC rates [59]. The increase could be linked to a higher prevalence of reproductive risk factors, as well as to other dietary and public health changes associated to faster growth rates and higher increases of body weight in adult population. The increases in mortality rates of BC in Japanese women show a cohort birth effect: a small increase occurred among women born around 1925 [60], suggesting that the fat consumption in adults does not influence substantially the risk of BC. In the same study, even though it could be argued that older women have not changed their lifestyle and diet, the notable increases in mortality due to colon cancer at all ages suggest that such explanation is unlikely.

Probably the most controversial side of the relationship between dietary fat and experimental mammary carcinogenesis is the relative importance of caloric intake. Since fat is the most dense macronutrient in terms of calories, diets which are fat-rich derive into higher intakes of calories, unless there is an adequate surveillance on having constant the energy. A considerably strong association between a high caloric intake and carcinogenesis has been observed in rats [61], as well as a powerful effect of caloric decrease in the tumour reduction, but no independent effect of fat related to body gain or tumour incidence was described [62].

The dietary fat could play some role in the development of BC through effects on the hormonal metabolism. The endogen estrogenic levels are considered to be related with the risk of BC. An increased exposure to sexual hormones, in particular estrogens, could lead to a situation of increased risk of BC through effects on the mammary proliferation. We analyzed thoroughly this issue in a recent review [63] and there is a background to discuss in the chapter on *Primary Prevention of Breast Cancer*. Vegetarian women, consuming higher amounts of fibre and lesser amounts of fat compared to non vegetarians, display lower blood levels and reduced urinary excretion of estrogens, apparently due to an increased faecal excretion [64].

Alternatively, any mechanism for a role of dietary fat in the BC can be less direct. For example, dietary styles which are fat-rich could lead to a larger body mass or also to obesity, a probable risk factor for BC in postmenopausal women. Also, a higher fat intake during childhood or adolescence could promote a faster growth and an earlier onset of menarche, both risk factors already established for BC, however, this relationship has not been still established. If diet at early and young ages is an important factor, this could be the explanation of why were reported so many inconsistent results from epidemiologic studies in which only adults' diet was measured.

TOTAL FAT-RICH DIETS POSSIBLY INCREASE THE RISK OF BREAST CANCER. THERE ARE INCONSISTENCIES IN RESULTS BUT THERE ARE PROPOSED BIOLOGICAL MECHANISMS, WHICH ARE PLAUSIBLE.

Saturated Fats

Its high caloric content is a reason why a fat-rich diet can imply a risk for the breast. In fact, a diet which is low in calories can protect against BC. But perhaps the main danger of saturated fats is in particular its capability to increase the insulin resistance. The main saturated fats are present in whole dairy foods and fatty red meats.

An analysis of seven cohort studies on BC [11] indicates that there were no associations between saturated or animal fat with the disease. Besides, other analysis of 12 case-control studies reported a risk increase for high intake of saturated fat among postmenopausal women (RR = 1.57), adjusted for total fat [13].

Most prospective and case-control studies have examined the intake of saturated or animal fat, and at the same time, most of them have displayed statistically non significant associations with BC, with Relative Risks in the range of 0.9–1.7 for the highest percentiles of intake. Five of 17 case-control studies which examined the intake of saturated fat reported a significant dose-response or a significant increase of risk for the highest consumption level, with RR between 1.8 and 3.6 for the highest intake levels. These studies were conducted in Canada, Hawaii, Italy, Argentina and France [6, 65–67]. Of all Relative Risks found in the 17 studies above quoted, five were between 1.6 and 1.9 and six were 2.0 or higher. When these data are compared with those on total fat, a higher proportion of data from saturated or animal fat suggest a strong increase in risk. In addition, there were no studies indicating a negative association, that is, some protective effect from the consumption of animal fat.

A Recent study [55] found an association between high saturated fat intake and greater breast cancer risk was found [HR=1.13 (95% CI 1.00, 1.27; p for trend=0.038)] but in menopausal women, the positive association with saturated fat was confined to nonusers of hormone therapy at baseline. Another recent European cohort study reported an increased risk of BC associated with high saturated fat intake [68].

DIETS HIGH IN SATURATED FATS PROBABLY INCREASE THE RISK OF BREAST CANCER, ALTHOUGH CERTAIN INCONSISTENCIES OF RESULTS TURN DIFFICULT A CONCLUSION.

Monounsaturated Fats

An analysis of seven cohort studies on BC [24] has not found associations between monounsaturated fat and the disease. In the same way that with saturated fats, an analysis of 12 case-control studies reported also an elevated risk of BC among post-menopausal women with high intake of monounsaturated fat (significant RR=1.4). In addition, the risk assessment in prospective studies is divided, in the sense of risk increase with high intake of monounsaturated fat, as well as a significant dose-response. Recent research reported no effect or even a positive association with BC [46–48, 69].

Some cohort studies reported a protective effect of monounsaturated fat intake on BC risk [49, 70–72]. There were also case-control studies in which an important number of investigations where no statistical associations between BC and the intake of monounsaturated fat were communicated, just the same as the findings of an international ecologic study which did not find correlation between monounsaturated fat intake and BC incidence [42].

Some ecologic studies which have analyzed the olive oil – where fat is almost exclusively monounsaturated oleic acid – showed protective associations. Since BC is less common in Mediterranean countries than in North America and North-Western Europe, there were authors proposing the more frequent intake of olive oil as a possible reason for such difference [73]. The evidence appears in three case-control studies expressed by a significant reduction in risk with high intake of the oil [74–76] and consistent with findings derived from previous animal experimentation [77]. Of the case-control studies, the findings in Greek women are remarkable, in view of a 25% risk reduction of BC among those ones whose intake of olive oil was more than once a day [76].

A recent study [78] reported that elevated adipose monounsaturated fatty acids and oleic acid (in gluteal adipose tissue) were found associated with reduced odds of BC (OR=0.15; 95% CI 0.03–0.64, and OR=0.18; 95% CI 0.04–0.71, respectively).

The belief that the protective effect of olive oil was based on its high average content (72%) of the monounsaturated fat oleic acid, as we mentioned before, has its weakness. Such fat is also found in the fat of a beefsteak, in chicken (also in the skin) in non negligible amounts (22–53%), as well as in other common vegetable oils as of corn, peanut, soy and sunflower, in the range of 23–50%. The point is that several other fats and oils which are rich in oleic acid are very associated with increased risk of BC and colon cancer in humans. Therefore, it is assumed that this monounsaturated fat cannot completely account for the protective effect or for the absence of promotion effect in the development of cancer [79]. Furthermore, a case-control study on individual storage of monounsaturated fatty acids in the adipose tissue in relation with BC in women indicated that the oleic acid in the olive oil did not show any protective property of this oil [80].

In the last years there is a substance that was proposed as the hypothetical responsible for the protective effect of olive oil: the ***squalene,*** a triterpene which is present up to a 0.7%, of particularly high concentration compared to other human and animal fats and oils [81, 82]. Sharks have highest known tissue concentration of squalene (40% or more in the liver oil) [82] and such concentration has been considered as an attribute for their particular resistance against cancer [83]. Squalene is an intermediate step in the way of steroid biosynthesis in plants and in animals, and a hypothetical mechanism for its antitumour activity was proposed [84].

Although theoretically a diet with an increase of dietary squalene could potentially increase the production of cholesterol and bile acids – and as a consequence being an enhancer for atherosclerosis –, on the contrary, the available data of human epidemiology derived from short-term studies on supplementation with squalene in humans, and experimental studies in animals suggest that an increased intake of squalene does not represent of hypercholesterolemia. Moreover, the high differences recognized in the average daily intake of squalene between Mediterranean countries and the United States (from 7 to 13 times higher in Europe) could be one of the factors which are related with a lower mortality of cancer in those populations sited at the Mediterranean basin [85].

DIETS RICH IN MONOUNSATURATED FAT COULD BE NOT RELATED WITH HIGH RISK OF BREAST CANCER. HOWEVER, A HIGH INTAKE OF OLIVE OIL PROBABLY REDUCES THE RISK THROUGH MECHANISMS NOT RELATED WITH OLEIC ACID.

Polyunsaturated Fatty Acids (PUFA) Ω-6 and Ω-3

Although in the previous years it was already recognized that the experimental evidence favoured the existence of a possible relation between BC and PUFA Ω-6 and Ω-3, the literature is not conclusive: there are works which show no association with the risk of the disease and the evidence is still not large. As it usually happens, different methodologies and estimations of the fat consumption could be underlying the different results that were observed.

In 2002 two studies [86, 87] measured the content of these fats in human mammary tissue, in patients with BC and in women without cancer: those afflicted with BC had a reduced content of Ω-3 and a higher content of Ω-6 compared with healthy women. Other epidemiologic studies have reported a risk reduction for a diet rich in Ω-3 or with an adequate Ω-6/Ω-3 ratio [88–90]. Nevertheless, more recent studies and reviews have not found association between the intake of PUFA and the risk of BC [91–93]. Since one of these papers [93] reported no association for any fatty acid in particular and also found a statistically significant interaction between Ω-6 PUFA intake, marine-derived Ω-3 PUFA may be more important for such risk than individual dietary amounts of these fatty acids.

Facing this evidence, the issue remains controversial since the experimental evidence in favour of the described associations is very important.

The possible role of essential PUFA (linoleic acid [LA] and α-linolenic acid [ALA]) [94] and the risk of BC was analyzed in Uruguayan population. PUFA were significantly and inversely associated with the risk of BC (OR = 0.38 for the group with highest intake), equivalent to a risk reduction of 62%. LA was associated with a significant risk reduction (OR = 0.24). On the contrary, ALA was significantly associated with a risk increase (OR = 2.76). Regarding this latter, it is worthy to remark that even though ALA is a Ω-3 PUFA, several animal and vegetables sources are its contributors. There were studies recognizing ALA as a marker of high intake of red meat, for example. There is no countersense if a high intake of this Ω-3 fatty acid is found positively associated with the risk of BC.

In particular, the final and long-chain PUFA (EPA and DHA) were also studied in the last decade among Uruguayan women [95]. A threefold risk of BC was found among those consumers of a ratio Ω-6/Ω-3 higher than 50, compared to those consumers of a low or modest ratio between both types of PUFA. Anyway, it should be recognized the fact that those populations who consume abundantly foods that are sources of Ω-3 PUFA, in Europe as well as in Asia and America, are not so afflicted by BC [96]. In this sense, experimental research conducted in the last years has found that the combination of high level of Ω-3 (in seafood and fishes), a low level of Ω-6 (in vegetable oils and fats) and a high intake of monounsaturated fats (in olive oil), which are present in the Mediterranean diet, is a powerful "anti-HER-2" cocktail [97].

THE EVIDENCE IS STILL NOT CONCLUSIVE, BUT IT SUGGESTS A POSITIVE RELATION OF Ω-6 FATS AND A NEGATIVE ONE OF Ω-3 FATS WITH BREAST CANCER.

TRANS Fatty Acids

The trans-fatty acids (TFA) are Ω-6 fatty acids, which have been chemically modified through a process of hydrogenation. They are artificially created and exist in those foods whose labels show the words "hydrogenated fats" or "partially hydrogenated fats". Their main application is to increase the conservation period of certain foods and to make the fat become more solid. They are constituents of French fries and other snack-type products, as well as in cookies, cakes, bakery and other popular sweetened products. These fats have influence on inflammation and endothelial biomarkers as Reactive C-Protein, IL-6 and others [98], something that locates these artificial products not only as potentially dangerous for the vascular structures but also from the metabolic and oncologic viewpoint.

There is conflicting evidence concerning the possible role of TFA in breast cancer. A cohort study on BC in the United States analyzed the intake of TFA and reported the absence of association, with a non significant RR = 0.9 for the highest intake level [71]. The issue is under continuous revision since some years and is still controversial [99]. However, the concentration of TFA in gluteal adipose tissue was positively associated (OR = 1.4) with the BC risk in European postmenopausal women [100] as part of the EURAMIC study (European Community Multicentre Study on Antioxidants, Myocardial Infarction, and Breast Cancer). The positive association was not attributable to differences in age, body mass index, exogenous hormone use, or socio-economic status.

TRANS-FATTY ACIDS POSSIBLY INCREASE THE RISK OF BREAST CANCER, BUT DATA DO NOT ENABLE US TO BE CONCLUSIVE.

Cholesterol

None of the 5 prospective studies on BC which examined the relationship with cholesterol intake did show any significant statistical association. In 4 of them, the RR for the level of highest consumption ranged between 0.7–1.2 and in the remaining study [43] the RR reached a value of 2.2. The analysis of 7 cohort studies conducted by Hunter et al. [45], already quoted, did not show an association with the intake of cholesterol.

Most case-control studies which examined the intake of cholesterol have not either reported any significant association, having found for the level of highest consumption a RR between 0.5 and 1.3 [101].

Regarding the role of mammographic density as a risk factor for BC, a recent study found no evidence indicating any association between dietary and serum cholesterol levels and mammographic density [102].

An experimental study examined the role of cholesterol in the regulation of tumour progression in a mouse model of mammary tumour formation [103], suggesting that cholesterol accelerates and enhances tumour formation. In addition, tumours were more aggressive, and tumour angiogenesis was enhanced. It was also observed that plasma cholesterol levels were reduced during tumour development but not prior to its initiation. These data provide new evidence for an increased utilization of cholesterol by tumours and for its role in tumour formation. Taken together, the results of this recent work imply that an increase in plasma cholesterol levels accelerates the development of tumours and exacerbates their aggressiveness.

As it will be shown further in the Uruguayan studies, the analysis of fats and risk of BC [94] showed that the highest consumers of cholesterol experienced significant increases of risk (OR = 4.3), stronger than for other fat components. We have suggested that the combination of high cholesterol intake together with an imbalance of Ω-6/Ω-3 PUFA is something characteristic of Western dietary styles [63] and it could increase the risk of BC since the latter imbalance makes difficult the bile elimination of cholesterol.

The estrogen action exerted by a hydroxylated derivative of cholesterol, in particular 25-hydroxycholesterol (25HC) may be considered as an additional factor involved in the progression of breast and ovarian tumours, according to an experimental research [104]. This study demonstrated that the α-estrogen receptor (α-ER) mediates gene expression changes and growth responses induced by 25HC in breast and ovarian cancer cells. These facts could explain partially the positive associations between BC and cholesterol that studies like the Uruguayan one have reported.

CHOLESTEROL-RICH DIETS COULD BE RELATED WITH THE RISK OF BREAST CANCER, BUT ANY STRONG STATEMENT IS STILL PREMATURE.

Proteins

Total Proteins

Since the research focused mainly on fat intake, protein consumption has been usually somehow underreported, in case-control as well as in cohort studies. A prospective cohort study of 1994 [44] which showed a risk increase related with meat consumption, did not reveal an influence of protein consumption, after adjusting for calories intake. An analysis of 12 case-control studies published two decades ago has not either shown any effect in the risk of BC from the intake of total protein, even if it was adjusted for fat intake [13].

Just as it happened with dietary fat, the ecologic studies exhibited strong correlations between consumption of total and animal protein and national mortality rates of BC (r = 0.6 and 0.9 respectively) [41]. A study on health in China has not found an association similar to the one before quoted [105]. The consumption levels along the 65 provinces included in this study were in general lower than those of countries belonging to the Western culture. Therefore, if a threshold effect exists, for which only intakes over a given and relatively high level affect the risk, an actual association could not become detectable within the studied Chinese populations.

CURRENTLY, ANY JUDGMENT ON POSSIBLE EFFECTS OF TOTAL PROTEINS IS NOT POSSIBLE TO BE ESTABLISHED. PROBABLY THEIR ANIMAL OR VEGETABLE SOURCE MEAN DIFFERENCES IN SUCH EFFECTS.

Animal Protein

At least four case-control studies on BC have analyzed the intake of animal protein. An Italian study showed a significant RR=2.9 for the level of highest consumption, an association which was evident for pre- as well as for postmenopausal women and remaining after adjustment for saturated fat intake [44]. A Hawaiian study also showed risk increase (a significant RR=1.6) only among Japanese but not in Caucasian women, and also among those who had had an early menarche [106]. Another two studies, performed in Asian populations as Singapore and Japan did not show significant associations in relation to the consumption of animal protein. In addition, the Japanese study did not show a relationship even when only the post-menopausal subset was considered. Differences between cases and controls were not either observed when the intake of foods which are sources of animal protein – such as meat, poultry, eggs and dairy – were analyzed.

International correlations between the intake of animal protein and rates of incidence and mortality of BC, as well as of other hormone-related cancers such as ovary, endometrium and prostate have been reported [41].

According to animal experimentation with rodents, diets with animal protein showed relationships with biological facts. When the intake level was notably low, the rates of body growth and sexual maturity were reduced and the tumour incidence also fell, when compared to the usual level of protein consumption on a basis of dairy casein [107]. The effect of tumour promotion derived from the dietary animal protein seems to be more pronounced during early stages of life, especially during sexual maturation and during the development of mammary glands, which are periods when hormonal activities are particularly significant [108].

THE EVIDENCE, ALTHOUGH STILL NOT ENOUGH, SUGGESTS THAT DIETS RICH IN ANIMAL PROTEIN COULD INCREASE THE RISK OF BREAST CANCER.

Vegetable Protein

An Italian case-control study reported a moderate reduction in the risk of BC (a significant RR=0.7) for the quartile with the highest intakes of protein having vegetal source [109]. As it was already quoted above, such study also showed a risk increase for animal protein. A case-control study in Singapore analyzed the intake of soy protein and found a strong association in the protective sense: a significant RR=0.4 for total soy protein and a significant RR=0.3 for the soy proportion in total protein [110].

BASED ON A SMALL EVIDENCE, IT IS STILL NOT POSSIBLE MAKE A JUDGEMENT ON THE ROLE OF VEGETABLE PROTEINS.

References

1. Key TJ, Spencer EA (2007) Carbohydrates and cancer: an overview of the epidemiological evidence. Eur J Clin Nutr 61(Suppl 1):S112–S121
2. Hems G (1978) The contributions of diet and childbearing to breast-cancer rates. Br J Cancer 37(6):974–982
3. Katsouyanni K, Trichopoulous A, Stuver S et al (1994) The association of fat and other macronutrients with breast cancer: a case-control study from Greece. Br J Cancer 70:537–541
4. Rohan TE, McMichael AJ, Baghurst PA (1988) A population-based case-control study of diet and breast cancer in Australia. Am J Epidemiol 128:478–489
5. Franceschi S, Favero A, Decarli A et al (1996) Intake of macronutrients and risk of breast cancer. Lancet 347:1351–1356
6. Iscovich J, Iscovich R, Howe J et al (1989) A case-control study of diet and breast cancer in Argentina. Int J Cancer 44:770–777
7. Rohan TE, Howe GR, Friedenreich CM et al (1993) Dietary fiber, vitamins A, C, and E, and risk of breast cancer: a cohort study. Cancer Causes Control 4:29–37
8. Van't Veer P, Kalb CM, Verhoef P et al (1990) Dietary fiber, beta-carotene and breast cancer: results from a case-control study. Int J Cancer 45:825–828
9. Wu AH, Yu MC, Tseng CC et al (2009) Dietary patterns and breast cancer risk in Asian American women. Am J Clin Nutr 89(4):1145–1154
10. Nielsen TG, Olsen A, Christensen J et al (2005) Dietary carbohydrate intake is not associated with the breast cancer incidence rate ratio in postmenopausal Danish women. J Nutr 135(1): 124–128
11. Graham S, Zielezny M, Marshall J et al (1992) Diet in the epidemiology of postmenopausal breast cancer in a New York State cohort. Am J Epidemiol 136:1327
12. Willett WC, Hunter DJ, Stampfer MJ et al (1992) Dietary fat and fiber to relation to risk of breast cancer: an eight year follow-up. JAMA 268:2037–2044
13. Howe GR, Hirohata T, Hislop TG et al (1990) Dietary factors and risk of breast cancer: combined analysis of 12 case-control studies. J Natl Cancer Inst 82:561–569
14. Zaridze D, Lifanova Y, Maximovitch D et al (1991) Diet, alcohol consumption and reproductive factors in a case-control study of breast cancer in Moscow. Int J Cancer 48:493–501
15. Yuan JM, Wang Q, Ross RK et al (1995) Diet and breast cancer in Shanghai and Tianjin, China. Br J Cancer 71:1353–1358
16. Freudenheim JL, Marshall JR, Vena JE et al (1996) Premenopausal breast cancer risk and intake of vegetables, fruits, and related nutrients. J Natl Cancer Inst 88:340–348
17. Sonestedt E, Borgquist S, Ericson U et al (2008) Plant foods and oestrogen receptor alpha- and beta-defined breast cancer: observations from the malmo diet and cancer cohort. Carcinogenesis 29(11):2203–2209
18. Cade JE, Burley VJ, Greenwood DC et al (2007) Dietary fibre and risk of breast cancer in the UK women's cohort study. Int J Epidemiol 36(2):431–438

19. De Stéfani E, Correa P, Ronco A et al (1997) Dietary fiber and risk of breast cancer. Nutr Cancer 28:14–19
20. Cohen LA, Kendall ME, Zang E et al (1991) Modulation of N-nitrosomethylurea-induced mammary tumor promotion by dietary fiber and fat. J Natl Cancer Inst 83:496–501
21. Adlercreutz H (2010) Can rye intake decrease risk of human breast cancer? Food Nutr Res 54:5231. doi:DOI: 10.3402/fnr.v54i0.5231
22. Goldin BR, Adlercreutz H, Gorbach SL et al (1982) Estrogen excretion patterns and plasma levels in vegetarian and omnivorous women. N Engl J Med 307:1542
23. Stoll BA (1996) Nutrition and breast cancer risk: can an effect via insulin resistance be demonstrated? Breast Cancer Res Treat 38:239–246
24. Franceschi S, Favero A, La Vecchia C et al (1995) Influence of food groups and food diversity on breast cancer risk in Italy. Int J Cancer 63(6):785–789
25. Katsouyanni K, Willett W, Trichopoulos D et al (1988) Risk of breast cancer among Greek women in relation to nutrient intake. Cancer 61:181–185
26. Ewertz M, Gill C (1990) Dietary factors and breast cancer risk in Denmark. Int J Cancer 46: 779–784
27. Seely S, Horrobin DF (1983) Diet and breast cancer: the possible connection with sugar consumption. Med Hypotheses 11(3):319–327
28. Bruning PF, Bonfrer JMG, Hart AAM et al (1992) Body measurements, estrogen availability and the risk of human breast cancer: a case-control study. Int J Cancer 51:14–19
29. Kazer RR (1995) Insulin resistance, insulin-like growth factor I and breast cancer: a hypothesis. Int J Cancer 62(4):403–406
30. Luceri C, Caderni G, Lodovici M et al (1996) Urinary excretion of sucrose and fructose as a predictor of sucrose intake in dietary intervention studies. Cancer Epidemiol Biomarkers Prev 5(3):167–171
31. Dal Maso L, La Vecchia C et al (2001) Dietary glycemic index and glycemic load, and breast cancer risk: a case-control study. Ann Oncol 12(11):1533–1538
32. Lajous M, Willett W, Lazcano-Ponce E et al (2005) Glycemic load, glycemic index, and the risk of breast cancer among Mexican women. Cancer Causes Control 16(10):1165–1169
33. Tavani A, Giordano L, Gallus S et al (2006) Consumption of sweet foods and breast cancer risk in Italy. Ann Oncol 17(2):341–345
34. Jonas CR, McCullough ML, Teras LR et al (2003) Dietary glycemic index, glycemic load, and risk of incident breast cancer in postmenopausal women. Cancer Epidemiol Biomarkers Prev 12(6):573–577
35. Holmes MD, Liu S, Hankinson SE et al (2004) Dietary carbohydrates, fiber, and breast cancer risk. Am J Epidemiol 159(8):732–739
36. Giles GG, Simpson JA, English DR et al (2006) Dietary carbohydrate, fibre, glycaemic index, glycaemic load and the risk of postmenopausal breast cancer. Int J Cancer 118(7):1843–1847
37. Higginbotham S, Zhang ZF, Lee IM et al (2004) Dietary glycemic load and breast cancer risk in the women's health study. Cancer Epidemiol Biomarkers Prev 13(1):65–70
38. Silvera SA, Jain M, Howe GR et al (2005) Dietary carbohydrates and breast cancer risk: a prospective study of the roles of overall glycemic index and glycemic load. Int J Cancer 114(4):653–658
39. Cho E, Spiegelman D, Hunter DJ et al (2003) Premenopausal dietary carbohydrate, glycemic index, glycemic load, and fiber in relation to risk of breast cancer. Cancer Epidemiol Biomarkers Prev 12(11 Pt 1):1153–1158
40. Tannenbaum A (1942) Genesis and growth of tumors. III. Effects of a high-fat diet. Cancer Res 2:468–475
41. Armstrong B, Doll R (1975) Environmental factors and cancer incidence and mortality in different countries, with special reference to dietary practices. Int J Cancer 15:617–631
42. Hursting S, Thornquist M, Henderson M (1990) Types of dietary fat and the incidence of cancer at 5 sites. Prev Med 19:242–253
43. Knekt P, Albanes D, Seppanen R et al (1990) Dietary fat and risk of breast cancer. Am J Clin Nutr 52:903–908

44. Toniolo P, Riboli E, Shore RE et al (1994) Consumption of meat, animal products protein, and fat and risk of breast cancer – a prospective cohort study in New York. Epidemiology 5:391–397
45. Hunter DJ, Spiegelman D, Adami HO et al (1996) Cohort studies of fat intake and the risk of breast cancer – a pooled analysis. N Engl J Med 334:356–361
46. Velie E, Kulldorff M, Schairer C et al (2000) Dietary fat, fat subtypes, and breast cancer in postmenopausal women: a prospective cohort study. J Natl Cancer Inst 92:833–839
47. Byrne C, Rockett H, Holmes MD (2002) Dietary fat, fat subtypes, and breast cancer risk: lack of an association among postmenopausal women with no history of benign breast disease. Cancer Epidemiol Biomarkers Prev 11:261–265
48. Kim EH, Willett WC, Colditz GA et al (2006) Dietary fat and risk of postmenopausal breast cancer in a 20-year follow-up. Am J Epidemiol 164:990–997
49. Lof M, Sandin S, Lagiou P et al (2007) Dietary fat and breast cancer risk in the Swedish women's lifestyle and health cohort. Br J Cancer 97:1570–1576
50. Holmberg L, Ohlander EM, Byers T et al (1994) Diet and breast cancer risk: results from a population-based, case-control study in Sweden. Arch Intern Med 154:1805–1811
51. La Vecchia C, Decarli A, Parazzini F et al (1987) General epidemiology of breast cancer in Northern Italy. Int J Epidemiol 16:347–355
52. Levi F, La Vecchia C, Gulie C et al (1993) Dietary factors and breast cancer risk in Vaud, Switzerland. Nutr Cancer 19:327–335
53. Boyd NF, Martin L, Noffel M et al (1993) A metaanalysis of studies of dietary-fat and breast-cancer risk. Br J Cancer 68:267–275
54. Boyd NF, Stone J, Vogt KN et al (2003) Dietary fat and breast cancer risk revisited: a meta-analysis of the published literature. Br J Cancer 89:1672–1685
55. Sieri S, Krogh V, Ferrari P et al (2008) Dietary fat and breast cancer risk in the European prospective investigation into cancer and nutrition. Am J Clin Nutr 88(5):1304–1312
56. Alexander DD, Morimoto LM, Mink PJ et al (2010) Summary and meta-analysis of prospective studies of animal fat intake and breast cancer. Nutr Res Rev 23(1):169–179
57. Wu AH (2000) Diet and breast carcinoma in multiethnic populations. Cancer 88(Suppl 5): 1239–1244
58. Rl P, Kakar F, Hursting S et al (1988) Aspects of the rationale for the women's health trial. J Natl Cancer Inst 80:802–814
59. Hirayama T (1978) Epidemiology of breast cancer with special reference to the role of diet. Prev Med 7:173–195
60. Aoki K, Hayakawa N, Kurihara M et al (1992) Death rates for malignant neoplasms for selected sites by sex and 5-year age group in 33 countries 1953–57 to 1983–87. UICC, Univ. of Nagoya Coop Press, Nagoya
61. Ip C, Chin SF, Scimeca JA et al (1991) Mammary cancer prevention by conjugated dienoic derivative of linoleic acid. Cancer 51:6118–6124
62. Welsch CW (1992) Relationship between dietary fat and experimental mammary tumorigenesis: a review and critique. Cancer Res 52(Suppl 7):2040s–2048s
63. Ronco AL, De Stéfani E, Stoll M (2010) Hormonal and metabolic modulation through nutrition: towards a primary prevention of breast cancer. Breast 19:322–332
64. Woods MN, Gorbach SL, Longcope C et al (1989) Low-fat, high-fiber diet and serum estrone sulfate in premenopausal women. Am J Clin Nutr 49:1179–1183
65. Hirohata T, Nomura AMY, Hankin JH et al (1987) An epidemiological study on the association between diet and breast cancer. J Natl Cancer Inst 78:595–600
66. Lubin JH, Burns PE, Blot WJ et al (1981) Dietary factors and breast cancer risk. Int J Cancer 28:685–689
67. Richardson S, Gerber M, Cenee S (1991) The role of fat, animal protein and some vitamin consumption in breast cancer: a case-control study in Southern France. Int J Cancer 48:1–9
68. Gonzalez CA, Riboli E (2010) Diet and cancer prevention: contributions from the European Prospective Investigation into Cancer and Nutrition (EPIC) study. Eur J Cancer 46(14): 2555–2562

69. Thiebaut AC, Kipnis V, Chang SC et al (2007) Dietary fat and postmenopausal invasive breast cancer in the National Institutes of health–AARP diet and health study cohort. J Natl Cancer Inst 99:451–462
70. Wolk A, Bergstrom R, Hunter D et al (1998) A prospective study of association of monounsaturated fat and other types of fat with risk of breast cancer. Arch Intern Med 158:41–45
71. Holmes MD, Hunter DJ, Colditz GA et al (1999) Association of dietary intake of fat and fatty acids with risk of breast cancer. JAMA 281:914–920
72. Voorrips LE, Brants HA, Kardinaal AF et al (2002) Intake of conjugated linoleic acid, fat, and other fatty acids in relation to postmenopausal breast cancer: the Netherlands cohort study on diet and cancer. Am J Clin Nutr 76:873–882
73. Rose DP, Boyar AP, Wynder EL (1986) International comparisons of mortality rates for cancer of the breast, ovary, prostate, and colon, and per capita food consumption. Cancer 58: 2263–2271
74. La Vecchia C, Negri E, Franceschi S et al (1995) Olive oil, other dietary fats, and the risk of breast cancer (Italy). Cancer Causes Control 6(6):545–550
75. Martin-Moreno JM, Willett W, Gorgojo L et al (1994) Dietary fat, olive oil intake and breast cancer risk. Int J Cancer 58:774–780
76. Trichopoulos A, Katsouyanni K, Stuver S et al (1995) Consumption of olive oil and specific food groups in relation to breast cancer risk in Greece. J Natl Cancer Inst 87:110–116
77. Welsch CW (1994) Interrelationship between dietary lipids and calories and experimental mammary gland tumorigenesis. Cancer 74(Suppl):1055–1062
78. Mamalakis G, Hatzis C, de Bree E et al (2009) Adipose tissue fatty acids in breast cancer patients versus healthy control women from Crete. Ann Nutr Metab 54(4):275–282
79. Newmark HL (1999) Squalene, olive oil, and cancer risk. In: Bradlow HL, Fishman J, Osborne MP (eds) Cancer prevention: novel nutrients and pharmaceutical developments, vol 889. Annals of the NewYork Academy Science, New York, pp 193–203
80. Simonsen N, Fernandez-Crehuet J, Martin-Moreno J et al (1997) Tissue stores of individual monounsaturated fats and breast cancer. FASEB J 11:A578
81. Becker R (1989) Preparation, composition and nutritional implications of amaranth seed oil. Cereal Foods World 34:950–953
82. Ck L, Ahrens EH, Schreibman H et al (1976) Measurement of squalene in human tissues and plasma: validation and application. J Lipid Res 17:38–45
83. Mathews J (1992) Sharks still intrigue cancer researchers. News report. J Natl Cancer Inst 84:1000–1002
84. Newmark HL (1997) Squalene, olive oil, and cancer risk: a review and hypothesis. Cancer Epidemiol Biomarkers Prev 6:1101–1103
85. Newmark HL (1999) Squalene, olive oil, and cancer risk. In: Bradlow HL, Fishman J, Osborne MP (eds) Cancer prevention: novel nutrients and pharmaceutical developments, vol 889. Annals of the New York Academy Science, New York, pp 193–203
86. Maillard V, Bougnoux P, Ferrari P et al (2002) N-3 and N-6 fatty acids in breast adipose tissue and relative risk of breast cancer in a case-control study in Tours, France. Int J Cancer 98(1): 78–83
87. Bagga D, Anders KH, Wang HJ et al (2002) Long-chain n-3-to-n-6 polyunsaturated fatty acid ratios in breast adipose tissue from women with and without breast cancer. Nutr Cancer 42(2):180–185
88. Tavani A, Pelucchi C, Parpinel M et al (2003) n-3 polyunsaturated fatty acid intake and cancer risk in Italy and Switzerland. Int J Cancer 105(1):113–116
89. Goodstine SL, Zheng T, Holford TR et al (2003) Dietary (n-3)/(n-6) fatty acid ratio: possible relationship to premenopausal but not postmenopausal breast cancer risk in U.S. women. J Nutr 133(5):1409–1414
90. Gago-Dominguez M, Yuan JM, Sun CL et al (2003) Opposing effects of dietary n-3 and n-6 fatty acids on mammary carcinogenesis: the Singapore Chinese Health Study. Br J Cancer 89(9):1686–1692

91. Engeset D, Alsaker E, Lund E et al (2006) Fish consumption and breast cancer risk. The European Prospective Investigation into Cancer and Nutrition (EPIC). Int J Cancer 119(1):175–182
92. MacLean CH, Newberry SJ, Mojica WA et al (2006) Effects of omega-3 fatty acids on cancer risk: a systematic review. JAMA 295(4):403–415
93. Murff HJ, Shu XO, Li H et al (2011) Dietary polyunsaturated fatty acids and breast cancer risk in Chinese women: a prospective cohort study. Int J Cancer 128(6):1434–1441
94. De Stéfani E, Deneo-Pellegrini H, Mendilaharsu M et al (1998) Essential fatty acids and breast cancer: a case-control study in Uruguay. Int J Cancer 76:491–494
95. Ronco A, De Stéfani E, Deneo-Pellegrini H (2006) Polyunsaturated fatty acids intake and risk of breast cancer: a case-control study. In: XIV World Congress on breast diseases, Zagreb, Croatia, May 18–21st 2006
96. Landa MC, Frago N, Tres A (1994) Diet and the risk of breast cancer in Spain. Eur J Cancer Prev 3:313–320
97. Menendez JA, Vazquez-Martin A, Ropero S et al (2006) HER2 (erbB-2)-targeted effects of the omega-3 polyunsaturated. Fatty acid alpha-linolenic acid (ALA; 18:3n-3) in breast cancer cells: the "fat features" of the "Mediterranean diet" as an "anti-HER2 cocktail". Clin Transl Oncol 8(11):812–820
98. Lopez-Garcia E, Schulze MB, Meigs JB et al (2005) Consumption of trans fatty acids is related to plasma biomarkers of inflammation and endothelial dysfunction. J Nutr 135(3):562–566
99. Kohlmeier L (1997) Biomarkers of fatty acid exposure and breast cancer risk. Am J Clin Nutr 66(6 Suppl):1548S–1556S
100. Kohlmeier L, Simonsen N, van 't Veer P et al (1997) Adipose tissue trans fatty acids and breast cancer in the European Community Multicenter study on antioxidants, myocardial infarction, and breast cancer. Cancer Epidemiol Biomarkers Prev 6(9):705–710
101. World Cancer Research Fund (1997) Food, nutrition and the prevention of cancer: a global perspective. American Institute for Cancer Research, Washington, DC, pp 252–287
102. Tamburrini AL, Woolcott CG, Boyd NF et al (2011) Associations between mammographic density and serum and dietary cholesterol. Breast Cancer Res Treat 125(1):181–189
103. Llaverias G, Danilo C, Mercier I et al (2011) Role of cholesterol in the development and progression of breast cancer. Am J Pathol 178(1):402–412
104. Lappano R, Recchia AG, De Francesco EM et al (2011) The cholesterol metabolite 25-Hydroxycholesterol activates estrogen receptor α-mediated signaling in cancer cells and in cardiomyocytes. PLoS One 6(1):e16631
105. Chen J, Campbell TC, Li J et al (1990) Diet, lifestyle and mortality in China. A study of the characteristics of 65 Chinese counties. Oxford Univ.Press/People's Medical Publishing House, Oxford/Beijing
106. Goodman MT, Nomura AMY, Wilkens LR et al (1992) The association of diet, obesity and breast cancer in Hawaii. Cancer Epidemiol Biomarkers Prev 1:269–275
107. Hawrylewicz EJ (1986) Fat-protein interaction, defined 2-generation studies. In: Ip C, Birt DF, Rogers AE (eds) Dietary fats and cancer, vol 222. Progress in clinical and biological research, Alan Liss Inc, New York, pp 403–434
108. Huang HH, Hawrylewicz EJ, Kissane JQ et al (1982) Effect of protein diet on release of prolactin and ovarian steroids in female rats. Nutr Rpts Int 26:807–820
109. Toniolo P, Riboli E, Protta F et al (1989) Calorie-providing nutrients and risk of breast cancer. J Natl Cancer Inst 81:278–86
110. Lee HP, Gourley L, Duffy SW et al (1991) Dietary effects on breast cancer risk in Singapore. Lancet 337:1197–1200

Chapter 5
Vitamins and Bioactive Substances

Vitamins

Carotenoids

The relationship between ß-carotene or carotenoids and the risk of BC has been assessed in different types of studies. Some cohort studies reported non significant RRs of 0.8–0.9 for the highest consumptions of carotenoids [1, 2]. A sample of women analyzed in the Women's Health Initiative study reported that the analyses of repeated measurements indicated that serum α-carotene and ß-carotene were inversely associated with BC [3].

A Swedish cohort study reported that dietary carotenoids were not significantly associated with the risk of BC overall or with any subtype defined by estrogen receptor (ER) and progesterone receptor (PR) status. However, dietary α-carotene and ß-carotene were inversely associated with the risk of ER-PR-BC among ever smokers [4]. No significant associations between BC risk and serum carotenoids were also reported in other European cohort study [5].

Of 14 case-control studies which examined the intake of carotenoids, 6 have communicated strong or moderate associations in a protective sense, with RRs ranging between 0.2 and 0.7 (three of them were significant) for the highest levels of intake. In addition, 4 studies reported a non significant RR = 0.8 and the rest reported risks between 1.0 and 1.2, which were not significant either [6].

A combined analysis of 8 case-control studies involving more than 6.000 cases found a weak but statistically significant protective association for the highest level of ß-carotene intake [7], an association which seemed to be limited only to postmenopausal women. Although such association is weak, it is consistent with the findings of the above quoted cohort studies.

A study in Uruguay [8] showed negative associations for the intake of all carotenoids and the risk of BC, but the most protective one was Lycopene (OR = 0.30) followed by α-Carotene and ß-Criptoxanthin, both with an OR = 0.52. In all cases, these estimates for the highest quartiles of consumption were statistically significant.

A.L. Ronco and E. De Stéfani, *Nutritional Epidemiology of Breast Cancer*,
DOI 10.1007/978-94-007-2397-9_5, © Springer Science+Business Media B.V. 2012

Dietary but not supplemental beta-carotene showed a protective effect against lobular BC (incidence rate ratio (IRR): 0.72, 95% CI 0.57–0.91) [9], albeit this study found no association between overall BC and any micronutrients. A study on nutrient patterns and BC [10] reported also a protective effect against non-ductal BC of the so-called "antioxidants" pattern, which displayed a high loading for carotenoids. Dietary ß-carotene was associated with a decreased risk in postmenopausal women with high alcohol intake [11]. No associations among premenopausal (OR = 1.04, 95% CI 0.85–1.27) or postmenopausal women (OR = 0.93, 95% CI 0.82–1.04) were found. In addition, a study restricted to invasive BC reported a significant and inverse association among premenopausal women for high levels of vitamin A, α-carotene, ß-carotene and lutein/zeaxanthin, whereas such inverse association was not observed among postmenopausal women [12].

Women with BC tended to have lower levels of plasma carotenoids than matched controls, but no significant associations were found among a multiethnic cohort [13]. Interestingly, the Nurses' Health Study reported that there was no inverse association between carotenoids and BC risk among women with low mammographic density, however, among women with high mammographic density, high levels of circulating alpha-carotene, beta-cryptoxanthin, lycopene, and lutein/zeaxanthin were associated with a significant 40–50% reduction in BC risk [14].

In addition, 2 studies of survival of BC have communicated that women with higher intakes of ß-carotene had a lower risk of dying because of their cancer, with a RR = 0.5 comparing the highest with the lowest level of intake [1, 15]. Besides, women with high plasmatic levels of carotenoids (specially eating more tomatoes, carrot, red pepper) reduced significantly their recurrence risk compared to those ones with low levels [16, 17]. The potential biologic mechanisms through which carotenoids could protect against BC include antioxidant activity, among others. Moreover, phase I enzyme inhibition and phase II enzyme induction were the underlying chemoprotective mechanisms of lycopene against Polycyclic Aromatic Hydrocarbons-induced toxicity, according to a recent experimental study [18].

HIGH DIETARY LEVELS OF CAROTENOIDS PROBABLY REDUCE THE RISK OF BREAST CANCER.

Vitamins B

Vitamins which belong to the B group such as folate, B-6 and B-12 work as coenzymes in one-carbon metabolism, which has been recognized as critical for DNA synthesis and methylation [19–22]. One-carbon metabolism is a network of interrelated biological reactions that provide essential cofactors for the production of S-adenosylmethionine, the primary methyl donor for methylation, as well as the methyl group in methylation of dUMP to dTMP for DNA synthesis [23]. The three vitamins are involved in different aspects of the metabolism of homocystein and therefore their deficiency may interfere with DNA methylation and synthesis, leading to aberrant gene expression and DNA instability and eventually the development of cancer [24, 25]. In addition to the quoted genetic risks, we should emphasize that DNA methylation involves potential epigenetic alterations, which could also be inherited.

Several studies have thoroughly analyzed the associations between folate, vitamin B-6, and vitamin B-12 and the risk of BC. Historically, an association between low plasmatic vitamin B-6 levels and BC was described more than three decades ago [26]. But a non significant increase of risk for high level of vitamin B-6 was also reported [27]. Some case-control studies have reported a negative association between dietary intakes of folate or other B vitamins and BC [8, 27–33].

Also part of the prospective cohort studies observed a negative association between folate intake and BC risk among alcohol consumers [34–38] and among current smokers [39]. Nevertheless, most of the studies have not found an overall association between intakes of folate or vitamins B-6 and B-12 [27, 34–41] neither of all B vitamins [42] and BC risk.

Data relating circulating concentrations of folate to BC risk are restricted to a few studies [43–46], where the three latter [44–46] suggested an inverse association between circulating folate concentrations and BC risk. Two recent meta-analysis studies concluded no clear association between folate intake and folate concentrations and BC risk [47, 48], suggesting that high folate status may be associated with little or no risk reduction of BC. On the other hand, also positive associations were seen in plasma folate and the risk of developing premenopausal BC and Estrogen Receptor (ER) positive or Progesterone Receptor (PR) positive breast tumors [27]. Other recent study [49] found a positive association between plasma folate concentration and ERbeta- BC but not in other BC groups defined by ER status.

Experimental animal research suggests that folate may have dual effects on BC development, depending on its timing [25]. Folate administration can prevent tumor development before the existence of preneoplastic lesions and increasing tumorigenesis once preneoplastic lesions are established. Experimental data suggest that the interaction between folate and estrogen is complex [50–53].

In addition, a randomized trial of folic acid supplementation during pregnancy reported that women who received such supplements had a non significantly increased risk of BC mortality compared with those in the placebo group [54]. Notably, in this study those women who received the highest dose (5 mg/day) had the highest mortality risk (RR=2.02; 95% CI 0.88–4.02), although the association was not statistically significant either.

Since alcohol is well recognized as a risk factor for BC [55], genetic polymorphisms in folate and alcohol metabolic pathways might influence the risk of the disease [56]. From a public heath perspective, it is important to identify risk factors, such as a low B vitamin consumption, that may guide an effective prevention strategy against the disease [57]. It should be also taken into account that food sources may have stronger anti-carcinogenic effects than the synthetic B vitamins found in supplements.

In spite of its main capabilities (DNA integrity and stability maintenance), the role of folate in cancer prevention deserves to be further reanalyzed. The question of folate intake through foods or supplements remains to be answered, and this is a pending issue to be solved.

A DEFINITE ROLE FOR FOLATE AND OTHER VITAMINS OF THE B GROUP HAS NOT BEEN ELUCIDATED REGARDING THEIR RELATIONS WITH THE RISK OF BREAST CANCER.

Vitamin C

Some prospective studies performed during the 90's in North America examined the intake of ascorbic acid (vitamin C). A null association or absence of association was reported in them, with RR = 1.0 or close to it [2, 58]. However, certain case-control studies [32, 59] and one meta-analysis [60] reported a significant inverse association for vitamin C intake.

On the other hand, some of the case-control studies have reported moderate protective associations or absence of association too [1, 61–67], as well as a non significant increase of risk [68, 69]. A combined analysis of 9 case-control studies which involved almost 7.000 cases, reported a significant RR = 0.69 for the highest quintile of vitamin C consumption [7]. This association remained after adjusting for intakes of fibre and ß-carotene (RR = 0.73). The BC risk was found not related to intakes of any vitamin supplement either [70–72].

Two survival studies on BC which were quoted above regarding carotenoid intake, revealed that women with the highest intake of vitamin C had less risks of dying because of their cancer (RR = 0.4–0.7) when the highest consumption was compared to the lowest [1, 14]. The levels of the antioxidant enzymes catalase, superoxide dismutase, glutathione peroxidase and glutathione-S-transferase were significantly normalized by vitamin C treatment [73], something that could partially explain the better survival of vitamin C-treated postmenopausal BC patients compared with normal individuals.

A recent cohort study [10] reported that dietary intake of vitamin C was not associated with BC risk in premenopausal (RR = 1.12, 95% CI 0.92–1.36) and postmenopausal women (RR = 0.98, 95% CI 0.87–1.11). However, in postmenopausal women using exogenous hormones, high intake of vitamin C (RR = 0.88, 95% CI 0.72–1.07, P-trend 0.05) was associated with reduced BC risk.

The experimental evidence is not consistent with the epidemiologic findings, since no effect was observed after the administration of vitamin C on the growth of induced or transplanted mammary tumours [74].

The potential biologic mechanisms through which vitamin C could protect against BC involve its roles as antioxidant, in the protein synthesis of conjunctive tissue and in the immunologic surveillance.

A HIGH DIETARY LEVEL OF VITAMIN C COULD REDUCE THE RISK OF BREAST CANCER, BUT MORE EVIDENCE IS STILL NECESSARY.

Vitamin D

Vitamin D (VD) is a powerful inhibitor of the cellular capability to divide itself and grow. It also helps mammary cells in the maturation process, with which they become less vulnerable to the action of harmful elements that have some participation in the development of BC. The major part of this hormone should proceed from foods and from the exposure to sunlight. Regarding this latter, it is accepted that an exposure of 15 min three times per week is a convenient degree, while it is unnecessary to remain exposed to the sun during a long time nor provoking a burning either.

Epidemiologic studies, in particular the ecologic ones, investigated correlations between incidence rates of BC [75] or mortality rates of the disease and the exposure levels to solar radiation [76]. On the base of such studies, the lack of solar exposure – which would mean a deficiency of VD – has been suggested as a possible risk factor for BC. Other studies found a strong inverse correlation between BC and the availability of solar radiation in an amount which is effective for the production of VD in the skin [77, 78]. When also is associated to a low average intake of VD, these authors suggested that an inadequate amount of VD could be a significant risk factor for BC. Data from the NHANES study support the hypothesis that sunlight and dietary VD reduce the risk of BC [79]. In addition, other ecologic study has found regional mortality rates of BC which were inversely correlated with the local intensity of sunlight, in other words, the more light less frequent cancer and vice versa [80].

The finding of low serum values of VD in Uruguayan women, following a seasonal fluctuation pattern [81], enabled the authors to suppose that in the latitude of temperate weather several population risks are present, such as of osteoporosis, colorectal cancer and eventually of BC too, if the results of the samples are extrapolated to the general population. Besides, a recent French study [82] reported that dietary and supplemental VD intakes were not associated with BC risk in regions with high ultraviolet radiation; nevertheless, the authors found a significantly lower BC risk among postmenopausal women with high dietary or supplemental VD intake when they were compared to women with the lowest VD intake.

A Norwegian study on breast, colon and prostate cancers found that adequate levels of VD3 at the moment of diagnosis (in Summer and Fall) and during the therapy were associated with lower risk of death [83]. An association of VD and calcium intake with the reduction of radiologic mammary density, suggests that both could reduce the risk of BC through an influence on the morphology of mammary tissue [84]. A more recent analysis, besides, recognized the potential role of VD in the prevention of BC [85, 151], although new studies are needed in order to find an optimal status of VD and to define its appropriate biomarkers in relation to the protection against BC [86]. Furthermore, a recent experimental research [87] reported that the addition of VD to tumour cell cultures induced the regression of certain typical morphologic features of more aggressive and of worse prognosis mammary cancers.

Besides, the incidence of BC in the Western world runs parallel to that of the major components of the insulin resistance syndrome, as hyperinsulinemia, dyslipidemia, hypertension, obesity and atherosclerosis. The growth of BC is enhanced by specific dietary fatty acids, visceral fat accumulation and insufficient physical activity, all of which are thought to interact in favouring the development of the insulin resistance syndrome.

The available literature enables the VD to be closely linked to some of the main features of the insulin resistance syndrome [88, 89]. A relationship between VD and insulin secretion was suggested more than two decades ago [90], and it was more recently analyzed [91–93]. Finally, the relationship with body fat content has been also investigated. Obesity increases the risk of VD deficiency [94]. Once VD is synthesized in the skin or ingested, it is deposited in body fat stores, making it less bioavailable to subjects having large of such fat stores.

All the preceding metabolic context gives us biologic bases to think that the frequent situation of insulin resistance, BC and low level of VD keep relationships among themselves. Since human mammary cells have receptors for VD, there is a plausible biologic base for the hypothesis that VD can contribute to the protection against BC.

THERE IS CURRENTLY IMPORTANT EPIDEMIOLOGIC AND EXPERIMENTAL EVIDENCE SUPPORTING A PREVENTIVE ROLE FOR VITAMIN D.

Vitamin E

Several types of studies have examined possible associations between the intake of α-tocopherol (vitamin E) and BC. Some prospective studies on BC have essentially reported an absence of association for dietary vitamin E [1, 58]. In one of them, a weakly protective association suggested initially disappeared completely when vitamin A was included in the analysis model [2]. Of five case-control studies, 3 communicated weak protective effects for the highest consumption [28, 95], and on the other hand 2 studies reported risk around 1 (no association) [69, 96].

A survival study reported that those women with the highest intakes of vitamin E previously to the onset of the disease, had a lower risk of dying of their cancer [15]. Some intervention studies from the 80's who used dietary supplements communicated the absence of effects of supplementation with vitamin E en prevalent cases of benign breast disease [97, 98].

A reviewed series of experimental studies performed in rats [99] showed combined results. Some of them revealed a protective effect, some absence of effects, but none showed a harmful effect. A study showed that vitamin E inhibited the BC when the experimental diet was rich in PUFA, however, other study did not confirm this finding. Several studies showed that the vitamin empowered the capability of selenium in inhibition of cancer development.

In the last years, additional evidence for the action of vitamin E in relation to BC has been produced. A review on the issue remarks that this vitamin can stimulate the apoptosis (programmed cell death) in tumour cells as well it can increase the anti-metastatic action of specific drugs [100], probably due to its anti-angiogenic capability [101]. Also chemical analogues of the vitamin have achieved an experimental reduction of metastatic capability of tumours [102]. Besides, its lack of relationship with the risk of BC in pre-menopausal women has been observed [39]. In addition, it does not seem recommendable its supplementation together with tamoxifen, due to the influence on estrogen receptors [103, 104].

A HIGH LEVEL OF DIETARY VITAMIN E COULD HAVE RELATIONSHIP WITH A LESSER RISK OF BREAST CANCER, BUT THE EVIDENCE IS STILL NOT SUFFICIENT.

Bioactive Substances

Phytoestrogens

Phytoestrogens are weak estrogens of mainly vegetable origin. They are present in particular in soybeans and in whole grain cereals, as well as in some seeds (flaxseed, specially). The major phytoestrogens are the isoflavones (daidzein, genistein), the coumestans and the lignans (enterolactone and enterodiol). Also cereals and dietary fibre constitute an important source of lignans, and is remarkable their high content in legumes. In Uruguay, the authors have investigated this issue [105], centered mainly in exploring lignans – which are the most common phytoestrogens in a Western diet like the Uruguayan. Lignans showed a strong reduction of risk of BC: the study reported a significant protection for the highest quartiles of intake of total lignans and enterodiol (OR = 0.43 for both substances), of enterolactone (OR = 0.55) and also of isoflavones (OR = 0.62). More recently, lignans appear as linked to the protection in postmenopausal ER- and PR + women [106].

The presence of non steroidal substances in certain plants having estrogenic activity was recognized since the 40's decade [107]. In those times, studies conducted in Western Australia [108] identified reproductive disruptions in sheep which were fed with a subterranean vegetable. Females experienced sterility and the cause was attributed to the intake of certain estrogenic substances in the clover. Since then, it has been recognized that hundreds of plants had compounds which expressed certain degree of estrogenic activity [109, 110]. The knowledge on the chemical structure, dietary sources and physiologic effects of phytoestrogens has grown considerably from that moment up to the present time [107, 111–113].

The potentially preventive actions of phytoestrogens (isoflavones and lignans) in BC have been intensely investigated in the past decade [111, 114–116]. Moreover, until 1996 there were no epidemiologic studies which have examined intakes of isoflavones or lignans per se. The literature has recently grown, suggesting mostly protective effects [117–121], albeit new revisions continue quoting the presence of controversial results [122–124]. Caution is required for the prescription under certain circumstances, since the effects could be opposite to those wanted [125].

A postulated anticarcinogenic mechanism involves a weak estrogenic activity of these compounds, estimated around a 0.1% of conjugated estrogens. Phytoestrogens can bind estrogen receptors without producing any major response, whereas they can block at the same time the binding of more powerful estrogens. These compounds are structurally similar to Tamoxifen, an antiestrogen used in hormonal therapy of BC and being assessed as an agent of primary prevention.

PHYTOESTROGEN-RICH DIETS PROBABLY REDUCE THE RISK OF BREAST CANCER.

Antocyanins

Not only vitamin E participates in the protection against angiogenesis. There is a group of substances among flavonoids called ANTOCYANINS, which have a powerful anti-angiogenic capability. They are components of a fruit group whose name ends in "berry". Probably the strawberry is better known than any other one, but there are also the elderberry, blueberry, bilberry, cranberry and raspberry. "Berries" are then fruits whose high content in antocyanin is beneficial for its antioxidant capability, because they help to prepare the cellular DNA and to protect its integrity [126]. The reduction of oxidative stress has also as collateral beneficial effects the improvement of neural and cognitive functions, thinking of the prevention of brain aging and of neurodegenerative pathologies.

Inositol Hexaphosphate

The inositol hexaphosphate (IP6), also known as phytic acid, is a polyphosphored carbohydrate which is naturally found in foods which are rich sources in fibre, as legumes, peas, integral cereals (oat, wheat, rye), wheat bran and soyfoods. The soybeans have the highest content known among legumes. IP6 is usually attached to the bran, the not soluble fibre, which is hard to digest. It is assumed that foods must be cooked to release IP6 from fibre and to allow it to be digested, however, the cooking process is thought that can destroy it.

In addition, IP6 is found not only in plants but in almost every cell of mammalians – although in much less amount – where is important for the regulation of vital cell functions just as signal transduction, cell proliferation and differentiation. During a long time, IP6 was recognized as a natural antioxidant, but it has also other beneficial qualities for human health, as the capability of enhancing the immune system, preventing the pathologic calcification and renal lithiasis, lowering the hypercholesterolemia and reducing the pathologic thrombocyte activity [127]. More recently, IP6 has received more attention for its role in cancer prevention and in the control of tumour growth, progression and metastasis at an experimental level [128]. As a consequence, it is currently defined as a substance with anti-angiogenic capability [129].

Its anticarcinogenic activity has been mainly observed at an experimental level in tumours of different sites: melanoma [130], colon [131, 132], prostate [133, 134], pancreas [135], soft tissue sarcomas [136] and breast [137–139]. In addition, an enhancement of antineoplastic activity of adriamicin and tamoxifen has been also reported [140].

Although its lack of clinical evidence, experimental findings have open a possibility for its therapeutic application, which could be assessed in the future. In the interim, its frequent inclusion in the diet seems recommendable, because it could be one of the possible explanations for the protective effect found in the intake of those foods which have it as a component.

Indol-3-Carbinol

Undoubtedly, there is a group of vegetables which notably outstands and they are the cruciferous (cauliflower, cabbage, broccoli, Brussels sprouts, i.e.). Cruciferous vegetables are a rich source of glucosinolates and their hydrolysis products. Isothiocyanates and indoles derived from the hydrolysis of glucosinolates, such as sulforaphane and indole-3-carbinol (I3C), have been implicated in a variety of anticarcinogenic mechanisms [141]. These hydrolysis products alter the metabolism or activity of sex hormones in ways that could inhibit the development of hormone-sensitive cancers, in particular enhancing the synthesis of "good" estrogens (the weak ones, from the group of 2-α-hydroxyestrogens). Few days after having a constant intake of these vegetables, the production level of the quoted hormones increases markedly [142]. Besides, the fact that the intake of vegetables correlates positively with the presence of carotenoids in serum and adipose tissue [143] supports the hypothesis of potential protection of these foods, perhaps through the combined effects of several components of vegetables.

Isothiocyanates

The isothiocyanates are non-nutrient substances which together with the indols derived from cruciferous have growth inhibitor activity and apoptosis inductor in cancerous cell lines, in vitro [144, 145]. The most known compound is Sulphoraphane. Among the capabilities of isothiocyanates at a molecular level is the induction of phase II enzymes (i.e. glutathione-S-transferases), the disruption of steroidal hormones metabolism, the regulation of responses of estrogen receptors and the stabilization of cell proliferation [146–149]. In addition, an anti-angiogenic capability has been lately described [150].

Their anticarcinogenic action is recognized for several types of cancers. They are described as associated to a BC risk reduction, as it was mentioned from the intake of cruciferous vegetables in case-control studies performed in the US, Sweden and China [146, 151, 152]. These studies found that measures of cruciferous vegetable intake were significantly lower in women diagnosed with BC than in cancer-free control groups. Nevertheless, cruciferous vegetable intake was not associated with BC risk in a pooled analysis of seven large prospective cohort studies [153]. Epidemiologic studies have indicated that the human exposure to isothiocyanates can reduce the risk of cancer, but the protective effects can be influenced by genetic variations (polymorphisms) in the metabolism and elimination from body of the isothiocyanates [141, 154].

References

1. Rohan TE, Howe GR, Friedenreich CM et al (1993) Dietary fiber, vitamins A, C, and E, and risk of breast cancer: a cohort study. Cancer Causes Control 4:29–37
2. Hunter DJ, Stampfer MJ, Colditz GA et al (1993) A prospective study of intake of vitamin C, E and A and the risk of breast cancer. N Engl J Med 329:234–240
3. Kabat GC, Kim M, Adams-Campbell LL et al (2009) Longitudinal study of serum carotenoid, retinol, and tocopherol concentrations in relation to breast cancer risk among postmenopausal women. Am J Clin Nutr 90(1):162–169
4. Larsson SC, Bergkvist L, Wolk A (2010) Dietary carotenoids and risk of hormone receptor-defined breast cancer in a prospective cohort of Swedish women. Eur J Cancer 46(6): 1079–1085
5. Maillard V, Kuriki K, Lefebvre B et al (2010) Serum carotenoid, tocopherol and retinol concentrations and breast cancer risk in the E3N-EPIC study. Int J Cancer 127(5):1188–1196
6. Garland M, Willett WC, Manson JE et al (1993) Antioxidant micronutrients and breast cancer. J Am Coll Nutr 12(4):400–411
7. Howe GR, Hirohata T, Hislop TG et al (1990) Dietary factors and risk of breast cancer: combined analysis of 12 case-control studies. J Natl Cancer Inst 82:561–569
8. Ronco AL, De Stéfani E, Boffetta P et al (1999) Vegetables, fruits, and related nutrients and risk of breast cancer: a case control study in Uruguay. Nutr Cancer 35(2):111–119
9. Roswall N, Olsen A, Christensen J et al (2010) Micronutrient intake and breast cancer characteristics among postmenopausal women. Eur J Cancer Prev 19(5):360–365
10. Ronco AL, De Stefani E, Aune D et al (2010) Nutrient patterns and risk of breast cancer in Uruguay. Asian Pac J Cancer Prev 11:519–524
11. Nagel G, Linseisen J, van Gils CH et al (2010) Dietary beta-carotene, vitamin C and E intake and breast cancer risk in the European Prospective Investigation into Cancer and Nutrition (EPIC). Breast Cancer Res Treat 119(3):753–765
12. Mignone LI, Giovannucci E, Newcomb PA et al (2009) Dietary carotenoids and the risk of invasive breast cancer. Int J Cancer 124(12):2929–2937
13. Epplein M, Shvetsov YB, Wilkens LR et al (2009) Plasma carotenoids, retinol, and tocopherols and postmenopausal breast cancer risk in the Multiethnic Cohort Study: a nested case-control study. Breast Cancer Res 11(4):R49
14. Tamimi RM, Colditz GA, Hankinson SE (2009) Circulating carotenoids, mammographic density, and subsequent risk of breast cancer. Cancer Res 69(24):9323–9329

15. Jain M, Miller AB, To T (1994) Premorbid diet and the prognosis of women with breast cancer. J Natl Cancer Inst 86(18):1390–1397
16. Rock CL, Flatt SW, Natarajan L et al (2005) Plasma carotenoids and recurrence-free survival in women with a history of breast cancer. J Clin Oncol 23(27):6631–6638
17. Rock CL, Natarajan L, Pu M et al (2009) Longitudinal biological exposure to carotenoids is associated with breast cancer-free survival in the Women's Healthy Eating and Living Study. Cancer Epidemiol Biomarkers Prev 18(2):486–494
18. Wang H, Leung LK (2010) The carotenoid lycopene differentially regulates phase I and II enzymes in dimethylbenz[a]anthracene-induced MCF-7 cells. Nutrition 26(11–12):1181–1187
19. Scott JM, Weir DG (1998) Folic acid, homocysteine and one-carbon metabolism: a review of the essential biochemistry. J Cardiovasc Risk 5:223–227
20. Ames BN (2001) DNA damage from micronutrient deficiencies is likely to be a major cause of cancer. Mutat Res 475:7–20
21. Mason JB, Choi SW (2000) Folate and carcinogenesis: developing a unifying hypothesis. Adv Enzyme Regul 40:127–141
22. Blount BC, Mack MM, Wehr CM et al (1997) Folate deficiency causes uracil misincorporation into human DNA and chromosome breakage: implications for cancer and neuronal damage. Proc Natl Acad Sci USA 94:3290–3295
23. Choi SW, Mason JB (2000) Folate and carcinogenesis: an integrated scheme. J Nutr 130: 129–132
24. Davis CD, Uthus EO (2004) DNA methylation, cancer susceptibility, and nutrient interactions. Exp Biol Med (Maywood) 229:988–995
25. Kim YI (2006) Does a high folate intake increase the risk of breast cancer? Nutr Rev 64: 468–475
26. Potera C, Rose DP, Brown RR (1977) Vitamin B6 deficiency in cancer patients. Am J Clin Nutr 30(10):1677–1679
27. Lin J, Lee IM, Cook NR et al (2008) Plasma folate, vitamin B-6, vitamin B-12, and risk of breast cancer in women. Am J Clin Nutr 87:734–743
28. Graham S, Hellmann R, Marshall J et al (1991) Nutritional epidemiology of postmenopausal breast cancer in western New York. Am J Epidemiol 134:552–566
29. Freudenheim JL, Marshall JR, Vena JE et al (1996) Premenopausal breast cancer risk and intake of vegetables, fruits, and related nutrients. J Natl Cancer Inst 88:340–348
30. Negri E, La Vecchia C, Franceschi S (2000) Re: dietary folate consumption and breast cancer risk. J Natl Cancer Inst 92:1270–1271
31. Shrubsole MJ, Jin F, Dai Q et al (2001) Dietary folate intake and breast cancer risk: results from the Shanghai Breast Cancer Study. Cancer Res 61:7136–7141
32. Levi F, Pasche C, Lucchini F et al (2001) Dietary intake of selected micronutrients and breast-cancer risk. Int J Cancer 91:260–263
33. Lajous M, Lazcano-Ponce E, Hernandez-Avila M et al (2006) Folate, vitamin B(6), and vitamin B(12) intake and the risk of breast cancer among Mexican women. Cancer Epidemiol Biomarkers Prev 15:443–448
34. Zhang S, Hunter DJ, Hankinson SE et al (1999) A prospective study of folate intake and the risk of breast cancer. JAMA 281:1632–1637
35. Sellers TA, Kushi LH, Cerhan JR et al (2001) Dietary folate intake, alcohol, and risk of breast cancer in a prospective study of postmenopausal women. Epidemiology 12:420–428
36. Rohan TE, Jain MG, Howe GR et al (2000) Dietary folate consumption and breast cancer risk. J Natl Cancer Inst 92:266–269
37. Baglietto L, English DR, Gertig DM et al (2005) Does dietary folate intake modify effect of alcohol consumption on breast cancer risk?Prospective cohort study. BMJ 331:807
38. Tjonneland A, Christensen J, Olsen A et al (2006) Folate intake, alcohol and risk of breast cancer among postmenopausal women in Denmark. Eur J Clin Nutr 60:280–286
39. Cho E, Spiegelman D, Hunter DJ et al (2003) Premenopausal intakes of vitamins A, C, and E, folate, and carotenoids, and risk of breast cancer. Cancer Epidemiol Biomarkers Prev 12: 713–720

40. Feigelson HS, Jonas CR, Robertson AS et al (2003) Alcohol, folate, methionine, and risk of incident breast cancer in the American Cancer Society Cancer Prevention Study II Nutrition Cohort. Cancer Epidemiol Biomarkers Prev 12:161–164
41. Ma E, Iwasaki M, Kobayashi M et al (2009) Dietary intake of folate, vitamin B2, vitamin B6, vitamin B12, genetic polymorphism of related enzymes, and risk of breast cancer: a case-control study in Japan. Nutr Cancer 61(4):447–456
42. Kabat GC, Miller AB, Jain M et al (2008) Dietary intake of selected B vitamins in relation to risk of major cancers in women. Br J Cancer 99:816–821
43. Wu K, Helzlsouer KJ, Comstock GW et al (1999) A prospective study on folate, B12, and pyridoxal 5'-phosphate (B6) and breast cancer. Cancer Epidemiol Biomarkers Prev 8:209–217
44. Zhang SM, Willett WC, Selhub J et al (2003) Plasma folate, vitamin B6, vitamin B12, homocysteine, and risk of breast cancer. J Natl Cancer Inst 95:373–380
45. Beilby J, Ingram D, Hahnel R et al (2004) Reduced breast cancer risk with increasing serum folate in a case-control study of the C677T genotype of the methylenetetrahydrofolate reductase gene. Eur J Cancer 40:1250–1254
46. Rossi E, Hung J, Beilby JP et al (2006) Folate levels and cancer morbidity and mortality: prospective cohort study from Busselton, Western Australia. Ann Epidemiol 16:206–212
47. Lewis SJ, Harbord RM, Harris R et al (2006) Meta-analyses of observational and genetic association studies of folate intakes or levels and breast cancer risk. J Natl Cancer Inst 98: 1607–1622
48. Larsson SC, Giovannucci E, Wolk A (2007) Folate and risk of breast cancer: a meta-analysis. J Natl Cancer Inst 99:64–76
49. Ericson U, Borgquist S, Ivarsson MI et al (2010) Plasma folate concentrations are positively associated with risk of estrogen receptor beta negative breast cancer in a Swedish nested case control study. J Nutr 140(9):1661–1668
50. Ross JF, Chaudhuri PK, Ratnam M (1994) Differential regulation of folate receptor isoforms in normal and malignant tissues in vivo and in established cell lines. Physiologic and clinical implications. Cancer 73:2432–2443
51. Kelley KM, Rowan BG, Ratnam M (2003) Modulation of the folate receptor alpha gene by the estrogen receptor: mechanism and implications in tumor targeting. Cancer Res 63:2820–2828
52. Hao H, d'Alincourt-Salazar M, Kelley KM et al (2007) Estrogen-induced and TAFII30-mediated gene repression by direct recruitment of the estrogen receptor and co-repressors to the core promoter and its reversal by tamoxifen. Oncogene 26:7872–7884
53. Hartmann LC, Keeney GL, Lingle WL et al (2007) Folate receptor overexpression is associated with poor outcome in breast cancer. Int J Cancer 121:938–942
54. Charles D, Ness AR, Campbell D et al (2004) Taking folate in pregnancy and risk of maternal breast cancer. BMJ 329:1375–1376
55. World Cancer Research Fund/American Institute for Cancer Research (2007) Food, nutrition, physical activity, and the prevention of cancer: a global perspective. American Institute for Cancer Research, Washington, DC
56. Sangrajrang S, Sato Y, Sakamoto H et al (2010) Genetic polymorphisms in folate and alcohol metabolism and breast cancer risk: a case-control study in Thai women. Breast Cancer Res Treat 123(3):885–893
57. Chen J, Gammon MD, Chan W et al (2005) One-carbon metabolism, MTHFR polymorphisms, and risk of breast cancer. Cancer Res 65(4):1606–1614
58. Graham S, Zielezny M, Marshall J et al (1992) Diet in the epidemiology of postmenopausal breast cancer in a New York state cohort. Am J Epidemiol 136:1327
59. Do MH, Lee SS, Jung PJ et al (2003) Intake of dietary fat and vitamin in relation to breast cancer risk in Korean women: a case-control study. J Korean Med Sci 18(4):534–540
60. Gandini S, Merzenich H, Robertson C et al (2000) Meta-analysis of studies on breast cancer risk and diet: the role of fruit and vegetable consumption and the intake of associated micronutrients. Eur J Cancer 36(5):636–646
61. Zaridze D, Lifanova Y, Maximovitch D et al (1991) Diet, alcohol consumption and reproductive factors in a case-control study of breast cancer in Moscow. Int J Cancer 48:493–501

62. Kushi LH, Fee RM, Sellers TA et al (1996) Intake of vitamins A, C, and E and postmenopausal breast cancer. The Iowa Women's Health Study. Am J Epidemiol 144(2):165–174
63. Jarvinen R, Knekt P, Seppanen R et al (1997) Diet and breast cancer risk in a cohort of Finnish women. Cancer Lett 114(12):251–253
64. Verhoeven DT, Assen N, Goldbohm RA et al (1997) Vitamins C and E, retinol, beta-carotene and dietary fibre in relation to breast cancer risk: a prospective cohort study. Br J Cancer 75: 149–155
65. Bohlke K, Spiegelman D, Trichopoulou A et al (1999) Vitamins A, C and E and the risk of breast cancer: results from a case-control study in Greece. Br J Cancer 79(1):23–29
66. Zhang S, Hunter DJ, Forman MR et al (1999) Dietary carotenoids and vitamins A, C and E and risk of breast cancer. J Natl Cancer Inst (Bethesda) 91:547–556
67. Wang C, Baumgartner RN, Yang D et al (2009) No evidence of association between breast cancer risk and dietary carotenoids, retinols, vitamin C and tocopherols in Southwestern Hispanic and non-Hispanic White women. Breast Cancer Res Treat 114(1):137–145
68. Katsouyanni K, Willett W, Trichopoulos D et al (1988) Risk of breast cancer among Greek women in relation to nutrient intake. Cancer 61:181–185
69. Toniolo P, Riboli E, Protta F et al (1989) Calorie-providing nutrients and risk of breast cancer. J Natl Cancer Inst 81:278–286
70. Moorman PG, Ricciuti MF, Millikan R et al (2001) Vitamin supplement use and breast cancer in a North Carolina population. Public Health Nutr 4(3):821–827
71. Michels KB, Holmberg L, Bergkvist L et al (2001) Dietary antioxidant vitamins, retinol, and breast cancer incidence in a cohort of Swedish women. Int J Cancer 91:563–567
72. Dorjgochoo T, Shrubsole MJ, Shu XO et al (2008) Vitamin supplement use and risk for breast cancer: the Shanghai Breast Cancer Study. Breast Cancer Res Treat 111(2):269–278
73. Muralikrishnan G, Amanullah S, Basha MI et al (2010) Effect of vitamin C on lipid peroxidation and antioxidant status in tamoxifen-treated breast cancer patients. Chemotherapy 56(4): 298–302
74. Abul-Hajj YJ, Kelliher M (1982) Failure of ascorbic acid to inhibit growth of transplantable and dimethylbenzanthracene induced rat mammary tumors. Cancer Lett 17:67–73
75. Gorham ED, Garland FC, Garland CF (1990) Sunlight and breast cancer incidence in the USSR. Int J Epidemiol 19(4):820–824
76. Garland FC, Garland CF, Gorham ED et al (1990) Geographic variation in breast cancer mortality in the United States: a hypothesis involving exposure to solar radiation. Prev Med 19:614–622
77. Ip C, Scimeca JA, Thompson H (1995) Effect of timing and duration of dietary conjugated linoleic acid on mammary cancer prevention. Nutr Cancer 24(3):241–247
78. Garland C, Garland F, Gorham E (1999) Epidemiology of cancer risk and vitamin D. In: Holick M (ed) Vitamin D: molecular biology, physiology, and applications. Humana Press, Totowa, pp 375–409
79. John EM, Schwartz GG, Dreon DM et al (1999) Vitamin D and breast cancer risk: the NHANES I Epidemiologic follow-up study, 1971–1975 to 1992. National Health and Nutrition Examination Survey. Cancer Epidemiol Biomarkers Prev 8(5):399–406
80. Grant WB (2002) An ecologic study of dietary and solar ultraviolet-B links to breast carcinoma mortality rates. Cancer 94(1):272–281
81. Mendoza B, Ronco AL, Mintegui G et al (2006) Serum vitamin D status among postmenopausal Uruguayan women. World Congress of the International Osteoporosis Foundation, Toronto
82. Engel P, Fagherazzi G, Mesrine S et al (2011) Joint effects of dietary vitamin D and sun exposure on breast cancer risk: results from the French E3N cohort. Cancer Epidemiol Biomarkers Prev 20(1):187–195
83. Robsahm TE, Tretli S, Dahlback A et al (2004) Vitamin D3 from sunlight may improve the prognosis of breast-, colon- and prostate cancer (Norway). Cancer Causes Control 15:149–158
84. Berube S, Diorio C, Verhoek-Oftedahl W et al (2004) Vitamin D, calcium, and mammographic breast densities. Cancer Epidemiol Biomarkers Prev 13(9):1466–1472

85. Zhang SM (2004) Role of vitamins in the risk, prevention, and treatment of breast cancer. Curr Opin Obstet Gynecol 16:19–25
86. Welsh J (2004) Vitamin D and breast cancer: insights from animal models. Am J Clin Nutr 80(Suppl):1721S–1724S
87. Pendas-Franco N, Gonzalez-Sancho JM, Suarez Y et al (2007) Vitamin D regulates the phenotype of human breast cancer cells. Differentiation 75(3):193–207
88. Krause R, Buhring M, Hopfenmuller W et al (1998) Ultraviolet B and blood pressure. Lancet 352(9129):709–710
89. Pfeifer M, Begerow B, Minne HW et al (2001) Effects of a short-term vitamin D(3) and calcium supplementation on blood pressure and parathyroid hormone levels in elderly women. J Clin Endocrinol Metab 86(4):1633–1637
90. Inomata S, Kadowaki S, Yamatani T et al (1986) Effect of 1 alpha (OH)-vitamin D3 on insulin secretion in diabetes mellitus. Bone Miner 1(3):187–192
91. Orwoll E, Riddle M, Prince M (1994) Effects of vitamin D on insulin and glucagon secretion in non-insulin-dependent diabetes mellitus. Am J Clin Nutr 59(5):1083–1087
92. Zeitz U, Weber K, Soegiarto DW et al (2003) Impaired insulin secretory capacity in mice lacking a functional vitamin D receptor. FASEB J 17(3):509–511
93. Borissova AM, Tankova T, Kirilov G et al (2003) The effect of vitamin D3 on insulin secretion and peripheral insulin sensitivity in type 2 diabetic patients. Int J Clin Pract 57(4):258–261
94. Arunabh S, Pollack S, Yeh J, Aloia JF (2003) Body fat content and 25-hydroxyvitamin D levels in healthy women. J Clin Endocrinol Metab 88(1):157–161
95. London SJ, Stein EA, Henderson IC et al (1992) Carotenoids, retinol, and vitamin E and risk of proliferative benign breast disease and breast cancer. Cancer Causes Control 3:503–512
96. Richardson S, Gerber M, Cenee S (1991) The role of fat, animal protein and some vitamin consumption in breast cancer: a case-control study in Southern France. Int J Cancer 48:1–9
97. Ernster VL, Goodson WH, Hunt TK et al (1985) Vitamin E and benign breast "disease": a double-blind, randomized clinical trial. Surgery 97:490–494
98. London SJ, Sundaram GS, Murphy L et al (1985) The effect of vitamin E on mammary displasia: a double-blind study. Obstet Gynecol 65:104–106
99. Knekt P, Aromaa A, Maatela J et al (1991) Vitamin E and cancer prevention. Am J Clin Nutr 53:2835–2865
100. Kline K, Yu W, Sanders BG (2004) Vitamin E and breast cancer. J Nutr 134(12 Suppl): 3458S–3462S
101. Schindler R, Mentlein R (2006) Flavonoids and vitamin E reduce the release of the angiogenic peptide vascular endothelial growth factor from human tumor cells. J Nutr 136(6):1477–1482
102. Hahn T, Szabo L, Gold M et al (2006) Dietary administration of the proapoptotic vitamin E analogue alpha}-tocopheryloxyacetic acid inhibits metastatic murine breast cancer. Cancer Res 66(19):9374–9378
103. Chamras H, Barsky SH, Ardashian A et al (2005) Novel interactions of vitamin E and estrogen in breast cancer. Nutr Cancer 52(1):43–48
104. Peralta EA, Viegas ML, Louis S et al (2006) Effect of vitamin E on tamoxifen-treated breast cancer cells. Surgery 140(4):607–614
105. Ronco AL, De Stéfani E (1999) Fitoestrógenos y riesgo de cáncer mamario: un estudio caso control. Rev Med Urug 15:94–102
106. Touillaud MS, Thiebaut AC, Fournier A et al (2007) Dietary lignan intake and postmenopausal breast cancer risk by estrogen and progesterone receptor status. J Natl Cancer Inst 99(6):475–486
107. Griffiths K, Adlercreutz H, Boyle P et al (1996) Nutrition and cancer. ISIS Medical Media, Oxford
108. Bennets HW, Underwood EJ, Sheir FL (1946) A specific breeding problem of sheep on subterranean clover pastures in Western Australia. Aust Vet J 22:2–12
109. Bradbury RB, White DC (1954) Oestrogens and related substances in plants. Vitam Horm 12: 207–233

110. Farnsworth NR, Bingel AS, Cordell GA et al (1975) Potential value of plants as sources of new anti fertility agents. J Pharm Sci 64:717–754
111. Horn-Ross PL (1995) Phytoestrogens, body composition, and breast cancer. Cancer Causes Control 6:567–573
112. Reinli K, Block G (1996) Phytoestrogen content of foods – a compendium of literature values. Nutr Cancer 26:123–148
113. Thompson LU, Robb P, Serraino M et al (1991) Mammalian lignan production from various foods. Nutr Cancer 16:43–52
114. Adlercreutz H (1990) Western diet and western diseases: some hormonal and biochemical mechanisms and associations. Scand J Clin Lab Invest 50(Suppl 201):3–23
115. Adlercreutz H, Markkanen H, Watanabe S (1993) Plasma concentrations of phytoestrogens in Japanese men. Lancet 342:1209–1210
116. Messina MJ, Persky V, Setchell KDR et al (1994) Soy intake and cancer risk: a review of the in vitro and in vivo data. Nutr Cancer 21:113–131
117. Piller R, Chang-Claude J, Linseisen J (2006) Plasma enterolactone and genistein and the risk of premenopausal breast cancer. Eur J Cancer Prev 15(3):225–232
118. McCann SE, Kulkarni S, Trevisan M et al (2006) Dietary lignan intakes and risk of breast cancer by tumor estrogen receptor status. Breast Cancer Res Treat 99(3):309–311
119. Ha TC, Lyons-Wall PM, Moore DE et al (2006) Phytoestrogens and indicators of breast cancer prognosis. Nutr Cancer 56(1):3–10
120. Bergman Jungestrom M, Thompson LU et al (2007) Flaxseed and its lignans inhibit estradiol-induced growth, angiogenesis, and secretion of vascular endothelial growth factor in human breast cancer xenografts in vivo. Clin Cancer Res 13(3):1061–1067
121. Verheus M, van Gils CH, Keinan-Boker L et al (2007) Plasma phytoestrogens and subsequent breast cancer risk. J Clin Oncol 25(6):648–655
122. Rice S, Whitehead SA (2006) Phytoestrogens and breast cancer – promoters or protectors? Endocr Relat Cancer 13(4):995–1015
123. Gikas PD, Mokbel K (2005) Phytoestrogens and the risk of breast cancer: a review of the literature. Int J Fertil Womens Med 50(6):250–258
124. Cassidy A, Albertazzi P, Lise Nielsen I et al (2006) Critical review of health effects of soyabean phyto-oestrogens in post-menopausal women. Proc Nutr Soc 65(1):76–92
125. Limer JL, Parkes AT, Speirs V (2006) Differential response to phytoestrogens in endocrine sensitive and resistant breast cancer cells in vitro. Int J Cancer 119(3):515–521
126. Bagchi D, Roy S, Patel V et al (2006) Safety and whole-body antioxidant potential of a novel anthocyanin-rich formulation of edible berries. Mol Cell Biochem 281(1–2):197–209
127. Vucenik I, Shamsuddin AM (2006) Protection against cancer by dietary IP6 and inositol. Nutr Cancer 55(2):109–125
128. Fox CH, Eberl M (2002) Phytic acid (IP6), novel broad spectrum anti-neoplastic agent: a systematic review. Complement Ther Med 10(4):229–234
129. Vucenik I, Passaniti A, Vitolo MI et al (2004) Anti-angiogenic activity of inositol hexaphosphate (IP6). Carcinogenesis 25(11):2115–2123
130. Rizvi I, Riggs DR, Jackson BJ et al (2006) Inositol hexaphosphate (IP6) inhibits cellular proliferation in melanoma. J Surg Res 133(1):3–6
131. Zhang Z, Song Y, Wang XL (2005) Inositol hexaphosphate-induced enhancement of natural killer cell activity correlates with suppression of colon carcinogenesis in rats. World J Gastroenterol 11(32):5044–5046
132. Weglarz L, Molin I, Orchel A et al (2006) Quantitative analysis of the level of p53 and p21(WAF1) mRNA in human colon cancer HT-29 cells treated with inositol hexaphosphate. Acta Biochim Pol 53(2):349–356
133. Singh RP, Sharma G, Mallikarjuna GU et al (2004) In vivo suppression of hormone-refractory prostate cancer growth by inositol hexaphosphate: induction of insulin-like growth factor binding protein-3 and inhibition of vascular endothelial growth factor. Clin Cancer Res 10(1 Pt 1):244–250

134. Singh RP, Agarwal R (2005) Prostate cancer and inositol hexaphosphate: efficacy and mechanisms. Anticancer Res 25(4):2891–2903
135. Somasundar P, Riggs DR, Jackson BJ et al (2005) Inositol hexaphosphate (IP6): a novel treatment for pancreatic cancer. J Surg Res 126(2):199–203
136. Vucenik I, Kalebic T, Tantivejkul K et al (1998) Novel anticancer function of inositol hexaphosphate. Inhibition of human rhabdomyosarcoma in vitro and in vivo. Anticancer Res 18:1377–1384
137. Vucenik I, Sakamoto K, Bansal M et al (1993) Inhibition of rat mammary carcinogenesis by inositol hexaphosphate (phytic acid). A pilot study. Cancer Lett 75(2):95–102
138. Shamsuddin AM, Vucenik I (1999) Mammary tumor inhibition by IP6: a review. Anticancer Res 19(5A):3671–3674
139. Tantivejkul K, Vucenik I, Shamsuddin AM (2003) Inositol hexaphosphate (IP6) inhibits key events of cancer metastasis: I. In vitro studies of adhesion, migration and invasion of MDA-MB 231 human breast cancer cells. Anticancer Res 23(5A):3671–3679 (a)
140. Tantivejkul K, Vucenik I, Eiseman J et al (2003) Inositol hexaphosphate (IP6) enhances the anti-proliferative effects of adriamycin and tamoxifen in breast cancer. Breast Cancer Res Treat 79(3):301–312
141. Higdon JV, Delage B, Williams DE et al (2007) Cruciferous vegetables and human cancer risk: epidemiologic evidence and mechanistic basis. Pharmacol Res 55(3):224–236
142. Bradlow HL, Sepkovic DW, Telang NT et al (1999) Multifunctional aspects of the action of Indole-3-carbinol as an antitumor agent. In: Bradlow HL, Fishman J, Osborne MP (eds) Cancer prevention. Novel nutrient and pharmaceutical developments, vol 889. Ann NY Acad Sci, New York, pp 204–213
143. Gomez-Arocena J, Bogers R, Van't Veer P et al (2003) Vegetable consumption and carotenoids in plasma and adipose tissue in Malaga, Spain. Int J Vitam Nutr Res 73(1):24–31
144. Pappa G, Strathmann J, Lowinger M et al (2007) Quantitative combination effects between sulforaphane and 3,3'-diindolylmethane on proliferation of human colon cancer cells in vitro. Carcinogenesis 28(7):1471–1477
145. Pledgie-Tracy A, Sobolewski MD, Davidson NE (2007) Sulforaphane induces cell type-specific apoptosis in human breast cancer cell lines. Mol Cancer Ther 6(3):1013–1021
146. Fowke JH, Chung FL, Jin F et al (2003) Urinary isothiocyanate levels, brassica, and human breast cancer. Cancer Res 63(14):3980–3986
147. Jackson SJ, Singletary KW (2004) Sulforaphane: a naturally occurring mammary carcinoma mitotic inhibitor, which disrupts tubulin polymerization. Carcinogenesis 25(2):219–227
148. Ji Y, Morris ME (2004) Effect of organic isothiocyanates on breast cancer resistance protein (ABCG2)-mediated transport. Pharm Res 21(12):2261–2269
149. Zhang S, Yang X, Morris ME (2004) Flavonoids are inhibitors of breast cancer resistance protein (ABCG2)-mediated transport. Mol Pharmacol 65(5):1208–1216
150. Xiao D, Singh SV (2007) Phenethyl isothiocyanate inhibits angiogenesis In vitro and Ex vivo. Cancer Res 67(5):2239–2246
151. Ambrosone CB, McCann SE, Freudenheim JL et al (2004) Breast cancer risk in premenopausal women is inversely associated with consumption of broccoli, a source of isothiocyanates, but is not modified by GST genotype. J Nutr 134(5):1134–1138
152. Terry P, Wolk A, Persson I et al (2001) Brassica vegetables and breast cancer risk. JAMA 285:2975–2977
153. Smith-Warner SA, Spiegelman D, Yaun SS et al (2001) Intake of fruits and vegetables and risk of breast cancer: a pooled analysis of cohort studies. JAMA 285:769–776
154. Seow A, Vainio H, Yu MC (2005) Effect of glutathione-S-transferase polymorphisms on the cancer preventive potential of isothiocyanates: an epidemiological perspective. Mutat Res 592(1–2):58–67

Chapter 6
Alcohol and Other Beverages

Alcohol Drinking

Around three decades ago, two case-control studies showed an association between high intake of alcohol and increased risk of breast cancer (BC) [1, 2]. Since then, the hypothesis postulating that the alcohol consumption increases the risk of BC has been intensely studied. According to expert opinions of an IARC Working Group on the Evaluation of Carcinogenic Risks to Humans more than 100 epidemiological studies – two thirds case–control and one third cohort – have evaluated the association between the consumption of alcoholic beverages and the risk for BC. In addition, two pooled analyses, the largest of which included data from more than 50 studies, have been conducted [3].

The Collaborative Group on Hormonal Factors on Breast Cancer made a pooled analysis of individual data from 53 studies on 58 515 women with BC, which compiled most of the evidence available worldwide a decade ago [4]. Results showed a linear increase in risk for BC with increasing levels of alcoholic beverage consumption, with a relative risk of 1.46 (95% CI, 1.34–1.60) for women who drank ≥45 g/day of alcohol (median 58 g/day) compared with non-drinkers. This corresponds to an increase of 7.1% (95% CI, 5.5–8.7%) per 10 g/day. This study also reported that the association of alcoholic beverages with the risk for BC was not modified by tobacco smoking, age at diagnosis, reproductive factors, a mother or sister with a history of BC, use of oral contraceptives or use of hormone replacement therapy.

The largest of the cohort studies comprised in the quoted technical monograph [3], which was conducted by the European Prospective Investigation into Cancer and Nutrition (EPIC) and based on 4300 cases, reported a significant 13% increase in risk for BC for intakes of ≥20 g/day of alcohol, which corresponds to an increase in risk of 3% per 10 g intake of alcohol per day (95% CI, 1–5%) [5]. On the other hand, according to the amount of alcohol intake per day, a higher amount (≥15.0 g/day) had no significant relation to BC risk (RR=0.87, 95% CI 0.40–1.91; P for trend=0.85) among Japanese women [6].

A. Ronco and E. De Stéfani, *Nutritional Epidemiology of Breast Cancer*,
DOI 10.1007/978-94-007-2397-9_6, © Springer Science+Business Media B.V. 2012

Concerning this point, although some information proceeding from international ecologic correlation studies exists, the experts agree in recognizing that they are not a considerable contribution in the particular case of alcohol intake among women [7]. A decade ago, the estimated age-adjusted attributable fraction for alcohol and BC was 2.1% among American women [8]. A recent study performed on the EPIC population, stated that 5% (2–8%) of cases of BC in women could be associated with total alcohol consumption [9]. Besides, Boffetta and Hashibe estimated that among women in Central and Eastern Europe, BC comprises 60% of alcohol attributable cancers [10]. These authors estimated in Europe in 2002 that 28,300 cases of BC, representing 7.7% of all BCs, were attributable to alcohol consumption. Concerning the attributable fraction of BC in France [11], 9.4% could be attributed to alcohol consumption, rather similarly to physical inactivity with 10.1% but almost doubling the estimate for changes in reproductive factors (5.4%).

More than two decades ago [12], a study reported that American women who had consumed alcohol before the age of 30 and afterwards ceased their intake experienced an elevation in their risk, which was similar to those ones who continued drinking. Another American study, but a cohort one [13] reported an increase of BC risk among former drinkers compared to non-drinkers (RR = 2.2), although the study lacked of age of quit.

Concerning intensity of intake, some studies have examined the effect of lifetime alcoholic beverage intake by total amount [4, 14–17] or by an intake of 10 g/day of alcohol [15, 18, 19] on the risk for BC. One large case–control study reported a 31% increase in risk for an alcohol intake of 13 g/day [15]. Conversely, the EPIC cohort found no association with lifetime alcoholic beverage intake after adjustment was made for current alcoholic beverage intake [5]. Most studies that examined the risk for BC and the age at which a woman began drinking reported no association [5, 14, 20–25].

The findings of a study on Mexican women support evidence that any alcohol intake increases risk of BC (ever vs. never drinking, OR = 1.25, 95% CI 0.99–1.58) [26]. Insufficient intake of folate may further elevate risk for developing BC among women who consume alcohol, according to this study (OR for lower folate intake = 1.99, 95% CI = 1.26–3.16).

Of some studies which examined the relationship of alcohol consumption and menopausal status of patients with BC, part suggested increased risk of BC in premenopausal but not in postmenopausal women [27], part suggested increased risk in both situations [28] and part suggested absence of relationship of any kind, or reduced risk among premenopausal women [29]. Therefore, clear evidence that some effect of alcohol is modified by menopausal status does not exist.

The types of alcoholic beverage were also studied, in order to clarify whether the increase of BC risk associated to increasing alcoholic consumption, occurred regardless of the beverage type [30]. Estimates from a pooled analysis of six cohort studies showed risks of 11%, 5% and 5% per 10 g intake of beer, wine and spirits per day, respectively [18], which suggested that the effect is mainly due to the presence of alcohol.

Tumour Type

Some studies examined whether the association between alcoholic beverage intake and risk for BC differed by estrogen receptor (ER) or progesterone receptor (PR) status. Three cohort studies [31–33] evaluated such association and all of them reported a significant association between alcoholic beverage consumption and risk for BC for the most common subgroup of ER+tumours; the small number of cases in the other subgroups may limit the power to detect significant differences between different tumour subtypes. The Iowa Women's Health Study [31, 34, 35] reported a higher risk with increasing alcoholic beverage intake for ER–/PR– tumours and the Swedish Mammography Cohort Study found a higher risk for ER+/PR+and ER+/PR– tumours [33]; both studies reported stronger associations for users of hormone replacement therapy compared with non-users, although these were based on small numbers of cases and caution is needed in the interpretation of results.

Of the case–control studies, only one reported a stronger association for ER+/PR+tumours than for ER–/PR– tumours in premenopausal women (RRs 1.4 and 0.9, respectively, for ≥3.5 drinks/week versus non-drinkers), although no significant difference was found in postmenopausal women [36].

More recently, the intake of ≥7 servings/week of alcohol represented a RR = 1.26 (95% CI 1.06–1.50) among triple-negative (ER-/PR-/Her2-) BC in a cohort of postmenopausal women [37]. Another study which made an analysis by cancer subtype reported that women who also consumed ≥7 servings/week of alcohol had a higher risk of hormone receptor-positive invasive lobular carcinoma (RR = 1.82, 95% CI 1.18–2.81) but not a statistically significant increased risk of hormone receptor-positive invasive ductal carcinoma (RR = 1.14, 95% CI 0.87–1.50) compared with never drinkers [38]. These authors conclude that alcohol use may be more strongly associated with risk of hormone-sensitive BCs than hormone-insensitive subtypes, suggesting different etiologic pathways for these two cancer subtypes.

In addition, in a large cohort study of postmenopausal women, alcohol intake was not associated either with risk of high-grade or low-/moderate-grade Ductal Carcinoma In Situ (RR=0.87, 95% CI 0.50–1.51) [39]. Besides, a recent study suggests that alcohol consumption does not appear to increase BC risk in women carrying a BRCA gene mutation [40], hence, there is a need of further studies to elucidate these points.

Primary prevention of the disease is not the only side of research on alcohol and BC: Consuming three to four alcoholic drinks or more per week after a BC diagnosis may increase risk of recurrence, particularly among postmenopausal and overweight/obese women, according to Kwan et al. [41].

Alcohol and Breast Cancer in Uruguayan Studies

We have performed a case-control study on a large database proceeding from the public hospitals healthcare system. The analyzed sample comprised 2.520 newly diagnosed BC cases and 2.434 hospitalized controls, admitted to the major public

Table 6.1 Alcohol consumption features of the studied population

Alcohol variable	Category	OR	95% CI
Alcohol drinking	Never drinkers	1.0	Reference
	1–30	1.24	0.94–1.65
	31+	1.26	1.02–1.55
	p-value for linear trend	0.01	
Alcohol duration	Never drinkers	1.0	Reference
	1-29	1.09	0.86–1.39
	30+	1.42	1.13–1.79
	p-value for linear trend	0.003	
Alcohol years	Never drinkers	1.0	Reference
	1–29	1.16	0.91–1.47
	30+	1.31	1.07–1.68
	p-value for linear trend	0.006	

hospitals in Montevideo, Uruguay during the years 1988–2004. More than half of cases as well as controls were residents in Montevideo (57% and 58% respectively). The urban fraction was 66.8% and 66.6% respectively for cases and controls. The logistic regression model included the following terms: age (continuous), residence (categorical), education (categorical), family history of BC (categorical), menopausal status (categorical), age at menarche (categorical), parity (categorical), smoking (categorical) and the alcohol variables.

In the following Table 6.1 the odds ratios of BC for intensity, years of drinking, and cumulative exposure to alcohol are shown:

Effect of Alcohol Duration in the Etiology of Breast Cancer

In the study conducted in Uruguay, years of drinking were directly associated with BC risk. It is noteworthy that most previous studies have focused on intensity of consumption of alcohol. Alcohol duration suggest that this risk factor is a marker of the stage of initiation of breast carcinogenesis. According to this hypothesis, alcohol consumption is a complete carcinogen, acting in the initiation and promotion of breast carcinogenesis.

The following variables could act as effect modifiers of the relationship between alcohol drinking and BC risk: menopausal status, age at menarche, parity, and family history of BC among first-degree relatives. In the following Table 6.2 the interaction between family history of BC and alcohol drinking are shown:

The findings for the interaction between parity and alcohol drinking are shown in Table 6.3.

The effect of alcohol drinking for different parity strata combined with family history of BC is shown in Table 6.4.

In spite of the additive or multiplicative nature of estimations, results suggest that nuliparae women having a family history of BC might constitute a potential high-risk subset of female population if in addition they are alcohol drinkers.

Table 6.2 Interactions between alcohol drinking and other menstrual variables and family history of breast cancer

Family history of BC					
No		Yes			
Alcohol drinking		Alcohol drinking		Total	
OR	95% CI	OR	95% CI	OR	95% CI
1.0	Reference	1.7	1.5–2.0	1.0	Reference
0.8	0.5–1.2	1.8	1.1–3.0	1.2	0.9–1.5
0.9	0.6–1.3	2.0	1.2–3.2	1.9	1.6–2.1
1.0	**Reference**	**1.9**	**1.6–2.1**	**Heterogeneity = 0.002**	

Table 6.3 Interactions between alcohol drinking and parity

Parity					
Para		Nuliparae			
Alcohol drinking		Alcohol drinking		Total	
OR	95% CI	OR	95% CI	OR	95% CI
1.0	Reference	1.0	0.8–1.2	1.0	Reference
0.8	0.5–1.2	1.3	0.7–2.5	1.2	0.9–1.5
0.9	0.6–1.3	2.1	1.2–3.7	1.4	1.4–1.7
1.0	**Reference**	**1.1**	**0.9–1.3**	**Heterogeneity = 0.02**	

Table 6.4 Effects of alcohol drinking stratified by parity and family history of breast cancer combined

		Alcohol drinking			
Parity	Family history	OR	95% CI	OR	95% CI
Para	No	0.7	0.4–1.1	0.7	0.4–1.2
	Yes	1.2	0.9–1.7	1.4	1.0–1.9
Nuliparae	No	1.3	0.4–3.8	1.9	0.7–5.1
	Yes	1.9	0.9–4.0	2.8	1.4–5.4

We also analyzed the possible interactions with red meat, white meat, total vegetables and fruit, raw vegetables, saturated fatty acids, fried red meat and benzopyrene, but there was no effect modification. All these foods and nutrients resulted in a modest attenuation concerning the risk of alcohol drinking in BC.

Postulated Mechanisms of Action

The biological mechanisms possibly involved in the development of BC are going to be elucidated. Several pathways have been proposed, including effects on the permeability of cell membranes in the breast, an increased hepatic metabolism of carcinogens by enzymes which are induced by ethanol, and inhibition of repair mechanisms of DNA. An influence on hormonal metabolism has been seen: alcohol increases the levels of endogenous estrogen in women, independently of menopausal status [42, 43]. Another study showed elevation of estrone sulphate, an indicator of estrogenic levels, among women which were regular alcohol drinkers [44]. The major source of postmenopausal estrogens is from the aromatization of androgens, and alcohol has been reported to increase the rate of aromatization [45]. A polymorphism in alcohol dehydrogenase type 3 (ADH3) affects the kinetics of alcohol oxidation and thereby could influence the effect of alcohol consumption on hormone levels [46]. Although elevated circulating prolactin levels have been suggested to be associated with BC [42], other authors [44] found no effect of alcohol consumption on plasma prolactin levels and in postmenopausal women.

Alcohol consumption was found associated with DNA methylation in postmenopausal breast tumors, suggesting that the association of alcohol and BC may be related, at least in part, to altered methylation, and may differ by drinking pattern [47]. Emerging data suggest that the epidermal growth factor receptor (EGFR) tyrosine kinase may contribute to BC genesis and progression [48].

Additionally, the effects of alcohol may be mediated through the production of prostaglandins, lipid peroxidation and the generation of free radical oxygen species. Reactive metabolites of alcohol, such as acetaldehyde may be carcinogenic: Cytosolic and microsomal in situ bioactivation of ethanol to acetaldehyde and free radicals and the resulting stimulation of oxidative stress could be a significant early event related to tumor promotion [49].

Aside from reactive oxygen species and other ethanol metabolites, studies using cultured human tumor cell lines have identified signaling molecules that may contribute to the effects of alcohol, including matrix metalloproteases, the ErbB2/Her2/Neu receptor tyrosine kinase, cytoplasmic protein kinases, adenylate cyclase, E-cadherins, estrogen receptor, and a variety of transcription factors [48]. Alcohol also acts as a solvent, enhancing penetration of carcinogens (like Benzo*a*Pyrenes) into cells. In vitro results showed that alcohol exposure increased the invasiveness of BC cells in a dose-dependent manner [50]. Exposure to ethanol drastically enhanced the adhesion of MCF(ErbB2) cells to fibronectin and increased the expression of focal adhesions [51], facilitating the metastasis process.

Anyway, no strong relations between genotype and environmental risk factors (comprising alcohol intake) were detected, suggesting that the low-penetrance susceptibility loci investigated in the Million Women Study do not generally affect BC risk through mechanisms involving these environmental factors [52].

Conclusions

There is a large body of evidence consistent with alcohol consumption increasing the risk of BC [3, 53]. Furthermore, there is also consistent evidence from large, prospective studies that even moderate alcohol consumption increases the risk of the disease [3], which was first shown by Willett almost 25 years ago [54]. Since the relative risk of BC associated with alcohol general consumption is quite small, and the level of alcohol intake among women is moderate in several countries, the proportion of BC attributable to alcohol intake is also small. Therefore, widespread efforts to reduce alcohol consumption appear as not having a potential substantial impact on BC rates in some populations.

ALCOHOL CONSUMPTION IS AN ESTABLISHED RISK FACTOR FOR BC. IT IS UNKNOWN AT THE PRESENT TIME WHETHER THE INCREASED RISK OF BC ASSOCIATED WITH ALCOHOL CONSUMPTION STOPS OR IS REDUCED.

Coffee

More than three decades ago a research reported that the elimination of caffein from diet led to the relief of symptoms in women afflicted with benign breast diseases [55], something which sparked the interest in caffein as a possible risk factor for BC. Since then began the study on the intake of coffee (main contributor of caffeine in several diets) as a potential risk factor for BC.

At the beginning of the 90's a work group of IARC [56] reviewed 7 case-control studies of BC which had examined the intake of coffee, concluding that all studies had risk estimates next to 1.0 and none suggested the existence of any association between the risk of BC and the intake of coffee. Moreover, there was no association either for instant coffee or for decaffeinated coffee, when results were presented separated. The final evaluation was that "there was evidence suggesting absence of carcinogenicity of the habit of coffee drinking on the female human breast".

Cohort studies performed in the United States and Norway have not shown relative risks far from 1.0 for the highest levels of intake. In a cohort of Norwegian women, while a clear association was not observed, an interaction with body mass did was seen, in such way that the coffee intake was associated with a reduced risk in women with small mass (significant RR=0.5), but increased in those with large body mass (non significant RR=2.1) [57].

During the decades of 80s and 90s case-control type studies were carried out in several countries (Canada, United States, New Zealand, United Kingdom, France, Israel, Italy, Japan, Spain, Sweden, Switzerland, Uruguay, among others), in which almost no report on the existence of any association between coffee and BC was made. When evaluating these studies and the rest of epidemiologic studies, 34 associations between BC and coffee were observed, independently from the statistic significance [58]. There were no risk estimates over 1.5, 30 were between 0.75 and 1.5 (or no association was concluded) and 4 were relative risks under 0.75. Therefore, the epidemiologic evidence, almost without exception, showed the absence of relationship between coffee intake and risk of BC.

An old international ecologic study reported that there was no correlation between BC mortality and coffee intake [59], whereas other study communicated a moderate positive correlation between coffee intake and BC incidence (non significant r=0.4) [60]. Finally, in experimental studies caffeine was observed stimulating as well as suppressing mammary tumours, depending on the involved animal species and the tumour phase in which the substance was administered.

THERE IS A CONVINCING EVIDENCE THAT THE INTAKE OF COFFEE DOES NOT KEEP RELATIONSHIP WITH THE RISK OF BREAST CANCER.

Black Tea

Tea consumption was also analyzed by the Work Group of IARC, who found that none of 5 epidemiologic studies on BC showed any association with such intake [56]. After that review from IARC, at least 4 prospective studies analyzed this possible association.

One of the studies in postmenopausal women reported the absence of association between the intake of black tea (RR = 1.1) for 2 or more daily cups, compared with a monthly intake or never [61]. A comprehensive study carried out in the United States, the Nurses Health Study, reported a moderate protective association (RR = 0.7) for 4 or more daily cups, compared to 1 or less.

Aside from the methylxantines (caffeine, theobromine) the tea has also variety of antioxidant polyphenols which were seen in animal experimentation and in vitro models, as having anticarcinogenic properties [62].

THE INTAKE OF BLACK TEA POSSIBLY DOES NOT HAVE ANY RELATIONSHIP WITH THE RISK OF BREAST CANCER.

Green Tea

Several epidemiologic and experimental studies, just in vitro as well as in vivo [63] have suggested that the intake of green tea can reduce the risk of several cancers, such as lung, prostate and breast. This preventive potential of green tea is attributed to biologically active flavonoids called catechines, which are chemically included as polyphenols. Of them, the most important is the EGC3G (epigallocatechine 3-o-galate) and it is a mediator of physiologic and pharmacologic actions which participate in tumour regression [64–67], apart from reducing the risk of cardiovascular diseases. Among the actions, it can be found the stimulus of tumour apoptosis and the inhibition of growth factors as Vascular Endothelial Growth Factor (VEGF). Thus, it could be summarized into a simultaneous antiproliferative and anti-angiogenic capability.

The evidence favouring a protection against BC has been accumulating in recent years, and although it is still not concluding, it is outstanding mainly in experimental studies [68–74] as well as in epidemiologic ones [75–79], usually with better results than with black tea [80, 81]. There are bases to think on green tea as having a probable coadjuvant therapeutic use, since it has been confirmed an inhibitor impact when there was overexpression of the Her-2-neu gene [82, 83], and also from a potential anti-angiogenic capability, working on the VEGF [84].

THE INTAKE OF GREEN TEA PROBABLY REDUCES THE RISK OF BREAST CANCER.

References

1. Williams RR, Horm JW (1977) Association of cancer sites with tobacco and alcohol consumption and socioeconomic status of patients: interview study from the third national cancer survey. J Natl Cancer Inst 58:525–547
2. Rosenberg L, Sloane D, Shapiro S et al (1982) Breast cancer and alcohol beverage consumption. Lancet 1:267–271
3. International Agency for Research on Cancer (2010) Alcohol consumption and ethyl carbamate. IARC monographs on the evaluation of carcinogenic risks to humans, vol 96. IARC, Lyon
4. Hamajima N, Hirose K, Tajima K et al (2002) Collaborative Group on hormonal factors in breast cancer. Alcohol, tobacco and breast cancer–collaborative reanalysis of individual data from 53 epidemiological studies, including 58,515 women with breast cancer and 95,067 women without the disease. Br J Cancer 87: 1234–1245
5. Tjønneland A, Christensen J, Olsen A et al (2007) Alcohol intake and breast cancer risk: the European Prospective Investigation into Cancer and Nutrition (EPIC). Cancer Causes Control 18:361–373
6. Kawai M, Minami Y, Kakizaki M et al (2011) Alcohol consumption and breast cancer risk in Japanese women: the Miyagi Cohort Study. Breast Cancer Res Treat 128:817–825
7. Longnecker MP (1994) Alcoholic beverage consumption in relation to risk of breast cancer: meta-analysis and review. Cancer Causes Control 5:73–82
8. Tseng M, Weinberg CR, Umbach DM et al (1999) Calculation of population attributable risk for alcohol and breast cancer (United States). Cancer Causes Control 10(2):119–123
9. Schütze M, Boeing H, Pischon T et al (2011) Alcohol attributable burden of incidence of cancer in eight European countries based on results from prospective cohort study. BMJ 342:d1584
10. Boffetta P, Hashibe M (2006) Alcohol and cancer. Lancet Oncol 7:149–156
11. Boffetta P, Tubiana M, Hill C et al (2009) The causes of cancer in France. Ann Oncol 20:550–555
12. Harvey EB, Schairer C, Brinton L (1987) Alcohol consumption and breast cancer. J Natl Cancer Inst 78:657–661
13. Hiatt RA, Klatsky AL, Armstrong MA (1988) Alcohol consumption and the risk of breast cancer in a prepaid health plan. Cancer Res 48:2284–2287
14. Freudenheim JL, Marshall JR, Graham S et al (1995) Lifetime alcohol consumption and risk of breast cancer. Nutr Cancer 23:1–11
15. Longnecker MP, Newcomb PA, Mittendorf R et al (1995) Risk of breast cancer in relation to lifetime alcohol consumption. J Natl Cancer Inst 87:923–929

16. Kinney AY, Millikan RC, Lin YH et al (2000) Alcohol consumption and breast cancer among black and white women in North Carolina (United States). Cancer Causes Control 11:345–357
17. Gammon MD, Neugut AI, Santella RM et al (2002) The Long Island Breast Cancer Study Project: description of a multi-institutional collaboration to identify environmental risk factors for breast cancer. Breast Cancer Res Treat 74:235–254
18. Smith-Warner SA, Spiegelman D, Yaun SS et al (1998) Alcohol and breast cancer in women: a pooled analysis of cohort studies. JAMA 279:535–540
19. Tjønneland A, Thomsen BL, Stripp C et al (2003) Alcohol intake, drinking patterns and risk of postmenopausal breast cancer in Denmark: a prospective cohort study. Cancer Causes Control 14:277–284
20. Holmberg L, Baron JA, Byers T et al (1995) Alcohol intake and breast cancer risk: effect of exposure from 15 years of age. Cancer Epidemiol Biomarkers Prev 4:843–847
21. Lenz SK, Goldberg MS, Labrèche F et al (2002) Association between alcohol consumption and postmenopausal breast cancer: results of a case-control study in Montreal, Quebec, Canada. Cancer Causes Control 13:701–710
22. Horn-Ross PL, Canchola AJ, West DW et al (2004) Patterns of alcohol consumption and breast cancer risk in the California Teachers Study cohort. Cancer Epidemiol Biomarkers Prev 13:405–411
23. Tjønneland A, Christensen J, Thomsen BL et al (2004) Lifetime alcohol consumption and postmenopausal breast cancer rate in Denmark: a prospective cohort study. J Nutr 134:173–178
24. Lin Y, Kikuchi S, Tamakoshi K et al (2005) Japan collaborative group. Prospective study of alcohol consumption and breast cancer risk in Japanese women. Int J Cancer 116:779–783
25. Terry MB, Zhang FF, Kabat G et al (2006) Lifetime alcohol intake and breast cancer risk. Ann Epidemiol 16:230–240
26. Beasley JM, Coronado GD, Livaudais J et al (2010) Alcohol and risk of breast cancer in Mexican women. Cancer Causes Control 21(6):863–870
27. Friedenreich CM, Howe GR, Miller AB et al (1993) A cohort study of alcohol consumption and risk of breast cancer. Am J Epidemiol 137:512–520
28. Martin-Moreno JM, Boyle P, Gorgojo L et al (1993) Alcoholic beverage consumption and risk of breast cancer in Spain. Cancer Causes Control 4(4):345–353
29. Ewertz M (1991) Alcohol consumption and breast cancer risk in Denmark. Cancer Causes Control 2(4):247–252
30. Singletary KW, Gapstur SM (2001) Alcohol and breast cancer: review of epidemiologic and experiment evidence and potential mechanisms. JAMA 286:2143–2151
31. Potter JD, Cerhan JR, Sellers TA et al (1995) Progesterone and estrogen receptors and mammary neoplasia in the Iowa Women's Health Study: how many kinds of breast cancer are there? Cancer Epidemiol Biomarkers Prev 4:319–326
32. Colditz GA, Rosner BA, Chen WY et al (2004) Risk factors for breast cancer according to estrogen and progesterone receptor status. J Natl Cancer Inst 96:218–228
33. Suzuki R, Ye W, Rylander-Rudqvist T et al (2005) Alcohol and postmenopausal breast cancer risk defined by estrogen and progesterone receptor status: a prospective cohort study. J Natl Cancer Inst 97:1601–1608
34. Gapstur SM, Potter JD, Drinkard C et al (1995) Synergistic effect between alcohol and estrogen replacement therapy on risk of breast cancer differs by estrogen/progesterone receptor status in the Iowa Women's Health Study. Cancer Epidemiol Biomarkers Prev 4:313–318
35. Sellers TA, Vierkant RA, Cerhan JR et al (2002) Interaction of dietary folate intake, alcohol, and risk of hormone receptor-defined breast cancer in a prospective study of postmenopausal women. Cancer Epidemiol Biomarkers Prev 11:1104–1107
36. Cotterchio M, Kreiger N, Theis B et al (2003) Hormonal factors and the risk of breast cancer according to estrogen- and progesterone-receptor subgroup. Cancer Epidemiol Biomarkers Prev 12:1053–1060
37. Kabat GC, Kim M, Phipps AI et al (2011) Smoking and alcohol consumption in relation to risk of triple-negative breast cancer in a cohort of postmenopausal women. Cancer Causes Control 22:775–783

38. Li CI, Chlebowski RT, Freiberg M et al (2010) Alcohol consumption and risk of postmenopausal breast cancer by subtype: the women's health initiative observational study. J Natl Cancer Inst 102(18):1422–1431
39. Kabat GC, Kim M, Shikany JM et al (2010) Alcohol consumption and risk of ductal carcinoma in situ of the breast in a cohort of postmenopausal women. Cancer Epidemiol Biomarkers Prev 19(8):2066–2072
40. Dennis J, Ghadirian P, Little J et al (2010) Alcohol consumption and the risk of breast cancer among BRCA1 and BRCA2 mutation carriers. Breast 19(6):479–483
41. Kwan ML, Kushi LH, Weltzien E et al (2010) Alcohol consumption and breast cancer recurrence and survival among women with early-stage breast cancer: the life after cancer epidemiology study. J Clin Oncol 28(29):4410–4416
42. Ginsburg ES, Walsh BW, Shea BF et al (1995) The effects of ethanol on the clearance of estradiol in postmenopausal women. Fertil Steril 63:1227–1230
43. Reichman ME, Judd JT, Longcope C et al (1993) Effects of alcohol consumption on plasma and urinary hormone concentration in premenopausal women. J Natl Cancer Inst 85:722–727
44. Hankinson SE, Willett WC, Manson JE et al (1995) Alcohol, height, and adiposity in relation to estrogen and prolactin levels in postmenopausal women. J Natl Cancer Inst 333(11):677–685
45. Gavaler JS, Love K, Van Thiel D et al (1991) An international study of the relationship between alcohol consumption and postmenopausal estradiol levels. Alcohol Alcohol 1:327–330
46. Hines LM, Hankinson SE, Smith-Warner SA et al (2000) A prospective study of the effect of alcohol consumption and ADH3 genotype on plasma steroid hormone levels and breast cancer risk. Cancer Epidemiol Biomarkers Prev 9(10):1099–1105
47. Tao MH, Marian C, Shields PG et al (2010) Alcohol consumption in relation to aberrant DNA methylation in breast tumors. Alcohol 17(7):930–931
48. Mill CP, Chester JA, Riese DJ (2009) EGFR may couple moderate alcohol consumption to increased breast cancer risk. Breast Cancer (London) 2009(1):31–38
49. Fanelli SL, Maciel ME, Díaz Gómez MI et al (2011) Further studies on the potential contribution of acetaldehyde accumulation and oxidative stress in rat mammary tissue in the alcohol drinking promotion of breast cancer. J Appl Toxicol 31(1):11–19
50. Hong J, Holcomb VB, Tekle SA et al (2010) Alcohol consumption promotes mammary tumor growth and insulin sensitivity. Cancer Lett 294(2):229–235
51. Xu M, Bower KA, Chen G et al (2010) Ethanol enhances the interaction of breast cancer cells over-expressing ErbB2 with fibronectin. Alcohol Clin Exp Res 34(5):751–760
52. Travis RC, Reeves GK, Green J et al (2010) Gene–environment interactions in 7610 women with breast cancer: prospective evidence from the million women study. Lancet 375(9732): 2143–2151
53. Boyle P, Boffetta P (2009) Alcohol consumption and breast cancer risk. Breast Cancer Res 11(Suppl 3):S3
54. Willett WC, Stampfer MJ, Colditz GA et al (1987) Moderate alcohol consumption and the risk of breast cancer. N Engl J Med 316:1174–1180
55. Minton JP, Foecking MK, Webster DJ et al (1979) Response of fibrocystic disease to caffeine withdrawal and correlation of cyclic nucleotides with breast disease. Am J Obstet Gynecol 135:157–158
56. International Agency for Research on Cancer, Tomatis L (eds) (1990) Cancer: causes, occurrence and control. International Agency for Research on Cancer, Lyon
57. Vatten LJ, Kvinnsland S (1990) Body mass index and risk of breast cancer. A prospective study of 23.826 Norwegian women. Int J Cancer 45:440–444
58. World Cancer Research Fund (1997) Food, nutrition and the prevention of cancer: a global perspective. American Institute for Cancer Research, Washington, DC, pp 252–287
59. Stocks P (1970) Cancer mortality in relation to national consumption of cigarettes, solid fuel, tea and coffee. Br J Cancer 24:215–225
60. Armstrong B, Doll R (1975) Environmental factors and cancer incidence and mortality in different countries, with special reference to dietary practices. Int J Cancer 15:617–631
61. Zheng W, Doyle TJ, Kushi LH et al (1996) Tea consumption and cancer incidence in a prospective study of postmenopausal women. Am J Epidemiol 144:175–182

62. Goldbohm RA, Hertog MGL, Brants HAM et al (1996) Consumption of black tea and cancer risk: a prospective cohort study. J Natl Cancer Inst 88:93–100
63. Ahmad N, Cheng P, Mukhtar H (2000) Cell cycle dysregulation by green tea polyphenol epigallocatechin-3-gallate. Biochem Biophys Res Commun 275(2):328–334
64. Gouni-Berthold I, Sachinidis A (2004) Molecular mechanisms explaining the preventive effects of catechins on the development of proliferative diseases. Curr Pharm Des 10(11):1261–1271
65. Doss MX, Potta SP, Hescheler J et al (2005) Trapping of growth factors by catechins: a possible therapeutical target for prevention of proliferative diseases. J Nutr Biochem 16(5):259–266
66. Beltz LA, Bayer DK, Moss AL et al (2006) Mechanisms of cancer prevention by green and black tea polyphenols. Anticancer Agents Med Chem 6(5):389–406
67. Stuart EC, Scandlyn MJ, Rosengren RJ (2006) Role of epigallocatechin gallate (EGCG) in the treatment of breast and prostate cancer. Life Sci 79(25):2329–2336
68. Kavanagh KT, Hafer LJ, Kim DW et al (2001) Green tea extracts decrease carcinogen-induced mammary tumor burden in rats and rate of breast cancer cell proliferation in culture. J Cell Biochem 82(3):387–398
69. Vergote D, Cren-Olive C, Chopin V et al (2002) (−)-Epigallocatechin (EGC) of green tea induces apoptosis of human breast cancer cells but not of their normal counterparts. Breast Cancer Res Treat 76(3):195–201
70. Sartippour MR, Pietras R, Marquez-Garban DC et al (2006) The combination of green tea and tamoxifen is effective against breast cancer. Carcinogenesis 27(12):2424–2433
71. Slivova V, Zaloga G, DeMichele SJ et al (2005) Green tea polyphenols modulate secretion of urokinase plasminogen activator (uPA) and inhibit invasive behavior of breast cancer cells. Nutr Cancer 52(1):66–73
72. Zhao X, Tian H, Ma X et al (2006) Epigallocatechin gallate, the main ingredient of green tea induces apoptosis in breast cancer cells. Front Biosci 11:2428–2433
73. Thyagarajan A, Zhu J, Sliva D (2007) Combined effect of green tea and Ganoderma lucidum on invasive behaviour of breast cancer cells. Int J Oncol 30(4):963–969
74. Thangapazham RL, Singh AK, Sharma A et al (2007) Green tea polyphenols and its constituent epigallocatechin gallate inhibits proliferation of human breast cancer cells in vitro and in vivo. Cancer Lett 245(1–2):232–241
75. Fujiki H (1999) Two stages of cancer prevention with green tea. J Cancer Res Clin Oncol 125(11):589–597
76. Inoue M, Tajima K, Mizutani M et al (2001) Regular consumption of green tea and the risk of breast cancer recurrence: follow-up study from the Hospital-based Epidemiologic Research Program at Aichi Cancer Center (HERPACC), Japan. Cancer Lett 167(2):175–182
77. Suzuki Y, Tsubono Y, Nakaya N et al (2004) Green tea and the risk of breast cancer: pooled analysis of two prospective studies in Japan. Br J Cancer 90(7):1361–1363
78. Seely D, Mills EJ, Wu P et al (2005) The effects of green tea consumption on incidence of breast cancer and recurrence of breast cancer: a systematic review and meta-analysis. Integr Cancer Ther 4(2):144–155
79. Zhang M, Holman CD, Huang JP et al (2007) Green tea and the prevention of breast cancer: a case-control study in southeast China. Carcinogenesis 28:1074–1078
80. Sun CL, Yuan JM, Koh WP et al (2006) Green tea, black tea and breast cancer risk: a meta-analysis of epidemiological studies. Carcinogenesis 27(7):1310–1315
81. Wu AH, Yu MC, Tseng CC et al (2003) Green tea and risk of breast cancer in Asian Americans. Int J Cancer 106(4):574–579
82. Guo S, Lu J, Subramanian A et al (2006) Microarray-assisted pathway analysis identifies mitogen-activated protein kinase signaling as a mediator of resistance to the green tea polyphenol epigallocatechin 3-gallate in her-2/neu-overexpressing breast cancer cells. Cancer Res 66(10): 5322–5329
83. Pianetti S, Guo S, Kavanagh KT et al (2002) Green tea polyphenol epigallocatechin-3 gallate inhibits Her-2/neu signaling, proliferation, and transformed phenotype of breast cancer cells. Cancer Res 62(3):652–655
84. Sartippour MR, Shao ZM, Heber D et al (2002) Green tea inhibits vascular endothelial growth factor (EGF) induction in human breast cancer cells. J Nutr 132(8):2307–2311

Chapter 7
Dietary Patterns

Most nutritional research has focused on the effects of individual foods and nutrients, as well as of food groups. However, from an epidemiologic viewpoint, foods and nutrients are never eaten isolated and their effects are likely to interact [1]. These facts have led to the acceptance of a more holistic approach to diet, which is implemented by the identification of patterns of dietary intake in order to represent the complex interactions between foods and nutrients and avoid confounding effects that may mask true associations [1]. Several studies have used factor analysis or principal components analysis to derive dietary patterns.

Definition of Factor Analysis

Factor analysis has been defined as a method which is used for reducing a large number of variables to a smaller number of factors for modeling purposes. In itself a dependent variable is not specified. The factors represent broad eating patterns of the population being studied.

Historical Perspective

Since the pioneer studies of Spearman [2] and Pearson [3], factor analysis has been employed in the fields of psychology and sociology. Later on, factor analysis was expanded in the fields of economy and other specialties. In 1992, Randall et al. [4] used for first time factor analysis aiming to clarify the relationship between colon cancer and factors (or patterns) derived from this method. After that, factor analysis was involved in numerous studies in cancer epidemiology and other chronic diseases.

Perhaps colon cancer was the main target but other malignancies like cancer of the breast, stomach, lung, esophagus (squamous cell carcinoma and adenocarcinoma), renal-cell, bladder, prostate, and larynx were submitted to factor analysis with rewarding results.

A.L. Ronco and E. De Stéfani, *Nutritional Epidemiology of Breast Cancer*,
DOI 10.1007/978-94-007-2397-9_7,

Table 7.1 Theoretical example of a factor loading matrix

Variable	Factor 1 *Western*	Factor 2 *Prudent*
Beef	**0.80**	0.01
Poultry	−0.10	**0.65**
Fish	0.02	**0.73**
Processed meat	**0.60**	−0.07
Vegetables and fruits	−0.05	**0.75**

Methodological Issues

Although this Chapter intentionally avoided the complexities of matrix analysis and algebraic foundations, we intend to define some important points. The factor loading matrix is an essential point. Whereas each row represents a variable, each column corresponds to a factor. Thus factor loading matrix could be represented as follows in Table 7.1:

This entirely hypothetical example displays a study in which factor analysis retained two factors (or patterns): the *Western* pattern and the *prudent* pattern. The first one is associated with an increased risk of a given malignancy, whereas the *prudent* pattern was strongly protective. Each cell is filled with a loading which varies in magnitude and, more important, loadings are clustered in each column. For example, the *Western* pattern showed high loadings for beef and processed meat, whereas the *prudent* pattern clusters white meat (poultry, fish) and vegetables and fruits.

Definition of High Loading

Although the criteria for defining a high loading is variable, loadings higher than 0.39 are considered as significant values and frequently are typed in bold. In the above example the *Western* pattern displayed high loadings for beef and processed meat, whereas the *prudent* pattern showed high loadings for poultry, fish, and total vegetables and fruits. It is important to avoid the frequent confusion between loading and correlation, since loading derive from the variance matrix.

Definition of Simple Structure

Thurstone [5] was responsible for the criterion of simple structure for the rotation of factors. Thurstone's criteria were as follows:

1. Each row of the rotated matrix should contain at least one zero.
2. In each factor the minimum number of zero loadings should be the number of factors in the rotation.

3. Simple structure factors are usually simple to interpret because they have only a few high loadings.
4. Simple structure factors are replicable (reproducible).

The Importance of Rotation

As a result of a factor analysis, the factor loading matrix results in non-rotated factors. Sometimes a non-rotated matrix is adequate, but in most instances rotation is needed in order to clarify the picture. On other words, rotation results in the clustering of related variables, which is easier and convenient for the interpretation of the factors as shown in the Table above. Essentially, there are two rotation methods (and infinite variants for each rotation): orthogonal rotation (usually called varimax rotation), and oblique rotation (usually called promax rotation). By far the varimax rotation is more frequently used, since oblique rotation implies that factors are correlated.

Foods and Nutrients

Foods or nutrients are employed in a given factor analysis. Most studies have used foods or food groups, being the use of food groups more frequent. Nevertheless, some recent studies have used individual foods [6, 7]. Some specialists have displayed some concerns about the use of nutrients for a factor analysis [8]. An Italian group has performed numerous studies on some cancers employing nutrients as variables for factor analysis [9]. An important drawback related with the use of nutrients is related with the difficulties in clarifying the meaning of nutrient factors.

Breast Cancer: An Important Field for Dietary Patterns

To our knowledge at least 28 studies [1, 9–35] have employed factor analysis in order to elucidate the etiology of BC. In first place we will use as examples the studies conducted by our group. The first of them was performed in 2006 with the objective of examine the role of red meat, vegetables and fruits in the etiology of BC [13]. Table 7.2 corresponds to the factor loading matrix (among controls):

Thus, the factor analysis retained six factors (patterns) namely *traditional, healthy, Western, stew, high-fat foods*, and *drinker*. Moreover the model explained 58.3% of the total variance. The patterns were scored using the regression method of Thomson [36] and applied to cases and controls. Then, they were analyzed by unconditional multiple logistic regression. Whereas the *healthy* and *traditional* were strongly protective, the *Western* pattern was directly associated with BC risk. The *stew* pattern was protective only among postmenopausal

Table 7.2 Factor loading matrix for the six factors retained among controls[a]

Food groups	Factor 1 traditional	Factor 2 healthy	Factor 3 Western	Factor 4 stew	Factor 5 high-fat foods	Factor 6 drinker	Communalities
Fried red meat	−0.04	0.04	**0.81**	−0.10	0.03	−0.07	0.68
Barbecue	0.30	−0.06	**0.66**	0.04	−0.12	0.05	0.56
Boiled meat	**0.51**	−0.12	0.01	**0.59**	−0.11	−0.03	0.64
White meat	0.02	**0.47**	−0.22	**−0.31**	**0.32**	0.15	0.49
Processed meat	0.15	0.26	**0.47**	0.24	0.22	0.18	0.45
Dairy foods	−0.05	0.06	−0.03	0.23	**0.70**	−0.23	0.61
Eggs	0.15	−0.19	0.04	−0.16	**0.61**	0.07	0.46
Desserts	0.16	0.36	0.15	0.24	**0.34**	0.21	0.40
Grains	**0.77**	−0.00	0.07	0.10	0.05	0.08	0.62
Raw vegetables	−0.07	**0.77**	0.01	0.09	−0.06	−0.06	0.61
Cooked vegetables	**0.51**	**0.48**	0.16	0.02	0.07	0.01	0.52
Total fruits	0.30	**0.51**	0.04	0.10	−0.09	−0.11	0.49
All tubers	**0.83**	0.05	0.05	0.02	0.02	−0.02	0.71
Legumes	0.02	0.11	−0.04	**0.84**	0.11	0.10	0.75
Alcohol	0.01	−0.02	−0.01	0.06	−0.06	**0.92**	0.86
Variance (%)	18.7	9.8	8.7	7.3	7.1	6.7	**58.3**[b]
N° of zeros	6	6	7	5	7	8	
N° of high loadings	4	4	3	3	4	1	

[a] Loadings higher than 0.39 are typed in bold
[b] Total variance explained by the model

women. Furthermore, the *high fatty foods* and the *drinker* patterns were not associated with risk of BC. The categorical OR's of *Western* and the *prudent* patterns are shown in Fig. 7.1.

The continuous estimates for the same dietary patterns, stratified by menopausal status are presented in Fig. 7.2.

The second study was conducted using nutrients [33] (Table 7.3).

The first factor was called *high-meat* nutrients, whereas the second pattern was labeled as the *antioxidants* one. Concerning the *high-meat* pattern, the higher loadings were observed for protein, saturated fat, monounsaturated fat, linoleic acid, α-linolenic acid, cholesterol, and the heterocyclic amines. The *antioxidants* pattern displayed high loadings for glucose, fructose, vitamin C, vitamin E, beta-carotene, other carotenoids, flavonoids, and phytosterols. The *high-meat* pattern was positively associated with BC (OR = 3.50), whereas the *antioxidants* pattern was inversely associated with risk of BC (OR = 0.44). In Fig. 7.3 the reader can find a graphic representation of the categorical estimates for both nutrient patterns. Concerning nutrients, linear trends as well as dose-response effect seemed to be better than the dietary patterns described before.

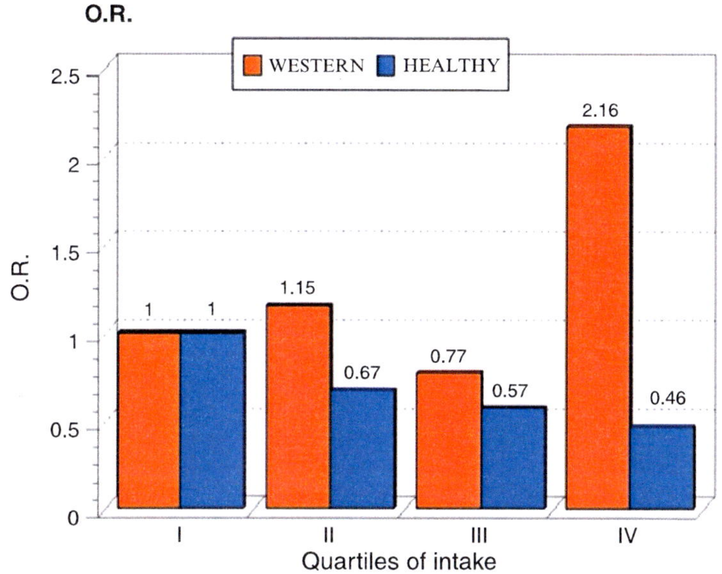

Fig. 7.1 Categorical odds ratios of BC for *Western* and *Prudent* patterns (Ref. [13])

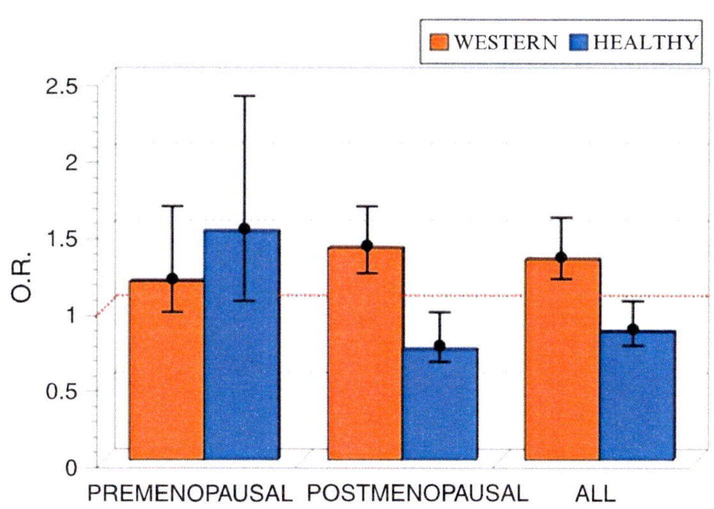

Fig. 7.2 Continuous odds ratios of BC for Western and Prudent patterns stratified by menopausal status (Ref. [13])

Finally, we conducted a factor analysis on ductal carcinoma of the breast [34]. In fact, this is the first study focused on the most frequent histologic type of BC. The most important conclusion is related with the similarities between this study and other studies which did not discriminate by histologic type. This study was

Table 7.3 Factor-loading matrix among controls[a, b]

Nutrient	Factor 1 high-meat	Factor 2 antioxidants	Communality
Protein	**0.68**	0.33	0.77
Saturated fat	**0.92**	0.05	0.88
Monounsaturated fat	**0.95**	0.02	0.91
Linoleic acid	**0.91**	0.03	0.85
Linolenic acid	**0.88**	0.11	0.87
Cholesterol	**0.77**	0.21	0.67
Glucose	−0.13	**0.85**	0.66
Fructose	−0.16	**0.82**	0.58
Vitamin C	0.03	**0.84**	0.73
Vitamin E	0.33	**0.71**	0.82
Beta-carotene	−0.03	**0.65**	0.41
Other carotenoids	−0.11	**0.78**	0.55
Flavonoids	0.16	**0.66**	0.55
Phytosterols	0.03	**0.73**	0.56
IQ[c]	**0.92**	−0.24	0.72
MeIQx[d]	**0.75**	−0.17	0.50
PhIP[e]	**0.79**	−0.13	0.56
Variance (%)	0.45	0.36	0.81[f]

[a] Loadings higher than 0.59 are typed in bold
[b] Sampling adequacy (KMO statistic) = 0.84
[c] (2-amino-3-methylimidazol[4,5-*f*]quinoline)
[d] (2-amino-3,8-dimethylimidazol[4,5-*f*]quinoxaline)
[e] (2-amino-1-methyl-6-phenylimidazol[4,5-*b*]pyridine)
[f] Total variance (including error variance): 81%

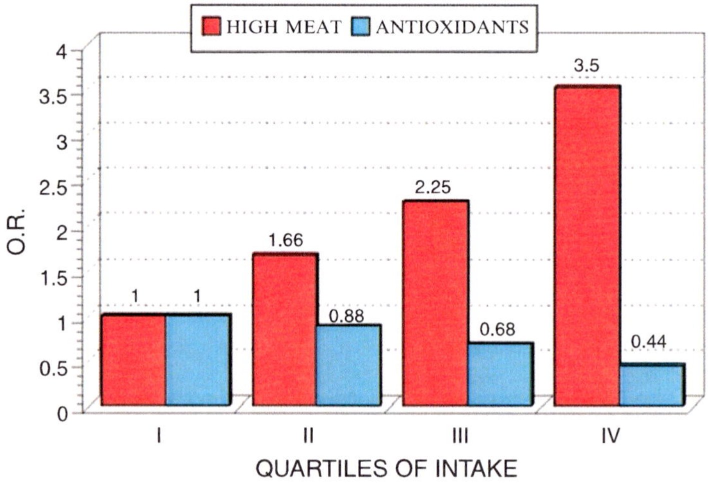

Fig. 7.3 Categorical odds ratios of BC for nutrient patterns (Ref. [33])

Table 7.4 Odds ratios of ductal carcinoma of the breast for dietary patterns (corresponding to Ref. [33])

Nutrient pattern	OR	95% CI	p-value
Low fat	0.73	0.58–0.93	0.001
Fried white meat	1.40	1.09–1.81	0.009
Non-alcoholic beverages	0.78	0.60–1.00	0.04
Western	1.44	1.10–1.89	0.03
Fatty cheese	1.64	1.24–2.16	<0.0001
Prudent	0.95	0.75–1.21	0.77

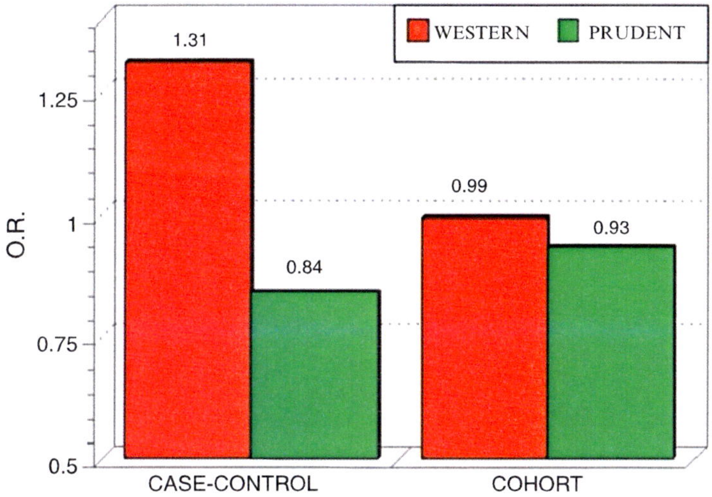

Fig. 7.4 OR's of both major patterns found in the existing literature, in pooled case-control and cohort studies

based on 111 cases and 222 controls. Importantly, the controls were healthy patients at difference with previous studies. The factor analysis retained six factors. These factors were labeled as follows: *low fat, fried white meat, non-alcoholic beverages, Western, fatty cheese*, and *prudent*. In the following Table 7.4, the risk of BC is shown:

As it was shown in a recent review [1] the results of most performed studies can be additionally summarized into two main patterns: The first one is the *Prudent/Healthy*, and the second one is the *Western/Unhealthy*. The former was associated to a risk reduction in case-control studies (OR = 0.84, 95% CI 0.67–1.04) and cohort studies (OR = 0.93, 95% CI 0.88–0.98) independently and combined (OR = 0.89, 95% CI 0.82–0.99). The latter displayed an increase of risk only in case-control studies (OR = 1.31, 95% CI 1.04–1.63) but lacked of association in cohort studies (OR = 0.99, 95% CI 0.90–1.08). When both types of studies were pooled, a non-significant increase in risk was found (OR = 1.09, 95% CI 0.98–1.22). The comparison of results belonging to both major patterns is shown in Fig. 7.4.

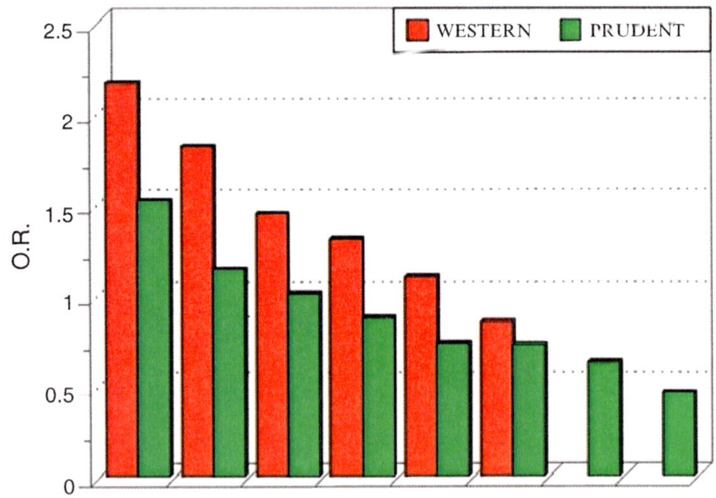

Fig. 7.5 Comparison of both major patterns found in pooled case-control studies

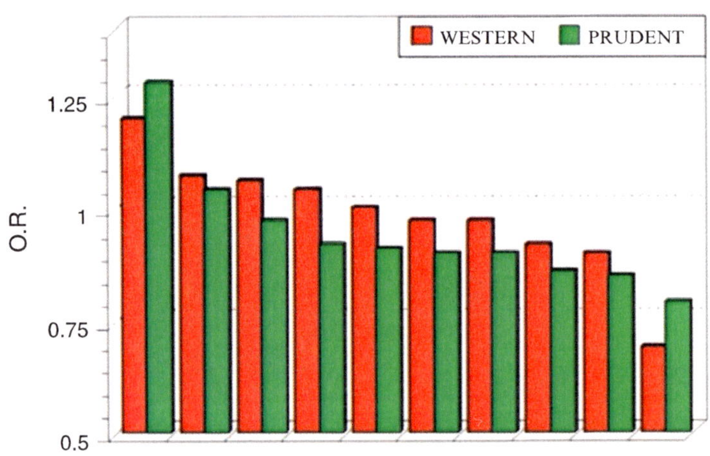

Fig. 7.6 Comparison of both major patterns found in pooled cohort studies

We have graphically expressed the risk estimations presented in the meta-analysis of Brennan [1], ordered from the highest to the lowest OR's. The comparison of results obtained by case-control studies displays evident differences (Fig. 7.5) for the two selected major patterns. On the contrary, cohort studies did not reveal differences between the patterns (Fig. 7.6), explaining why there was no association found.

Despite the methodological issues involved in such different estimates from case-control and cohort studies, which could explain partially the results, each of the two major patterns found have common items to be remarked. The *Prudent/ healthy* pattern had high loadings for plant foods and low loadings for red meat and processed meat. On the other hand, the *Western/ Unhealthy* pattern showed high loadings for meat and fatty foods. The preparation and cooking methods could be very different among populations and this fact might explain the unexpected lack of association found.

In conclusion, we can say that Factor analysis is considered as a powerful statistical method and it has been reported as more efficient than the traditional reductionist approach [37]. This type of analysis has shed some light on the links between diet and BC, in part differing from what the panel of experts stated before in the World Cancer Research Fund report [38] about the insufficiency of evidence for dietary patterns. While there is no clear evidence that any specific dietary component can effectively reduce BC risk [39], the fact that several foods have convergence on a few dietary patterns – and probably beyond these latter could be even fewer nutrient patterns [33] – is something we could probably profit from, thinking of recommendations for potential nutritional prevention such as those we have recently proposed [40].

References

1. Brennan SF, Cantwell MM, Cardwell CR, Valentzis LS, Woodside JV (2010) Dietary patterns and breast cancer risk: a systematic review and meta-analysis. Am J Clin Nutr 91:1294–1302
2. Spearman C (1904) General intelligence, objectively determined and measured. Am J Psychol 15:201–293
3. Pearson K (1901) On lines and planes of closest fit to systems of points in space. Phil Mag 6:559–572
4. Randall E, Marshall JR, Brasure J et al (1992) Dietary patterns and colon cancer in Western New York. Nutr Cancer 18:265–276
5. Thurstone LL (1947) Multiple factor analysis: a development and expansion of vectors of the mind. University of Chicago Press, Chicago
6. Dixon LB, Balder HF, Virtanen MJ et al (2004) Dietary patterns associated with colon and rectal cancer: results from the Dietary Patterns and Cancer (DIETSCAN) project. Am J Clin Nutr 80(4):1003–1011
7. De Stefani E et al. Unpublished results on foods and esophagus cancer.
8. Martínez ME, Marshall JR, Scherest L (1998) Invited commentary: factor analysis and the search for objectivity. Am J Epidemiol 148:17–19
9. Edefonti V, Decarli A, La Vecchia C et al (2008) Nutrient dietary patterns and the risk of breast and ovarian cancers. Int J Cancer 122:609–613
10. Terry P, Suzuki R, Hu FB et al (2001) A prospective study of major dietary patterns and the risk of breast cancer. Cancer Epidemiol Biomarkers Prev 10:1281–1285
11. Sieri S, Krogh V, Pala V et al (2004) Dietary patterns and risk of breast cancer in the ORDET cohort. Cancer Epidemiol Biomarkers Prev 13:567–572
12. Fung TT, Hu FB, Holmes MD et al (2005) Dietary patterns and the risk of postmenopausal breast cancer. Int J Cancer 116:116–121
13. Ronco AL, De Stefani E, Boffetta P et al (2006) Food patterns and risk of breast cancer: a factor analysis study in Uruguay. Int J Cancer 119:1672–1678
14. Männisto S, Dixon LB, Balder HF et al (2005) Dietary patterns and breast cancer risk: results from three cohort studies in the DIETSCAN project. Cancer Causes Control 16:725–733
15. Sant M, Allemani C, Sieri S et al (2007) Salad vegetables dietary pattern protects against HER-2 positive breast cancer: a prospective Italian study. Int J Cancer 121:911–914
16. Prentice RL, Caan B, Chlebowski RT et al (2006) Low-fat dietary pattern and risk of invasive breast cancer: the women's health initiative randomized controlled dietary modification. JAMA 295:629–642

17. Lee MM, Shen JM (2008) Dietary patterns using traditional Chinese medicine principles in epidemiological studies. Asian Pac J Clin Nutr 18:79–81
18. Ibiebele TI, van der Pols JC (2008) Dietary pattern predicts breast cancer risk-evidence from the EPIC-Potsdam study. Br J Cancer 100:925–926
19. Kroenke TI, Fung TT, Hu FB et al (2005) Dietary patterns after breast cancer diagnosis. J Clin Oncol 23:9295–9303
20. McCann SE, McCann WE, Hong CC et al (2007) Dietary patterns related to glycemic index and load and risk of premenopausal and postmenopausal breast cancer in the Western New York exposure and breast cancer study. Am J Clin Nutr 86:465–471
21. Schulz M, Hoffmann K, Weikert C et al (2008) Identification of a dietary pattern characterized by high-fat food choices associated with increased risk of breast cancer: the European prospective Investigation into cancer and nutrition (EPIC)-Potsdam study. Br J Cancer 100:942–946
22. Engeset D, Dyachenko A, Ciampi A et al (2009) Dietary patterns and risk of cancer in various sites in the Norwegian European prospective investigation into cancer and nutrition cohort: the Norwegian women and cancer study. Eur J Cancer Prev 18:69–75
23. Adebamowo CA, Hu FB, Cho E et al (2005) Dietary patterns and the risk of breast cancer. Ann Epidemiol 15:789–795
24. Velie EM, Schairer C, Flood A et al (2005) Empirically derived dietary patterns and risk of postmenopausal breast cancer in a large prospective cohort study. Am J Clin Nutr 82:1308–1319
25. Cui X, Dai Q, Tseng M et al (2007) Dietary patterns and breast cancer risk in the Shanghai breast cancer study. Cancer Epidemiol Biomarkers Prev 16:1443–1448
26. Hirose K, Matuso K, Iwata H et al (2007) Dietary patterns and the risk of breast cancer in Japanese women. Cancer Sci 98:1431–1438
27. Murtaugh MA, Sweeney C, Giuliano AR et al (2008) Diet patterns and breast cancer risk in Hispanic and non-Hispanic white women: the four-corners breast cancer study. Am J Clin Nutr 87:978–984
28. Wu AH, Yu MC, Tseng C-C et al (2009) Dietary patterns and breast cancer risk in Asian American women. Am J Clin Nutr 89:1145–1154
29. Cottet V, Touvier M, Fournier A et al (2009) Premenopausal breast cancer risk and dietary patterns in the E3N-EPIC prospective cohort study. Am J Epidemiol 170:1257–1267
30. Agurs-Collins T, Rosenberg L, Makambi K et al (2009) Dietary patterns and breast cancer risk in women participating in the black women's health study. Am J Clin Nutr 90:621–628
31. De Stefani E, Deneo-Pellegrini H, Boffetta P et al (2009) Dietary patterns and risk of cancer: a factor analysis in Uruguay. Int J Cancer 124:1391–1397
32. Edefonti V, Randi G, La Vecchia C et al (2009) Dietary patterns and breast cancer: a review with focus on methodological issues. Nutr Rev 67:297–314
33. Ronco AL, De Stefani E, Aune D et al (2010) Nutrient patterns and risk of breast cancer in Uruguay. Asian Pac J Cancer Prev 11:519–524
34. Ronco AL, De Stefani E, Deneo-Pellegrini H et al (2010) Dietary patterns and risk of ductal carcinoma of the breast: a factor analysis in Uruguay. Asian Pac J Cancer Prev 11:1187–1193
35. Buck K, Vrieling A, Flesch-Janys D et al (2010) Dietary patterns and the risk of postmenopausal breast cancer in a German case-control study. Cancer Causes Control 22:273–282
36. Thomson GH (1939) The factorial analysis of human ability. Houghton Mifflin, Oxford, England
37. Slattery ML, Boucher KM, Caan BJ et al (1998) Eating patterns and risk of colon cancer. Am J Epidemiol 148:4–16
38. World Cancer Research Fund / American Institute for Cancer Research (2007) Food, nutrition, physical activity, and the prevention of cancer: a global perspective. American Institute for Cancer Research, Washington DC
39. Mahoney MC, Bevers T, Linos E et al (2008) Opportunities and strategies for breast cancer prevention through risk reduction. CA Cancer J Clin 58:347–371
40. Ronco AL, De Stéfani E, Stoll M (2010) Hormonal and metabolic modulation through nutrition: towards a primary prevention of breast cancer. Breast 19:322–332

Chapter 8
Omega-3 and Omega-6 Fatty Acids and Breast Cancer

The Ω-6 and Ω-3 polyunsaturated fatty acids (Ω-6 and Ω-3 PUFA) became in the last years co-responsible of one the most important advances in the medical knowledge, in our opinion. Undoubtedly, the responsibility attributed to these fatty acids in the genesis of several and important chronic non-communicable diseases, which have high impact in modern society, is high [1]. A high Ω-6/Ω-3 ratio, as is found in current Western diets, promotes the pathogenesis of many diseases, including cardiovascular disease, cancer, osteoporosis, arthritis, inflammatory and autoimmune diseases, whereas increased levels of Ω-3 PUFA (a lower Ω-6/Ω-3 ratio), exert suppressive effects. The relationships between breast cancer (BC) and the quoted PUFA will be analyzed in this chapter.

Numerous scientific (anthropologic, nutritional, genetic) studies indicate that humans' dietary patterns have experienced great changes over the last thousands of years [2–4]. Ω-3 PUFA have been a part of the human diet for millennia. It has been estimated that the Ω-6/Ω-3 ratio in the diet of early humans was 1:1 [1]. Instead of a balanced 1/1 Ω-6/Ω-3 ratio (as with wild animals and presumably in humans during their long evolution of millions of years), this ratio rises to 10/1, 15/1 or even higher. Probably the main changes took place along the past decades, specifically from the middle of the twentieth century under the influence of the food industrialization and the agribusiness, which provided the economic stimulus for such changes [2–4]. It has been estimated that the present Western diet is "deficient" in Ω-3 PUFA.

The primary, short-chain Ω-6 and Ω-3 PUFA belong to the group of essential fatty acids (EFA), that is, the human organism does not produce them. Therefore, their intake must be done by an exogenous way, usually through foods. Linoleic acid (LA) is the essential Ω-6 EFA and α-linolenic acid (ALA) is the essential Ω-3 EFA and their long-chain derivatives are important components of animal and plant cell membranes. LA is abundant in nearly all commonly available vegetable oils, including corn, sunflower, safflower and in lesser amounts, in olive oil. Sources of ALA include soybeans, walnuts, dark green leafy vegetables such as kale, spinach, broccoli and Brussels sprouts, and seeds or their oils such as linseed, flaxseed, mustard seed and canola; however, it is important to remark that most of these oils are also rich in LA.

A.L. Ronco and E. De Stéfani, *Nutritional Epidemiology of Breast Cancer*,

DOI 10.1007/978-94-007-2397-9_8, © Springer Science+Business Media B.V. 2012

These two types of EFA are not interconvertible, are metabolically and functionally distinct, and often have important opposing physiological functions.

The human body has mechanisms to take and convert the ALA into the active Ω-3 PUFA, the DHA (docosahexaenoic acid) and EPA (eicosapentaenoic acid), but there are very long and not efficient processes from a biochemical viewpoint which feature mammalian organisms. It is recognized that the human organism can achieve a conversion of around 0.05–0.2% [5]. This means, for example, that an intake of 100 g of linseeds would become around 50 mg of DHA or 200 mg of EPA. The conversion is adequately performed by other animals belonging to different steps of the animal scale, for example insects which eat green leaves (where plant Ω-3 is), and poultry and other animals which eat vegetable seeds (where plant Ω-6 is) as well as those insects fed with Ω-3. In addition, mammalian cells cannot convert Ω-6 to Ω-3 PUFA because they lack the converting enzyme, Ω-3 desaturase. On the other hand, the conversion from LA to arachidonic acid (AA), the long-chain active Ω-6 PUFA, is easily performed in the human organism.

On this basis, the best would be the intake of DHA and EPA from the original sources which have the highest contents, from blue fishes as salmon, tuna, sardines, codfish and hering, for example. When humans ingest fish or fish oil, the EPA and DHA from the diet partially replace the Ω-6 fatty acids, especially AA, in the membranes of probably all cells, but especially in the membranes of platelets, erythrocytes, neutrophils, monocytes, and liver cells [6], due to the mutual competition that both Ω-6 and Ω-3 PUFA have for the same receptors or points of action, like for example Phospholipase A2, Cyclooxygenase (COX) and Lypooxygenase (LOX) enzymes. On the contrary, diets rich in common vegetable oils (such as sunflower, soybean, corn), margarines and poultry fed with seeds of those plants, derive into an overwhelming amount of Ω-6 PUFA, breaking the Ω-6/Ω-3 ratio.

Just in the same way that there are balances between "good" and "bad" substances, as cholesterol lipoproteins and estrogens, the Ω-6 and Ω-3 PUFA produce some substances that according to scientific knowledge, could be classified like them. The human organism needs both of these fatty acids. Such substances are called **eicosanoids**. They are hormones derived from the PUFA of 20 carbons (the prefix "eicosa" means 20) after the action of COX and LOX on the former Ω-6 and Ω-3 PUFA and are the final effectors of the functions that feature their role. Eicosanoids influence many physiological processes, including calcium transport across cell membranes, angiogenesis, apoptosis, cell proliferation, and immune cell function [7]. The Ω-6 are mainly "bad" and the Ω-3 are mainly "good" due to the type of eicosanoids derived from them [8]. Because of the increased amounts of Ω-6 PUFA in the Western diet, the eicosanoid metabolic products from AA, specifically prostaglandins, thromboxanes and leukotrienes are synthesized in larger quantities than those formed from Ω-3 PUFA [1].

The eicosanoids from AA are biologically active in very small quantities and, if they are formed in large amounts, they contribute to the formation of a chronic inflammatory status. In the course of inflammatory activation, pro-inflammatory eicosanoids of AA metabolism are released from membrane phospholipids. This status is expressed among others by thrombus and atheromas, allergies, chronic pain, autoimmune activity and cell proliferation, increasing the risk of developing a cancer. As a consequence, inflammation is now recognized as a central causative event for several of the most common human diseases prevailing in the developed world, such as atherosclerosis, cancer, asthma, autoimmune diseases, caries, and various neuropathological disorders such as stroke, Alzheimer's, and Parkinson diseases [9].

In particular, inflammation is intimately associated with cancer initiation and cancer progression [10, 11]. Cytokines, growth factors and mediators released in the above quoted chronic diseases and the developing tissue microenvironment, such as Interleukin-1b, Prostaglandin E2, Tumour Necrosis Factor-α, and Tumour Growth Factor b, have been found to have deleterious properties that pave the way for epithelial mesenchymal transition, prevent apoptosis and lead to the destruction of specific host cell-mediated immune responses against tumour antigens.

DIET SHOULD NOT HAVE AN EXCESS OF Ω-6 PUFA, SINCE THEIR EICOSANOIDS CONTRIBUTE TO THE DEVELOPMENT OF CHRONIC DISEASES AS BREAST CANCER.

Though we cannot state that there is a strong evidence to suggest an association between cancer incidence and intake of Ω-3 PUFA [12], according to some human studies of different geographic origins a high dietary intake of Ω-3 PUFA present in fish and other marine products as well as some vegetable oils (e.g. canola and linseed oils) can reduce the risk of developing BC [13–16] and inhibit metastasis [17]. The data on the geographic variation in the risk for cancer development suggest a strong association of fish oil diet in preventing BC: for example, BC incidence is 4–7 fold higher in North American women than in Chinese or Japanese ones [18]. In addition, a higher incidence of BC in Japanese women years ago correlates with decreased consumption of fish and increased intake of vegetable oil rich in Ω-6 PUFA [19].

Besides, fatty acid composition in breast adipose tissue was used as a qualitative biomarker of past dietary intake of fatty acids. There were findings showing that Ω-3 PUFA levels in adipose tissue are inversely linked to BC risk [20, 21], which is consistent with epidemiologic findings. Maillard et al. [21] reported that women in the highest tertile of ALA had a reduced risk when compared to women in the lowest tertile (OR = 0.39, 95% CI 0.19–0.78). In the same way, the highest tertile of DHA was also negatively associated (OR = 0.31, 95% CI 0.13–0.75). The dose of fish-oil/Ω-3 PUFA needed to achieve maximal target tissue effects for BC prevention remains undefined, but it has been recently shown that body mass index and baseline fatty acid concentrations modulated the dose-response effects of Ω-3 PUFA supplements on serum EPA and DHA and breast adipose tissue DHA [22].

Nevertheless, there are studies that report either no change or even a significant increase in BC risk among women who consumed high levels of Ω3 PUFA [23–26]. In one study [25] women in the highest quartile of fish intake had an increased risk of BC relative to women in the lowest quartile of fish intake (RR = 1.47; 95% CI 1.10–1.98). The Nurses Health Study also compared the effect of marine omega-3 FA on pre- and postmenopausal women [27]. In this study, a small increased risk of

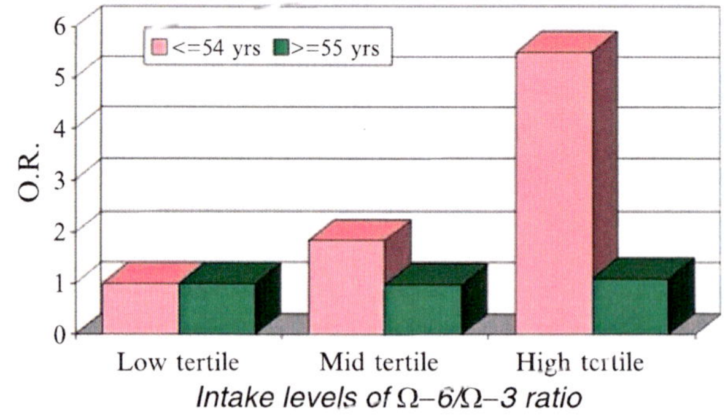

Fig. 8.1 Estimated OR's of dietary Ω-6/Ω-3 ratio according to age groups (Extracted from Ref. [28])

BC was observed in postmenopausal women (RR = 1.09; 95% CI 1.02–1.17), but no significant association was seen overall or for premenopausal women.

A study in Uruguay reported a negative association for the consumption of Ω-3 PUFA and the risk of BC [28]. This association was stronger and significant in the younger subset, under age 54 (OR = 0.20, 95% CI 0.04–0.96) than for the older one (OR = 0.67, 95% CI 0.26–1.76). In the same direction, the risk for the highest tertile of intake of Ω-6 PUFA was also higher among the younger subset than the older one (OR = 7.20, 95% CI 1.45–35.7 vs. OR = 4.05, 95% CI 1.65–9.94 respectively). As a consequence, the highest tertiles of Ω-6/Ω-3 ratio also displayed a significant positive association among pre-menopausal women (OR = 5.51, 95% CI 1.77–17.2), but no statistical association was found among postmenopausal ones (OR = 1.09, 95% CI 0.55–2.13) (Fig. 8.1). The evidence suggested a risk association of Ω-6 PUFA and a protective effect of Ω-3 PUFA with the risk of BC among Uruguayan women, but in this case the finding was especially within a subpopulation like the younger women in which is usually hard to find nutritional links with the risk of BC. The point appears as an interesting issue which deserves to be further explored.

It should be taken into account that cooking methods involving frying may partially explain the association of Ω-6 PUFA to fish, with which the Ω-6/Ω-3 PUFA ratio would lead to values that are potentially deleterious, specially when lean fish species are those implied, having a low level of Ω-3 in their flesh. A simple calculation

Estimated OR's of Ω-6/Ω-3 ratio according to age groups

Tertile	≤=54 year	≥=55 year
I	1.0 –	1.0 –
II	1.8 (0.5–6.6)	1.0 (0.5–1.9)
III	5.5 (1.8–17.2)	1.1 (0.5–2.1)

would lead us to know that there would be some grams of Ω-6 PUFA per fried piece, which would not be counterbalanced by some tens of milligrams of Ω-3 PUFA present in such species. In addition, the low content of Ω-3 is even reduced by the heating process implied in frying the fish.

The risk associations with the intake of essential PUFA (the short-chain ones like LA and ALA) seem to be controversial. The study in Uruguay [29] reported an increase of risk associated to high intake of ALA (OR=2.76, 95% CI 1.08–7.03) and also a risk reduction for high intake of LA (OR=0.24, 95% CI 0.12–0.45), which appear to be contrary to the expected results. Besides, a recent French study [30] communicated an inverse association of BC risk with ALA intake from fruit and vegetables (OR=0.74, 95% CI 0.63–0.88) and from vegetable oils (OR=0.83, 95% CI 0.71–0.97). Conversely, BC risk was positively associated to ALA intake from nut mixes (p trend 0.004) and processed foods (p trend 0.068), as was total ALA intake among women in the highest quintile of dietary vitamin E (p trend 0.036). The authors emphasize the need to consider food sources, as well as interactions between fatty acids and with antioxidants, when evaluating associations between PUFA intakes and risk of BC.

One study analyzed the relationship among BC incidence, marine Ω-3 PUFA intake, and Ω-6 PUFA intake [31]. In this study, among subjects in the lowest quartile of marine Ω-3 consumption, BC risk increased significantly with increasing levels of Ω-6 consumption (p for trend=0.08). Relative to women in the lowest quartile of both Ω-6 and marine Ω-3 consumption, the odds of developing BC for women in both the lowest quartile of Ω-3 consumption and the highest quartile of Ω-6 consumption was 1.87 (95% CI 1.06–3.27).

Prepubertal dietary exposure to Ω-3 PUFAs could affect later susceptibility to BC [32]. Plausible mechanisms explaining at an experimental level why rats fed prepubertally a low fat Ω-3 PUFA diet are at reduced BC risk and why those fed a high fat Ω-3 PUFA diet are at an increased risk were studied recently [33].

Experimental research on rodents showed some years ago that the generation delivered by mothers which had been fed with Ω-6 PUFA rich diets had: (a) a puberty onset at a younger age; (b) more terminal end buds in their glands; (c) more dense glands; (d) a higher frequency of BC than those ones fed with a standard diet; and (e) the lowest survival for those cancer cases [34]. Conversely, diets that were supplemented with Ω-3 PUFA reduced the cancer risk in the next generation, showing more mammary gland differentiation [35] (Fig. 8.2). Extrapolating from the animal model to humans led us to think that the potentiality of risk increase or reduction to develop BC from intrauterine life is something feasible and it might be modulated beginning with a given dietary style. Probably adult intake of some bioactive dietary components reduces cancer risk increased by early life dietary exposure, or inhibits tumour growth by reversing epigenetic changes in various molecular targets [36, 37].

Animal studies showed that a high maternal consumption of corn oil consisting mainly of LA, an EFA, increases both circulating estradiol (E2) levels during pregnancy and the risk of developing carcinogen-induced mammary tumors among the female rat offspring [38], possibly by altering mammary gland morphology and expression of fat- and/or estrogen-regulated genes. The Ω-6 PUFA-induced increase in maternal E2 levels indicates a mechanistic link among diet, mammary parenchymal patterns, puberty onset, and BC risk [34]. Accepting the hypothesis that prenatal exposure to endocrine disruptors might cause cancer, the field of Ω-6 and Ω-3 PUFA brings interesting points to be considered, in the same way that different individual agents were analyzed [39].

A recent review [40] suggests that Ω-3 PUFA EPA and DHA found mainly in oily fish have potent anti-angiogenic effects inhibiting production of many important

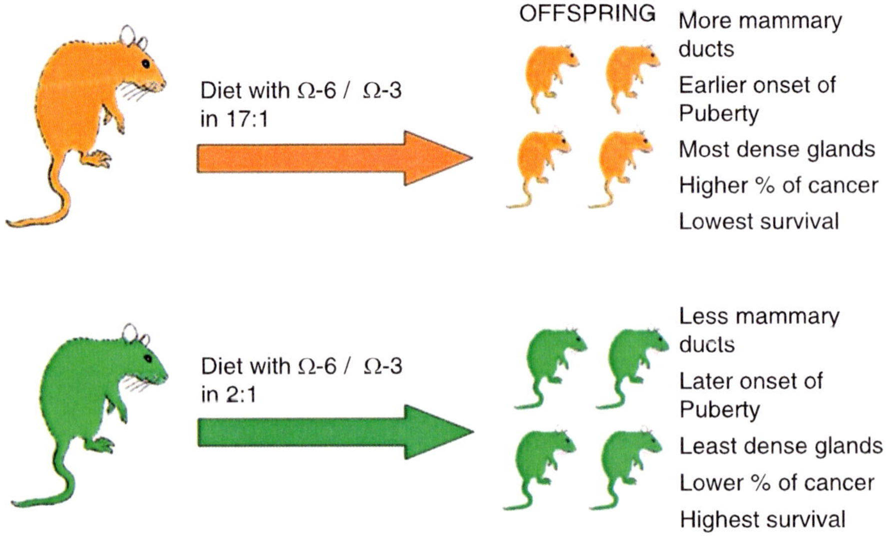

Fig. 8.2 Dietary Ω-6/Ω-3 ratio and experimental breast cancer (Adapted from results of Refs. [34, 35])

angiogenic mediators namely: Vascular Endothelial Growth Factor (VEGF), Platelet-Derived Growth Factor (PDGF), Platelet-Derived Endothelial Cell Growth Factor (PDECGF), cyclo-oxygenase 2 (COX-2), prostaglandin-E2 (PGE2), nitric oxide, Nuclear Factor Kappa Beta (NFKB), matrix metalloproteinases and beta-catenin.

The combination of epidemiological evidence together with the demonstrated effects of Ω-3 PUFA on cancer in animal and cell culture models, has motivated the development of clinical interventions using Ω-3 PUFA in the prevention and treatment of cancer, as well as for nutritional support of cancer patients to reduce weight loss and modulate the immune system [41]. Nowadays, sufficient evidence is available to suggest that major clinical trials with these natural compounds as adjuncts to standard therapies should be undertaken as a priority [42]. Therefore, from the prevention up to therapeutics and thinking specifically about BC, a place for cooperation as anti-cancer agents arises for the quoted Ω-3 PUFA.

References

1. Simopoulos AP (2006) Evolutionary aspects of diet, the omega-6/omega-3 ratio and genetic variation: nutritional implications for chronic diseases. Biomed Pharmacother 60:502–507
2. Eaton SB, Konner M (1985) Paleolithic nutrition. A consideration of its nature and current implications. N Engl J Med 312:283–289
3. Simopoulos AP, Childs B (eds) 1990 Genetic variation and nutrition. World Rev Nutr Diet, vol 63. Karger, Basel

4. Simopoulos AP, Ordovas J (eds) 2004 Nutrigenetics and nutrigenomics. World Rev Nutr Diet, vol 93. Karger, Basel
5. Pawlosky RJ, Hibbeln JR, Novotny JA et al (2001) Physiological compartmental analysis of alphalinolenic acid metabolism in adult humans. J Lipid Res 42:1257–1265
6. Simopoulos AP (1991) Omega-3 fatty acids in health and disease and in growth and development. Am J Clin Nutr 54:438–463
7. Avula CPR, Lawrence RA, Jolly CA et al (2000) Role of n-3 polyunsaturated fatty acids (PUFA) in autoimmunity, inflammation, carcinogenesis, and apoptosis. Recent Res Dev Lipids 4:303–319
8. Karmali RA (1987) Eicosanoids in neoplasia. Prev Med 16:483–502
9. Gallin JL, Snyderman R (1999) Inflammation. Basic principles and clinical correlates. Lippincott Williams & Wilkins, Philadelphia
10. Coussens LM, Werb Z (2002) Inflammation and cancer. Nature 420:860–867
11. Rakoff-Nahoum S (2006) Why cancer and inflammation? Yale J Biol Med 79:123–130
12. MacLean CH, Newberry SJ, Mojica WA et al (2006) Effects of omega-3 fatty acids on cancer risk: a systematic review. JAMA 295(4):403–415
13. Trichopoulou A, Katsouyanni K, Stuver S et al (1995) Consumption of olive oil and specific food groups in relation to breast cancer risk in Greece. J Natl Cancer Inst 87:110–116
14. Kaizer L, Boyd NF, Kriukov V et al (1989) Fish consumption and breast cancer risk: an ecological study. Nutr Cancer 12:61–68
15. Lund E, Bonaa KH (1993) Reduced breast cancer mortality among fishermen's wives in Norway. Cancer Causes Control 4:283–287
16. Key TJ, Sharp GB, Appleby PN (1999) Soya foods and breast cancer risk: a prospective study in Hiroshima and Nagasaki, Japan. Br J Cancer 81:1248–1256
17. Bougnoux P, Koscielny S, Chajes V et al (1994) Alpha-Linolenic acid content of adipose breast tissue: a host determinant of the risk of early metastasis in breast cancer. Br J Cancer 70:330–334
18. Kelsey JL, Horn-Ross PL (1993) Breast cancer: magnitude of the problem and descriptive epidemiology. Epidemiol Rev 15(1):7–16
19. Lands WE, Hamazaki T, Yamazaki K et al (1990) Changing dietary patterns. Am J Clin Nutr 51(6):991–993
20. Klein V, Chajes V, Germain E et al (2001) Low alpha-linolenic acid content of adipose breast tissue is associated with an increased risk of breast cancer. Eur J Cancer 36:335–340
21. Maillard V, Bougnoux P, Ferrari P et al (2002) N-3 and N-6 fatty acids in breast adipose tissue and relative risk of breast cancer in a case-control study in Tours, France. Int J Cancer 98:78–83
22. Yee LD, Lester JL, Cole RM et al (2010) Omega-3 fatty acid supplements in women at high risk of breast cancer have dose-dependent effects on breast adipose tissue fatty acid composition. Am J Clin Nutr 91(5):1185–1194
23. Goodstine SL, Zheng T, Holford TR et al (2003) Dietary (n-3)/(n-6) fatty acid ratio: possible relationship to premenopausal but not postmenopausal breast cancer risk in U.S. women. J Nutr 133:1409–1414
24. Caygill CP, Hill MJ (1995) Fish, n-3 fatty acids and human colorectal and breast cancer mortality. Eur J Cancer Prev 4:329–332
25. Stripp C, Overvad K, Christensen J et al (2003) Fish intake is positively associated with breast cancer incidence rate. J Nutr 133:3664–3669
26. Zhu ZR, Agren J, Mannisto S et al (1995) Fatty acid composition of breast adipose tissue in breast cancer patients and in patients with benign breast disease. Nutr Cancer 24:151–160
27. Holmes MD, Hunter DJ, Colditz GA et al (1999) Association of dietary intake of fat and fatty acids with risk of breast cancer. JAMA 281(10):914–920 [comment]
28. Ronco A, De Stéfani E, Deneo-Pellegrini H et al (2005) Consumo de grasas poliinsaturadas y riesgo de cáncer de mama: un estudio caso-control. Rev Bras Nutr Clin 20(Supl.1):S1–SS8, p.12
29. De Stéfani E, Deneo-Pellegrini H, Mendilaharsu M et al (1998) Essential fatty acids and breast cancer: a case-control study in Uruguay. Int J Cancer 76:491–494

30. Thiébaut AC, Chajès V, Gerber M et al (2009) Dietary intakes of omega-6 and omega-3 polyunsaturated fatty acids and the risk of breast cancer. Int J Cancer 124(4):924–931
31. Gago-Dominguez M, Yuan JM, Sun CL et al (2003) Opposing effects of dietary n-3 and n-6 fatty acids on mammary carcinogenesis: the Singapore Chinese health study. Br J Cancer 89(9):1686–1692
32. Olivo SE, Hilakivi-Clarke L (2005) Opposing effects of prepubertal low- and high-fat n-3 polyunsaturated fatty acid diets on rat mammary tumorigenesis. Carcinogenesis 26(9):1563–1572
33. Olivo-Marston SE, Zhu Y, Lee RY et al (2008) Gene signaling pathways mediating the opposite effects of prepubertal low and high fat n-3 polyunsaturated fatty acid diets on mammary cancer risk. Cancer Prev Res (Phila) 1(7):532–545
34. Hilakivi-Clarke L, Clarke R, Onojafe I et al (1997) Maternal diet high in n-6 polyunsaturated fats alters mammary gland development, puberty onset, and breast cancer risk among female rat offspring. Proc Natl Acad Sci USA 94:9372–9377
35. Hilakivi-Clarke L, Cho E, Cabanes A et al (2002) Dietary modulation of pregnancy estrogen levels and breast cancer risk among female rat offspring. Clin Cancer Res 8:3601–3610
36. Hilakivi-Clarke L (2007) Nutritional modulation of terminal end buds: its relevance to breast cancer prevention. Curr Cancer Drug Targets 7:465–474
37. Maclennan M, Ma DW (2010) Role of dietary fatty acids in mammary gland development and breast cancer. Breast Cancer Res 12(5):211
38. Hilakivi Clarke L, Clarke R, Lippman M (1999) The influence of maternal diet on breast cancer risk among female offspring. Nutrition 15(5):392–401
39. Soto AM, Vandenberg LN, Maffini MV et al (2008) Does breast cancer start in the womb? Basic Clin Pharmacol Toxicol 102(2):125
40. Spencer L, Mann C, Metcalfe M et al (2009) The effect of omega-3 FAs on tumour angiogenesis and their therapeutic potential. Eur J Cancer 45(12):2077–2086
41. Berquin IM, Edwards IJ, Chen YQ (2008) Multi-targeted therapy of cancer by omega-3 fatty acids. Cancer Lett 269(2):363–377
42. Shaikh IA, Brown I, Wahle KW et al (2010) Enhancing cytotoxic therapies for breast and prostate cancers with polyunsaturated fatty acids. Nutr Cancer 62(3):284–296

Chapter 9
Insulin Resistance and Metabolic Syndrome

Metabolic syndrome or insulin resistance syndrome, first described by Reaven in 1988 [1] as syndrome X, is characterized by abdominal obesity, dyslipidemia (high triglycerides and low HDL-cholesterol levels), high fasting blood glucose and high blood pressure levels. Several studies [2–16] have suggested a direct association between components of metabolic syndrome and breast cancer (BC) risk. Therefore, low HDL-cholesterol [2], high blood glucose [3], high triglycerides [4], postmenopausal overweight [5], abdominal obesity [6], hypertension [7], high levels of insulin [8], C peptide [9], and insulin-like growth factor I (IGF-I) [10], have all been associated with increased BC risk. Metabolic and hormonal factors related to metabolic syndrome have also been implicated in BC prognosis [11–15]. Furthermore, the increase in BC incidence has occurred in parallel with a steady increase in the frequency of type 2 diabetes and metabolic syndrome [16].

Interestingly, the metabolic syndrome was also found associated with a decreased risk of incident BC in women below age 50 with high body mass index, and with an increased risk of BC mortality in women above 60, according to a European study [17]. New evidence emphasizes that metabolic syndrome increases the risk mainly in postmenopausal women [18] and it has been found as significantly more prevalent in triple-negative BC patients as opposed to non-triple-negative patients [19].

A case-control study designed in order to explore the associations among anthropometry, some specific items of medical history related to metabolic syndrome (diabetes, hypertension, dyslipidemias, hyperuricemia) and the risk of BC in Uruguayan women was recently performed [20]. The study reported that a personal history of diabetes was positively associated to the risk of BC (OR = 1.64 [95% CI 0.99–2.70]), being higher and significant only among postmenopausal women (OR = 1.92 [95% CI 1.04–3.54]). Among overweight postmenopausal women having history of dislypidemia we found an OR = 7.82 (95% CI 1.46–41.9) in diabetic compared to non diabetic ones. Diabetes was also significantly associated in overweight postmenopausal women with hypertension (OR = 4.95 [95% CI 1.38–17.8]) as well as with a strongly endomorphic

A.L. Ronco and E. De Stéfani, *Nutritional Epidemiology of Breast Cancer*,
DOI 10.1007/978-94-007-2397-9_9,

Table 9.1 Features of the IR–CH syndrome

Insulin resistance – compensatory hyperinsulinemia	
Abdominal obesity	Increase of PAI-1
Postprandial hyperglycemia	Increase of fibrinogen
Intolerance to carbohydrates	Blood hypertension
Type 2 Diabetes	Infertility
Increase of triglycerides	Hyperandrogenism
Decrease of HDL2 cholesterol	Decrease of SHBG
Increase of LDL type B cholesterol	PCOS (Polycystic Ovary Syndrome)
Postprandial hyperlipidemia	
Hyperuricemia	

SHBG Sex hormone-binding globulins

somatotype (adipose distribution prevailing in abdomen, buttocks and lower limbs) (OR = 7.59 [CI 95% 1.71–33.6]). The risk of BC in postmenopausal women with overweight/obesity, dislypidemia, hypertension and diabetes compared to those postmenopausal ones being normoweight and without any history of dislypidemia, hypertension nor diabetes was very high (OR = 19.1 [95% CI 1.48–93.8]). We suggested that the quoted results could contribute to define new groups and individuals of high risk – for primary as well as for secondary prevention- if further studies confirm the reported findings, since this pathologic pattern linked to the metabolic syndrome is usually not taken into account for BC prevention.

There are several possible mechanisms by which metabolic syndrome may influence the natural history of cancer and in particular may promote the development of postmenopausal BC. Although they are not completely understood, the mechanisms probably include the effect of insulin on the bioavailability of sex hormones and growth factors [21–23] and the effect of overweight and insulin resistance on metabolism and on the bioavailability of inflammatory cytokines [24], as major reasons. We will herewith summarize both suggested mechanisms.

First of all, metabolic syndrome should be recognized as an insulin resistance syndrome. Insulin resistance (IR) could be defined when a lower biologic response is given by a normal level of the hormone. The tissues which present higher IR are skeletal muscle, adipose tissue (mainly the visceral one) and the liver. Not all tissues will present IR, therefore, the concept of compensatory hyperinsulinemia (CH) deserves an important merit to be acknowledged. It is clear that during the situation of peripheral IR the pancreas increases its insulin secretion in order to maintain a normal glycemia, to beat such resistance and to incorporate the glucose into the interior of each cell. This CH will overexpress their effects on the tissues that remain sensitive to insulin. It is the genesis of multiple alterations which characterize the syndrome of IR-CH. The syndrome features are shown in Table 9.1. The mammary tissue is sensitive to the action of insulin and it will become hyperestimulated in the quoted syndrome.

The Impact on Bioavailability of Sex Hormones and Growth Factors

Several studies have implicated insulin in BC development [23]. The C-peptide serum level – which is an indicator of pancreatic insulin production – is associated with increased BC risk among postmenopausal women [9]. Besides, high serum insulin is associated with worse prognosis in BC patients [11]. Among other ones, insulin has a gonadotropic effect [25], stimulating the ovarian stroma to produce androgens, whose aromatization in peripheral tissues is the main source of estrogens after menopause [26, 27]. In addition, insulin upregulates aromatase activity too [28]. Therefore, both necessary conditions for the estrogen synthesis are modulated by insulin. Most estrogens are produced in abdominal, breast, thigh and buttock adipose tissue [29]. Abdominal adipose, in particular, is an important source of both androgens and estrogens [30]. Obese postmenopausal women produce high levels of estrogens, which provide a wide basis of association of obesity with BC [31]. A recent study, however, reported that obesity was not associated with BC risk, suggesting that metabolic syndrome has an effect that is independent of obesity [14]. Insulin also lowers liver production of sex hormone-binding globulin (SHBG), thereby increasing sex hormone bioavailability [32] and metabolic syndrome is associated with increased circulating levels of both total [13] and free [22] testosterone, which in turn are associated with increased BC risk [33, 34].

A further mechanism by which insulin may increase BC risk is through its effect on the bioavailability of insulin-like growth factor I (IGF-I). The overabundance of insulin, called hyperinsulinemia, amplifies the bioavailability of IGF-I. Insulin decreases hepatic production of two IGF-binding proteins, IGFBP1 and IGFBP2 [35, 36], thereby increasing IGF-I bioavailability, and stimulates the synthesis of Growth Hormone (GH)-receptor [37, 38] thus allowing GH to promote IGF-I synthesis. Both insulin [39] and IGF-I co-operate with estrogens to stimulate the proliferation of breast epithelium cells [10], an effect that could enhance migration and invasion [40, 41]. Several prospective studies have examined the relationship of BC with prediagnostic serum levels of IGF-I, achieving inconsistent results [10]. The first studies found a positive association only in premenopausal women [3, 42, 43]; more recent studies on larger cohorts, however, did not confirm an association among premenopausal women, but highlighted a significant positive association in postmenopausal ones [44, 45].

Besides, there is good evidence that a negative energy balance is associated with a hormonal and/or metabolic milieu that would be predicted to reduce BC risk [46, 47]. For example, restricted energy intake has been associated with reduced insulin, and bioavailable IGF-1 (e.g., IGF-1/IGF Binding Protein-3 ratio). Body mass index (BMI) and waist-to-hip ratio (WHR) were significantly positively correlated with IGFBP-3 and C-peptide while adult exercise/sports activity and occupational activity were significantly negatively correlated with IGF-1 [48, 49]. These findings suggest that the association between positive energy balance and BC may be partially explained by the high concentrations of these biomarkers.

Exercise training also results in increased insulin sensitivity and decreased insulin concentrations [50]. A possible mechanism for the effect of physical activity on incidence of BC is mediated by an increased capacity for glucose transport into the muscle and adipose tissue in response to insulin stimulation. It is likely that physical activity is associated with decreased BC risk via multiple interrelated biologic pathways that may involve adiposity, sex hormones, insulin resistance, adipokines, and chronic inflammation. Exercise-induced myokines appear to be involved in mediating both systemic as well as local anti-inflammatory effects [51]. Recent reviews [52, 53] remark that the associations were strongest for recreational activity, for activity sustained over the lifetime or done after menopause, and for activity that is of moderate to vigorous intensity and performed regularly. According to the quoted authors, there is also some evidence for a stronger effect of physical activity among postmenopausal women, women who are normal weight, have no family history of BC, and are parous.

The Impact on Metabolism and Bioavailability of Inflammatory Cytokines

According to Kabat [54], hyperinsulinemia may provide the unifying mechanism by which the metabolic syndrome might be associated with increased BC risk [16, 55, 56]. Insulin has mitogenic activity in addition to metabolic effects and can promote cell proliferation in normal mammary epithelial cells and BC cell lines [57, 58]. Theoretically, high glucose levels could also increase the risk of postmenopausal BC by conferring a selective growth advantage on malignant cells [59], since high rates of glucose uptake and glycolysis are a common feature of malignant growth [60]. In addition to its association with IR and the metabolic syndrome, abdominal obesity is associated with the release of non-esterified fatty acids from adipose tissue and their accumulation in muscle and liver, leading to dyslipidemia [55].

Adipose tissue in obese subjects displays abnormalities in the production of several adipokines. Metabolic syndrome is associated with increasing levels of inflammatory cytokines and plasminogen activator inhibitor (PAI)-1 [61] and leptin [62], which can promote cell proliferation through various mechanisms [24, 63], and is inversely associated with adiponectin [64], which downregulates tumour cell proliferation and upregulates apoptosis [24]. Therefore, in addition to the effects of insulin and glucose, low-grade chronic inflammatory effects associated with the metabolic syndrome may be relevant to breast carcinogenesis [65]. Although hypertension associated with the metabolic syndrome seems to be secondary to the effects of IR-CH on the sympathoadrenal system [66], BC and hypertension may share common pathways involving inflammation and hormone synthesis and metabolism [16, 67, 68].

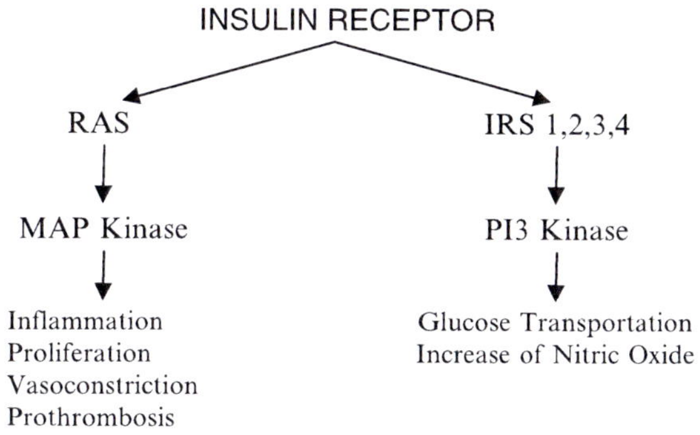

Fig. 9.1 Simplification of the insulin receptor and its two pathways: metabolic (PI3 Kinase) and mitogenic (MAP Kinase). In the insulin resistance the metabolic pathway is blocked and the mitogenic one is enhanced

The Insulinic Action in the IR-CH Syndrome

The insulin receptor belongs to the family of tirosin kinase receptors. Once it is activated two ways of action are clearly defined [69] (Fig. 9.1): (a) A metabolic pathway, the PI-3 Kinase way mainly destined to glucose transportation and the promotion of nitric oxide; (b) A mitogenic pathway, way of the MAPK destined to the promotion of growth factors, inflammatory factors, prothrombotic factors and vasoconstrictor factors. In sensible tissues such as the mammary ones, the IR-CH could determine a prevalence of the mitogenic pathway over the metabolic one, expressed by the promotion of IGF-1 and inflammatory factors [70].

The metabolic situation comprised into the IR-CH, that is the promotion of growth and inflammatory factors, could activate the transformation of an in situ mammary carcinoma towards infiltration and expansion. The hyperestrogenemia could also determine this transformation [71]. The body fat gain, very frequent during climacterics, could favour both situations [72].

The relationships between IR syndrome and climacterics have been analyzed [73]. During the latter, the fall of the hormonal axes and the fact that lipogenic hormones prevail over lipolytic ones, combined with sedentariness promote the gain of visceral fat. This fat generates a flux of free fatty acids and cytokines, just as TNF-α, all of which are able to generate IR through post-receptor actions on the PI-3 Kinase metabolic pathway, the one which regulates glucose transportation. An excessive adipose tissue, through the aromatase P450 enzymatic system, determines then a relative increase of estrogens, as it was already quoted. Through an overexpression of its mitogenic pathway activating the MAP Kinase, enhancing the effect of growth factors like IGF-1, inflammatory factors, and sharing an enhancement of the mitogenic action of estrogens, the CH facilitates an appropriate environment for the growth and invasion of BC. This situation takes places often during the post-menopause.

Table 9.2 Conditions associated to IR–CH and breast cancer

Conditions associated to IR–CH and breast cancer	
Saturated fats	Elevated triglycerides
Carbohydrates of high glycemic index	Elevated estradiol
Obesity	Elevated free testosterone
Waist circumference	Decreased SHBG
Hirsutism	Elevated IGF-1 and 2
Acantosis nigricans	Increased IGF-1 receptors
PCOS	Reduced IGF-BP3
Type 2 diabetes	
Glucose intolerance	
Elevated basal insulin	

SHBG Sexual Hormone Binding Globulin, *IGF* Insulin like growth factor, *BP* Binding protein

In the pre-menopause, certain conditions which generate an empowerment of the IR syndrome just as the PCOS (it adds another genetic factor in the expression of insulin resistance) [74] could determine a precocious presentation of BC. The PCOS is an important risk factor for BC in pre- as well as in post-menopausal women [75], due to its frame of severe IR-CH. The quoted conditions relating BC and these metabolic abnormalities are shown in Table 9.2.

Recent population studies have given information pointing to the concept that insulin sensitizers as Metformin could be associated to a reduced incidence and a better prognosis in certain cancers [76]. Metformin is an activator of AMP-activated protein kinase which inhibits protein synthesis and gluconeogenesis during cellular stress. Furthermore, metformin can induce cell cycle arrest and apoptosis and can reduce growth factor signalling. This drug has been widely used in the therapy of type 2 Diabetes, since it lowers the glycemia and reduces the hyperinsulinemia that is associated with IR. It has been experimentally demonstrated that Metformin works as a growth inhibitor as well as insulin sensitizer for epithelial cells [77]. Recently, metformin has been shown to inhibit BC stem cell growth and to synergize with chemotherapy in suppression of tumour growth and prolongation of survival of breast tumour-bearing animals [78].

Emerging evidence suggests that certain cancer therapies might increase patients' risk of developing metabolic syndrome secondary to the oncologic treatments. As the number of cancer survivors continues to grow, treating physicians must be aware of the potential risks facing patients who have been treated with anti-estrogen therapy [79, 80]. The expected consequences of a more frequent use of insulin sensitizers as a preventive tool as well as in patients already diagnosed with BC seem to be very favourable, looking to the future [81].

The analysis of the current knowledge gives us a broad view of the relationship with BC, leading to think that prevention or reversal of metabolic syndrome by lifestyle changes may be effective in preventing BC, mainly in postmenopausal women.

References

1. Reaven GM (1988) Banting lecture 1988. Role of insulin resistance in human disease. Diabetes 37:1595–1607
2. Furberg AS, Veierod MB, Wilsgaard T et al (2004) Serum high-density lipoprotein cholesterol, metabolic profile, and breast cancer risk. J Natl Cancer Inst 96:1152–1160
3. Muti P, Quattrin T, Grant BJ et al (2002) Fasting glucose is a risk factor for breast cancer: a prospective study. Cancer Epidemiol Biomarkers Prev 11:1361–1368
4. Potischman N, McCulloch CE, Byers T et al (1991) Associations between breast cancer, plasma triglycerides, and cholesterol. Nutr Cancer 15:205–215
5. World Cancer Research Fund/American Institute for Cancer Research (2007) Food, nutrition, physical activity, and the prevention of cancer: a global perspective. AICR, Washington DC
6. Connolly BS, Barnett C, Vogt KN et al (2002) A meta-analysis of published literature on waist-to-hip ratio and risk of breast cancer. Nutr Cancer 44:127–138
7. Soler M, Chatenoud L, Negri E et al (1999) Hypertension and hormone related neoplasms in women. Hypertension 34:320–325
8. Hirose K, Toyama T, Iwata H et al (2003) Insulin, insulin-like growth factor-I and breast cancer risk in Japanese women. Asian Pac J Cancer Prev 4:239–246
9. Verheus M, Peeters PH, Rinaldi S et al (2006) Serum C-peptide levels and breast cancer risk: results from the European Prospective Investigation into Cancer and Nutrition (EPIC). Int J Cancer 119:659–667
10. Campagnoli C, Pasanisi P, Peris C et al (2008) Insulin-like growth factor-I and breast cancer: epidemiological and clinical data. In: Pasqualini JR (ed) Breast cancer: prognosis, treatment and prevention, 2nd edn. Informa Healthcare, New York
11. Goodwin PJ, Ennis M, Pritchard KI et al (2002) Fasting insulin and outcome in early-stage breast cancer: results of a prospective cohort study. J Clin Oncol 20:42–51
12. Rock CL, Demark-Wahnefried W (2002) Can lifestyle modification increase survival in women diagnosed with breast cancer? J Nutr 132:3504S–3507S
13. Pasanisi P, Berrino F, De Petris M et al (2006) Metabolic syndrome as a prognostic factor for breast cancer recurrences. Int J Cancer 119:236–238
14. Agnoli C, Berrino F, Abagnato CA et al (2010) Metabolic syndrome and postmenopausal breast cancer in the ORDET cohort: a nested case-control study. Nutr Metab Cardiovasc Dis 20(1):41. doi:10.1016/j.numecd.2009.02.006
15. Tsugane S, Inoue M (2010) Insulin resistance and cancer: epidemiological evidence. Cancer Sci 101(5):1073–1079
16. Xue F, Michels KB (2007) Diabetes, metabolic syndrome, and breast cancer: a review of the current evidence. Am J Clin Nutr 86:s823–s835
17. Bjørge T, Lukanova A, Jonsson H et al (2010) Metabolic syndrome and breast cancer in the me-can (metabolic syndrome and cancer) project. Cancer Epidemiol Biomarkers Prev 19(7):1737–1745
18. Capasso I, Esposito E, Pentimalli F et al (2011) Metabolic syndrome affects breast cancer risk in postmenopausal women: National Cancer Institute of Naples experience. Cancer Biol Ther 10(12):1240–1243
19. Maiti B, Kundranda MN, Spiro TP et al (2010) The association of metabolic syndrome with triple-negative breast cancer. Breast Cancer Res Treat 121(2):479–483
20. Ronco AL, De Stéfani E (2010) Diabetes, overweight and risk of breast cancer: a case-control study in Uruguay. XVI world congress on breast diseases, Valencia, 20–22 Oct 2010
21. Berrino F, Villarini A, De Petris M et al (2006) Adjuvant diet to improve hormonal and metabolic factors affecting breast cancer prognosis. Ann N Y Acad Sci 1089:110–118
22. Golden SH, Ding J, Szklo M et al (2004) Glucose and insulin components of the metabolic syndrome are associated with hyperandrogenism in postmenopausal women: the atherosclerosis risk in communities study. Am J Epidemiol 160:540–548

23. Kaaks R (1996) Nutrition, hormones, and breast cancer: is insulin the missing link? Cancer Causes Control 7:605–625
24. Vona-Davis L, Howard-McNatt M, Rose DP (2007) Adiposity, type 2 diabetes and the metabolic syndrome in breast cancer. Obes Rev 8:395–408
25. Poretsky L, Cataldo NA, Rosenwaks Z et al (1999) The insulin-related ovarian regulatory system in health and disease. Endocr Rev 20:535–582
26. Berrino F, Muti P, Micheli A et al (1996) Serum sex hormone levels after menopause and subsequent breast cancer. J Natl Cancer Inst 88:291–296
27. Nelson LR, Bulun SE (2001) Estrogen production and action. J Am Acad Dermatol 45:S116–S124
28. McTernan PG, Anwar A, Eggo MC et al (2000) Gender differences in the regulation of P450 aromatase expression and activity in human adipose tissue. Int J Obes Relat Metab Disord 24:875–881
29. Grodin JM, Siiteri PK, MacDonald PC (1973) Source of estrogen production in postmenopausal women. J Clin Endocrinol Metab 36:207–214
30. Cauley JA, Gutai JP, Kuller LH et al (1989) The epidemiology of serum sex hormones in postmenopausal women. Am J Epidemiol 129:1120–1131
31. Key TJ, Appleby PN, Reeves GK et al (2003) Body mass index, serum sex hormones, and breast cancer risk in postmenopausal women. J Natl Cancer Inst 95:1218–1226
32. Sherif K, Kushner H, Falkner BE (1998) Sex hormone-binding globulin and insulin resistance in African-American women. Metabolism 47:70–74
33. Kaaks R, Rinaldi S, Key TJ et al (2005) Postmenopausal serum androgens, oestrogens and breast cancer risk: the European prospective investigation into cancer and nutrition. Endocr Relat Cancer 12:1071–1082
34. Key T, Appleby P, Barnes I et al (2002) Endogenous sex hormones and breast cancer in postmenopausal women: reanalysis of nine prospective studies. J Natl Cancer Inst 94:606–616
35. Brismar K, Hilding A, Lindgren B (1995) Regulation of IGFBP-1 in humans. Prog Growth Factor Res 6:449–456
36. Norat T, Dossus L, Rinaldi S et al (2007) Diet, serum insulin-like growth factor-I and IGF-binding protein-3 in European women. Eur J Clin Nutr 61:91–98
37. Hanaire-Broutin H, Sallerin-Caute B, Poncet MF et al (1996) Insulin therapy and GH-IGF-I axis disorders in diabetes: impact of glycaemic control and hepatic insulinization. Diabetes Metab 22:245–250
38. Tollet P, Enberg B, Mode A (1990) Growth hormone (GH) regulation of cytochrome P-450IIC12, insulin like growth factor-I (IGF-I), and GH receptor messenger RNA expression in primary rat hepatocytes: a hormonal interplay with insulin, IGF-I, and thyroid hormone. Mol Endocrinol 4:1934–1942
39. Panno ML, Salerno M, Pezzi V et al (1996) Effect of oestradiol and insulin on the proliferative pattern and on oestrogen and progesterone receptor contents in MCF-7 cells. J Cancer Res Clin Oncol 122:745–749
40. Sachdev D, Yee D (2001) The IGF system and breast cancer. Endocr Relat Cancer 8:197–209
41. Macaulay VM (1992) Insulin-like growth factors and cancer. Br J Cancer 65:311–320
42. Hankinson SE, Willett WC, Colditz GA et al (1998) Circulating concentrations of insulin-like growth factor-I and risk of breast cancer. Lancet 351:1393–1396
43. Toniolo P, Bruning PF, Akhmedkhanov A et al (2000) Serum insulin like growth factor-I and breast cancer. Int J Cancer 88:828–832
44. Baglietto L, English DR, Hopper JL et al (2007) Circulating insulin-like growth factor-I and binding protein-3 and the risk of breast cancer. Cancer Epidemiol Biomarkers Prev 16:763–768
45. Rinaldi S, Peeters PH, Berrino F et al (2006) IGF-I, IGFBP-3 and breast cancer risk in women: the European Prospective Investigation into Cancer and Nutrition (EPIC). Endocr Relat Cancer 13:593–605
46. Loucks AB (2003) Energy availability, not body fatness, regulates reproductive function in women. Exerc Sport Sci Rev 31:144–148

47. De Souza MJ, Van Heest J, Demers LM et al (2003) Luteal phase deficiency in recreational runners: evidence for a hypometabolic state. J Clin Endocrinol Metab 88:337–346
48. Chadan SG, Dill RP, Vanderhoek K et al (1999) Influence of physical activity on plasma insulin-like factor 1 and insulin-like binding proteins in healthy older women. Mech Ageing Dev 109:21–34
49. Fair AM, Dai Q, Shu XO et al (2007) Energy balance, insulin-resistance biomarkers and breast cancer risk. Cancer Detect Prev 31(3):214–219
50. Westerlind KC (2003) Physical activity and cancer prevention –mechanisms. Med Sci Sports Exerc 35:1834–1840
51. Brandt C, Pedersen BK (2010) The role of exercise-induced myokines in muscle homeostasis and the defense against chronic diseases. J Biomed Biotechnol 2010:520258
52. Friedenreich CM (2011) Physical activity and breast cancer: review of the epidemiologic evidence and biologic mechanisms. Recent Results Cancer Res 188:125–139
53. Lynch BM, Neilson HK, Friedenreich CM (2011) Physical activity and breast cancer prevention. Recent Results Cancer Res 186:13–42
54. Kabat GC, Kim M, Chlebowski RT et al (2009) A longitudinal study of the metabolic syndrome and risk of postmenopausal breast cancer. Cancer Epidemiol Biomarkers Prev 18(7):2046–2053
55. Morimoto LM, White E, Chen Z et al (2002) Obesity, body size, and risk postmenopausal breast cancer: the women's health initiative (United States). Cancer Causes Control 13:741–751
56. Strickler HD, Wylie-Rosett J, Rohan T et al (2001) The relation of type 2 diabetes and cancer. Diabetes Technol Ther 3:263–275
57. Milazzo G, Giorgino F, Damante F et al (1992) Insulin receptor expression and function in human breast cancer cell lines. Cancer Res 52:3924–3930
58. Cullen KJ, Yee D, Sly WS et al (1990) Insulin like growth factor receptor expression and function in human breast cancer. Cancer Res 50:48–53
59. Warburg O (1956) On the origin of cancer cells. Science 123:309–314
60. Dang CV, Semenza GL (1999) Oncogenic alterations of metabolism. Trends Biochem Sci 24:68–72
61. Rose DP, Haffner SM, Baillargeon J (2007) Adiposity, the metabolic syndrome, and breast cancer in African-American and white American women. Endocr Rev 28:763–777
62. Sieminska L, Wojciechowska C, Foltyn W et al (2006) The relation of serum adiponectin and leptin levels to metabolic syndrome in women before and after the menopause. Endokrynol Pol 57:15–22
63. Purohit A, Newman SP, Reed MJ (2002) The role of cytokines in regulating estrogen synthesis: implications for the etiology of breast cancer. Breast Cancer Res 4:65–69
64. Ryo M, Nakamura T, Kihara S et al (2004) Adiponectin as a biomarker of the metabolic syndrome. Circ J 68:975–981
65. Dossus L, Kaaks R (2008) Nutrition, metabolic factors and cancer risk. Best Pract Res Clin Endocrinol Metab 22:551–571
66. Reaven GM, Lithell H, Landsberg L (1996) Hypertension and associated metabolic abnormalities – the role of insulin resistance and the sympathoadrenal system. N Engl J Med 334:374–381
67. Balkwill F, Charles KA, Mantovani A (2005) Smoldering and polarized inflammation in the initiation and promotion of malignant disease. Cancer Cell 7:211–217
68. Cheng Z, Vapaatalo H, Mervaala E (2005) Angiotensin II and vascular inflammation. Med Sci Monit 11:RA194–RA205
69. Hunter SJ, Garvey WT (1998) Insulin action and insulin resistance: diseases involving defects in insulin receptors, signal transduction, and the glucose transport effector system. Am J Med 105(4):331–345
70. Kaaks R (2001) Plasma insulin.IGF-I and breast cancer. Gynecol Obstet Fertil 29(3):185–191
71. Nagata C, Shimizu H, Takami R et al (2000) Relations of insulin resistance and serum concentrations of estradiol and sex hormone-binding globulin to potential breast cancer risk factors. Jpn J Cancer Res 91(9):948–953

72. Jernstrom H, Barrett-Connor E (1999) Obesity, weight change, fasting insulin, proinsulin, C-peptide, and insulin-like growth factor-1 levels in women with and without breast cancer: the Rancho Bernardo study. J Womens Health Gend Based Med 8(10):1265–1272
73. Pisabarro R (2000) Metabolismo y Climaterio: la visión de un Endocrinólogo. Rev Med Uruguay 16:144–151
74. Dunaif A (1999) Insulin action in the polycystic ovary syndrome. Endocrinol Metab Clin North Am 28(2):341–359
75. Solomon CG (1999) The epidemiology of polycystic ovary syndrome: prevalence and associated disease risk. Endocrinol Metab Clin North Am 28(2):247–263
76. Jalving M, Gietema JA, Lefrandt JD et al (2010) Metformin: taking away the candy for cancer? Eur J Cancer 46(13):2369–2380
77. Zakikhani M, Dowling R, Fantus IG et al (2006) Metformin is an AMP kinase-dependent growth inhibitor for breast cancer cells. Cancer Res 66(21):10269–10273
78. Wysocki PJ, Wierusz-Wysocka B (2010) Obesity, hyperinsulinemia and breast cancer: novel targets and a novel role for metformin. Expert Rev Mol Diagn 10(4):509–519
79. Thomson CA, Thompson PA, Wright-Bea J et al (2009) Metabolic syndrome and elevated C-reactive protein in breast cancer survivors on adjuvant hormone therapy. J Womens Health (Larchmt) 18(12):2041–2047
80. Redig AJ, Munshi HG (2010) Care of the cancer survivor: metabolic syndrome after hormone-modifying therapy. Am J Med 123(1):87.e1–6
81. Gonzalez-Angulo AM, Meric-Bernstam F (2010) Metformin: a therapeutic opportunity in breast cancer. Clin Cancer Res 16(6):1695–1700

Part II
The Research in Uruguay

Chapter 10
General Features and Methodology

The history of epidemiologic research on the role of nutritional elements and BC in Uruguay is brief and its beginning was two decades ago [1]. During the years 1994–2010 the authors have produced more than 50 scientific works on the area [2–52]. A high fraction of them were case-control type studies, lately not only carried out following conventional analysis but also factor analysis in search of nutritional patterns [26, 36, 43, 51, 52]. They were mostly performed in population admitted to public hospitals (who belong to low socio-economic strata) coming from the whole country but we also analyzed a population sample belonging to the private healthcare system (mid-to-high socio-economic strata) in the capital city, Montevideo, in order to cover different risk populations. Our studies have given to the medical literature their usually original contributions, whose publication in specialized scientific journals and presentations in congresses have allowed an adequate international dissemination of their results, also cited nowadays in Internet. Of special interest for us were also the papers referred to selection of risk population using dietary information [11–13, 16–19], and more recently those reporting the results of anthropometric [24, 25, 29, 30, 33, 34, 44, 45] and other epidemiologic research [35], including a review [47]. Finally, some recent multisite analyses have brought additional information on specific items related to BC [36–42]. The most relevant features of our work are herewith summarized.

Methodology

The research was carried out based on population subsets belonging to one of the existing healthcare systems. Cases were women with certified BC with a recent diagnosis, residents in Uruguay for 10 or more years and of ages between 24 and 84 years old.

(a) The public system. Patients were admitted to the major hospitals in Montevideo: Instituto Nacional de Oncología, Hospital de Clínicas, Hospital Pasteur, Hospital Maciel and Hospital Pereira Rossell. Controls were patients not

A.L. Ronco and E. De Stéfani, *Nutritional Epidemiology of Breast Cancer*,
DOI 10.1007/978-94-007-2397-9_10, © Springer Science+Business Media B.V. 2012

afflicted with cancer, with nutritional, hormonal or gynecologic diseases. The most common diseases were: bone fractures, eye disturbances, abdominal hernia and traumas. The studies focusing on anthropometry involved control women having a recent normal mammogram (labeled as BI-RADS 1).

(b) The private system. Patients were affiliated to a medical institution (IMPASA) representative of the private healthcare system, all residents in Montevideo or neighbour locations. Of them, controls were women having a recent normal mammogram (labeled as BI-RADS 1).

Questionnaire

All patients were face-to-face interviewed with a structured questionnaire shortly after admittance to the hospitals. The questionnaire included sections on (i) socio-demographic variables (age, residence, urban/rural status and hospital), (ii) a complete history of tobacco smoking (age at start, age of quit, average number of cigarettes per day, type of tobacco and type of cigarette), (iii) a complete history of alcohol drinking (age at start, age of quit, number of glasses drunk per day and type of beverage), (iv) a section on occupational exposures based on job titles and its duration, (v) menstrual and reproductive variables (age at menarche, age at menopause, number of live births, age at first live birth, age at last live birth, breastfeeding, spontaneous abortions, induced abortions, use of exogenous hormones and use of contraceptive drugs), (vi) self reported height and weight 5 years before the interview, (vii) family history of cancer in first- and second-degree relatives and (viii) a food frequency questionnaire (FFQ) representative of the Uruguayan diet, including intake of soft drinks, coffee, tea, mate and vitamins supplementation. Studies at public hospitals involved a FFQ on 64 foods and at the private centre on 120 foods. Each FFQ asked about food consumption 5 years prior to diagnosis in cases and prior to the interview in controls, taking into account that within a period of few years diet may be recalled with acceptable levels of misclassification. The FFQ was not validated, but was tested for reproducibility with reasonably good results [26]. The questionnaire of 120 items was a modification of the previous one, having added some details concerning selected items not only of nutritional interest but also of epidemiologic interest. Furthermore, it allowed the estimation of total energy intake of each subject. For each one of the dietary items, a serving size was estimated, based on the tables of nutrients we consulted. All dietary questions of our semi-quantitative questionnaire were open-ended, in order to manage each food as a continuous variable. They were converted into servings/year, multiplying by the most adequate time units each answer deserved. We have considered this type of registration of information as the best expression of the true intake, instead of forcing answers within pre-existing categories. In order to calculate daily nutrients or energy, we compiled an analysis program which made the sum of all individual values, each one obtained after multiplying the number of servings/year by the ratio nutrient content or calories of the serving/100 g of each individual food, divided by 365 days. Most typical or average servings of solid foods are within the range of 100–150 g, and fluid foods are included in a cup of 200 ml.

Statistical Analysis

The distribution of all study subjects was categorized into tertils, quartils or quintils (depending on the circumstances) for each food, food group or nutrient. Crude and adjusted Relative risks (RR) were estimated through the application of unconditional logistic regression [53]. Potential confounding factors were included in the multivariate models. They were usually: age, residence, education level, family history of BC, body mass index. In each study, other variables which could be correlated with the interest variables were also entered in the regression models. The trend after adjustment by covariates was determined by chi2 test. The 95% confidence intervals for every RR were calculated. Most calculations were performed with the STATA software [54].

Results

The Uruguayan studies which were carried out on diet and BC have reported information about meats and their preparation, heterocyclic amines, fatty foods, vegetables, fruits, fibre, types of fats, phytoestrogens, macronutrients, selected bioactive substances, dietary patterns and their relationship with this type of cancer. Regarding the other arm of nutrition, that is, anthropometry, our studies focused their interest on two particular aspects: fat and muscle fractions and body shape. For these studies we have applied original techniques as body composition and somatotype. In the following chapters the most relevants points of each research study are presented.

References

1. Fierro L, De Stéfani E, Larrinaga MT et al (1992) Tabaco, alcohol y riesgo de cáncer de mama en Uruguay. Arch Med Int Urug XIV:81–90
2. Ronco AL, Carámbula JA (1994) Tiempo perdido en el cáncer de mama. Arch Med Int Urug (N° especial) 14
3. Ronco AL, De Stéfani E (1994) Dieta y Cáncer de Mama. Arch Med Int Urug (N° especial) 14
4. Ronco AL, Mendilaharsu M, De Stéfani E. (1995) Meat, fat and risk of breast cancer. In: Proceedings of the 1995 annual meeting of the international association of cancer registries, Rio de Janeiro, 30 Oct –1 Nov, p 5
5. Ronco AL, Cornélissen G, Halberg F et al (1995) About-half-yearly pattern in the incidence of hormone-related cancers in Uruguay. Abstract N° 314, Anticancer Res 15(5A): 1753

6. Ronco AL, De Stéfani E, Deneo-Pellegrini H et al. (1996) Factores dietarios de riesgo para cáncer de mama en Uruguay: un estudio caso-control. Arch Med Int (N° especial), p 44
7. Ronco AL, De Stéfani E, Mendilaharsu M et al (1996) Meat, fat and the risk of breast cancer: a case-control study from Uruguay. Int J Cancer 65:328–331
8. De Stéfani E, Correa P, Ronco A et al (1997) Dietary fiber and risk of breast cancer. Nutr Cancer 28:14–19
9. De Stéfani E, Ronco AL, Mendilaharsu M et al (1997) Meat intake, heterocyclic amines, and risk of breast cancer: a case-control study in Uruguay. Cancer Epidemiol Biomarkers Prev 6:573–581
10. De Stéfani E, Deneo-Pellegrini H, Mendilaharsu M et al (1998) Essential fatty acids and breast cancer: a case-control study in Uruguay. Int J Cancer 76:491–494
11. Ronco AL, Carámbula JA (1998) The breast cancer risk score: in search of high-risk premenopausal women for screening. Breast J 4(Suppl 1):S17
12. Ronco AL (1998) Evaluation of classificatory capabilities of an artificial neural network in search of breast cancer risk populations: a pilot study. Breast J 4(Suppl 1):S22
13. Ronco AL, Carámbula JA (1998) Classificatory improvement of a breast clinical screening programme by application of an artificial neural network: a pilot study. Breast J 4(Suppl 1):S21
14. Ronco AL, De Stéfani E, Boffetta P et al (1999) Vegetables, fruits, and related nutrients and risk of breast cancer: a case control study in Uruguay. Nutr Cancer 35(2):111–119
15. Ronco AL, De Stéfani E (1999) Fitoestrógenos y riesgo de cáncer mamario: un estudio caso control. Rev Med Urug 15:94–102
16. Ronco AL (1999) Use of artificial neural networks in modeling associations of discriminant factors: towards an intelligent selective breast cancer screening. Artif Intell Med 16(3):299–309
17. Ronco AL (1999) Artificial intelligence-based screening for breast cancer: a pilot project. In: Proceedings of the I conference on screening and early detection of cancer, development of a European strategy, Vienna, 18–19 Nov, 1999. Abstract 9001, p 37
18. Ronco AL (1999) Discriminating breast cancer high-risk individuals with artificial neural networks: a novel approach to selective screenings. In: Proceedings of the I conference on screening and early detection of cancer, development of a European strategy, Vienna, 18–19 Nov 1999. Abstract 9030, p 51
19. Ronco AL, De Stéfani E (1999) Role of classical and dietary discriminant factors for classification of breast cancer high-risk populations: a study with neural networks. Cancer Strateg 1:203–209
20. Ronco AL, De Stéfani E, Dáttoli R (2002) Dairy foods and risk of breast cancer: a case-control study in Montevideo, Uruguay. Eur J Cancer Prev 11(5):457–463
21. Ronco AL, De Stéfani E, Fabra A (2003) White meat intake and the risk of breast cancer: a case-control study in Montevideo, Uruguay. Nutr Res 23(2):151–162
22. Ronco AL, De Stefani E, Deneo-Pellegrini H et al (2005) Consumo de frutas y riesgo de cáncer de mama: un estudio caso-control. Rev Bras Nutr Clin 20(Suppl 1):S1–SS8, p 13
23. Ronco A, De Stéfani E, Deneo-Pellegrini H (2005) Consumo de grasas poliinsaturadas y riesgo de cáncer de mama: un estudio caso-control. Rev Bras Nutr Clin 20(Suppl 1):S1–SS8, p 12
24. Ronco AL, Varas X, Leborgne F et al (2005) Composición corporal y Cáncer de mama: el rol del status menopáusico. XIII Congreso Latinoamericano de Mastología, Santiago de Chile, 16–19 Nov 2005
25. Ronco AL, Varas X, Jaumandreu S et al (2005) Somatotipo y Cáncer de mama en premenopáusicas: un estudio piloto. XIII Congreso Latinoamericano de Mastología, Santiago de Chile, 16–19 Nov 2005
26. Ronco AL, De Stefani E, Boffetta P et al (2006) Food patterns and risk of breast cancer: A factor analysis study in Uruguay. Int J Cancer 19(1):1672–1678
27. Ronco A, De Stéfani E, Deneo-Pellegrini H (2006) Polyunsaturated fatty acids intake and risk of breast cancer: a case-control study. XIV world congress on breast diseases, Zagreb, 18–21 May 2006

28. Ronco AL, De Stefani E, Deneo-Pellegrini H (2006) Fruit consumption and risk of breast cancer: a case-control study. In: Flaps P (ed) New developments in nutrition research. Nova Science Publishers, New York
29. Ronco AL, Varas X, Febles G et al (2006) Body composition and breast cancer: the role of menopausal status. XIV world congress on breast diseases, Zagreb, 18–21 May 2006
30. Ronco AL, Varas X, De Stéfani E et al (2006) Somatotype and breast cancer in premenopausal women: a pilot study. XIV world congress on breast diseases, Zagreb, 18–21 May 2006
31. Ronco AL, De Stéfani E, Deneo-Pellegrini H (2008) Fruit intake and risk of breast cancer: a case-control study. In: Fortugno LP (ed) Frontiers in breast cancer research. Nova Science Publishers, New York, pp 175–186
32. Ronco AL, De Stéfani E, Deneo-Pellegrini H et al (2008) Epidemiología Nutricional del Cáncer de Mama. Ediciones de la Plaza, Montevideo
33. Ronco AL, Mendoza B, Varas X et al (2008) Somatotype and risk of breast cancer: a case-control study in Uruguay. Braz J Epidemiol 11(2):215–227
34. Ronco AL, Boeing H, De Stéfani E et al (2009) A case-control study on fat to muscle ratio and risk of breast cancer. Nutr Cancer 61(4):466–474
35. Ronco AL, Stoll M, De Stéfani E et al (2009) Rh factor, family history and risk of breast cancer: a case-control study in Uruguay. Cancer Detect Prev 32:277–285
36. De Stéfani E, Deneo-Pellegrini H, Boffetta P et al (2009) Dietary patterns and risk of cancer: a factor analysis in Uruguay. Int J Cancer 124(6):1391–1397
37. Aune D, De Stéfani E, Ronco AL et al (2009) Meat consumption and the risk of cancer: a case-control study in Uruguay. Cancer Ther 7:174–187
38. Aune D, De Stéfani E, Ronco AL et al (2009) Legume intake and the risk of cancer: a multisite case–control study in Uruguay. Cancer Causes Control 20(9):1605–1615
39. Aune D, De Stéfani E, Ronco AL et al (2009) Fruits, vegetables and the risk of cancer: a multisite case-control study in Uruguay. Asian Pac J Cancer Prev 20:419–428
40. Aune D, De Stéfani E, Ronco AL et al (2009) Egg consumption and the risk of cancer: a multisite case-control study in Uruguay. Asian Pac J Cancer Prev 10(5):869–876
41. De Stéfani E, Aune D, Boffetta P et al (2009) Salted meat consumption and the risk of cancer: a multisite case-control study in Uruguay. Asian Pac J Cancer Prev 10(5):853–857
42. Aune D, Deneo-Pellegrini H, Ronco AL et al (2011) Dietary folate intake and the risk of 11 types of cancer: a case–control study in Uruguay. Ann Oncol 22(2):444–451
43. Ronco AL, De Stéfani E, Aune D et al (2010) Nutrient patterns and risk of breast cancer in Uruguay. Asian Pac J Cancer Prev 11(2):519–524
44. Ronco AL, Quarneti A, Febles G et al (2010) Anthropometric variables as risk classificators of breast cancer: comparing neural networks and logistic regressions. In: Proceedings of the XVI world congress of the senologic international society. Valencia, 20–22 Oct 2010
45. Ronco AL, De Stéfani E (2010) Interrelationships between body composition and somatotype and the risk of breast cancer. In: Proceedings of the XVI world congress of the senologic international society. Valencia, 20–22 Oct 2010
46. Ronco AL, Maisonneuve J, Stoll M et al (2010) The Breast Cancer Risk Profile Report: development of a personalized preventive tool. In: Proceedings of the XVI world congress of the senologic international society. Valencia, 20–22 Oct 2010.
47. Ronco AL, De Stéfani E, Stoll M (2010) Hormonal and metabolic modulation through nutrition: towards a primary prevention of breast cancer. Breast 19:322–332
48. Ronco AL, Gibbons J, Caserta B et al (2010) Anthropometry, hormonal receptors and Her-2-neu gene expressions among Uruguayan women. In: Proceedings of the XVI world congress of the senologic international society. Valencia, 20–22 Oct 2010
49. Ronco AL, Stoll M, Maisonneuve J et al (2010) Rhesus factor and family breast cancer: a case-control study in Uruguay. In: Proceedings of the XVI world congress of the senologic international society. Valencia, 20–22 Oct 2010
50. Ronco AL, De Stéfani E (2010) Diabetes, overweight and risk of breast cancer: a case-control study in Uruguay. In: Proceedings of the XVI world congress of the senologic international society, Valencia, 20–22 Oct 2010

51. Ronco AL, De Stéfani E, Aune D et al (2010) Nutrient patterns and risk of breast cancer: a case-control-study in Uruguay. In: Proceedings of the XVI world congress of the senologic international society, Valencia, 20–22 Oct 2010
52. Ronco AL, De Stéfani E, Deneo-Pellegrini H et al (2010) Dietary patterns and risk of ductal carcinoma of the breast: a factor analysis in Uruguay. Asian Pac J Cancer Prev 11(5):1187–1193
53. Breslow NE, Day NE (1980) Statistical methods in cancer research. Vol. 1. The analysis of case-control studies, IARC ScientificPublication 32. IARC, Lyon
54. STATA (2007) Stata User's Guide and Reference Manual. Release 10. Stata Press, College Station

Chapter 11
The Role of Foods

Meats

Some international studies which were already quoted (Chapter on *Foods and Breast Cancer*) had shown inconsistent increases in the risk associated with the intake of fats. Besides, the intake of meats – considered as a marker of the fats intake – has been associated with an increased risk of BC. Years ago it was suggested that heterocyclic amines derived from the cooking process of meats played a role as a potential carcinogen through the character of cancer initiator. The identification of a possible independent effect of meat was something of considerable practical importance, indeed.

The main results of our initial study on meats, fats and BC [1] are shown in Table 11.1. Both, total meat and red meat were associated with a monotonic increase in the risks, having significant dose-response patterns. The ORs for total meat were 3.34 and for red meat 4.16. White meat (poultry and fish together) showed an inverse association with a 40% reduction in the risk of BC. No associations were observed with processed meats. The effects of total meat and red meat remained unchanged after the adjustment by fat intake.

In Table 11.2 are also shown the ORs for meats according to cooking methods. A strong positive association between fried meat (milanesa, panned) and BC risk was observed in this study (OR for the highest quartile = 5.31, significant) after adjusting by potential confounding factors. A significantly increased risk was observed for barbecued and grilled meat, however no effect was detected for boiled meat.

Table 11.3 shows the results of the analysis performed in a further study [2], where the effects were discriminated taking into account the menopausal status of interviewed patients. The Ors for total meat, red meat and white meat were significant in all women and in postmenopausal ones. In the same way, a risk increase in high consumers of beef and lamb as well a risk decrease in high intake of fish were significant among postmenopausal women. This suggested a possible accumulative effect, in which duration in addition to intensity of intake could be playing an important role, given the higher mean age of postmenopausal women compared to premenopausal ones.

A.L. Ronco and E. De Stéfani, *Nutritional Epidemiology of Breast Cancer*,
DOI 10.1007/978-94-007-2397-9_11,

Table 11.1 Relative risks of BC for meat consumption

	Quartiles of consumption				
Dietary item	I	II	III	IV	p-value for trend
Total meat	1.0	1.12	1.42	3.34*	0.001
Red meat	1.0	1.29	2.03*	4.16*	0.001
White meat	1.0	0.61	0.58*	0.60	0.07
Processed meat	1.0	0.75	0.70	1.24	0.59

Adjusted by family history of BC, BMI, parity, age at menarche, menopausal status and total energy intake
* = statistically significant

Table 11.2 Relative risks of BC for cooking methods of meats

	Quartiles of consumption				
Dietary item	I	II	III	IV	p-value for trend
Fried meat	1.0	1.49	1.53	5.31*	<0.001
Barbecued/grilled meat	1.0	1.10	1.05	2.21*	0.02
Boiled meat	1.0	1.08	0.99	1.02	0.92

Adjusted by family history of BC, BMI, parity, age at menarche, menopausal status and total energy intake
* = statistically significant

Vegetables and Fruits

We have already seen in the respective chapter related to international literature that diets rich in vegetables and fruits probably reduce the risk of BC [3, 4]. Foods belonging to these groups are a rich source of nutrients, bioactive substances and non-nutritional substances which are probably anticarcinogens [5, 6], among which carotenoids, vitamin C, vitamin E and flavonoids were found as associated with a risk reduction for several types of cancer.

We have extracted the following results from one of the research papers related to diet and BC which were published by us [7]. Table 11.4 shows the ORs of vegetables and fruits for BC. The intake of total vegetables was inversely associated with the risk of BC (RR = 0.41, IC al 95% 0.26–0.65), while the intake of total fruits displayed a RR = 0.57 (IC 0.36–0.89). Total vegetables and fruits combined showed a significant protective effect of 58%.

Raw and green-leaf vegetables were strongly protective (RR = 0.36 for the latter) and also cooked vegetables displayed a negative association (RR = 0.58). Finally, whereas legumes were also negatively associated with the risk of BC, cruciferous vegetables did not show an association. Results are expressed in the following graphic (Fig. 11.1).

Table 11.3 Relative risks of BC associated with meat variables and according to menopausal status

	Quartiles of consumption					
Dietary item	Menopausal status	I	II	III	IV	p-value for trend
Total meat	All	1.0	1.29	1.63	2.26*	0.006
	Pre	1.0	0.90	1.27	2.42	0.11
	Post	1.0	1.33	1.58	2.19*	0.03
Red meat	All	1.0	1.25	1.76	2.62*	0.001
	Pre	1.0	1.41	2.13	3.01	0.09
	Post	1.0	1.29	1.57	2.79*	0.006
White meat	All	1.0	0.67	0.60*	0.59*	0.02
	Pre	1.0	0.62	1.36	0.28	0.31
	Post	1.0	0.60	0.48*	0.63*	0.03
Processed meat	All	1.0	0.80	0.85	0.88	0.64
	Pre	1.0	0.66	0.48	1.30	0.56
	Post	1.0	0.80	0.91	0.73	0.38
Beef	All	1.0	1.23	2.09*	3.84*	<0.001
	Pre	1.0	1.91	2.41	2.60	0.16
	Post	1.0	1.15	2.02*	4.75*	<0.001
Lamb	All	1.0	1.05	2.38*		0.01
	Pre	1.0	1.32	1.45		0.53
	Post	1.0	0.88	2.90*		0.02
Poultry	All	1.0	0.75	0.78		0.18
	Pre	1.0	0.62	0.32		0.06
	Post	1.0	0.73	0.85		0.35
Fish	All	1.0	0.76	0.64		0.06
	Pre	1.0	1.97	0.54		0.65
	Post	1.0	0.62*	0.63		0.04

Adjusted by age, residence, family history of BC in first degree relatives, parity, age at menarche, prior history of benign breast diseases, total calories, vegetables intake and fat intake. Lamb, poultry and fish were analyzed by tertiles
* = statistically significant

Table 11.4 Relative risks of breast cancer for vegetables and fruits intake

	Quartiles of consumption				
Dietary item	I	II	III	IV	p-value (trend)
Total vegetables	1.0	0.52	0.45	0.41	0.004
Total fruits	1.0	1.01	0.86	0.57	0.05
Vegetables & fruits	1.0	0.61	0.46	0.42	0.005
Raw vegetables	1.0	0.64	0.58	0.51	<0.001
Cooked vegetables	1.0	1.02	0.67	0.58	0.009
Green-leaf vegetables	1.0	0.56	0.53	0.36	<0.001
Legumes	1.0	0.84	0.91	0.42	0.004
Cruciferous vegetables	1.0	2.16	1.07		0.12

Adjusted by age, residence, urban/rural status, family history of BC in 1° relatives, body mass index, age at menarche, parity, menopausal status and total calories consumption

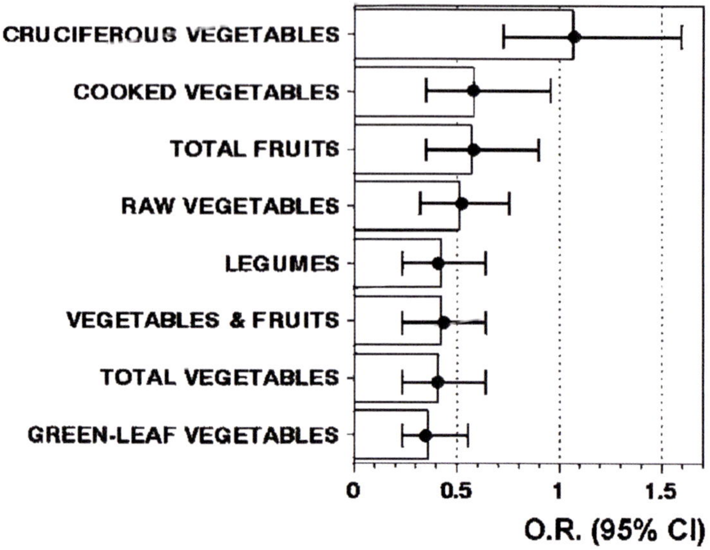

Fig. 11.1 Relative risks of breast cancer for vegetables and fruits intake

Besides, tomatoes and tomato-derived foods were found as protective. Raw tomatoes were associated with a moderate and not significant risk reduction (RR = 0.62, IC 0.36–1.06), foods dressed with tomato sauce displayed a strong protective and significant effect (RR = 0.30, IC 0.17–0.52).

Since lycopene has been one of the most protective nutrients and it would explain partially the effect of total vegetables, and also considering that this carotenoid is the one prevailing in tomatoes, we examined the risk associated with tomatoes and tomato-rich foods (pasta and polenta, which are commonly accompanied by tomato sauce), and the results are shown in Table 11.5. The protective effect observed for lycopene remained after adjusting by total vegetables and other antioxidants. In Uruguay, the richest sources of lycopene are tomatoes and tomato products like sauce. Besides, it has been reported that lycopene is better absorbed from oil-cooked tomato products than from raw tomatoes [8].

Dairy Foods

Our study [9] analyzed the following dairy products: whole milk, skimmed milk, chocolate milk, whole milk, ricotta cheese, mozzarella cheese, quartirolo cheese, Parmesan cheese, gruyere cheese, total cheese, whole yoghurt, skimmed yoghurt, total yoghurt, total liquid dairy (total milk + total yoghurt), butter, chantilly cream, ice cream and total dairy. The intake of milk and butter at age 18 was also queried.

Table 11.5 Relative risks of breast cancer for tomatoes and tomato-rich foods intake

Dietary item	RR	(95% IC)	
Tomatoes (servings/week)			
<=0.5	1.0		
0.6–1.5	0.58*	0.40–0.86	
1.6–2.5	0.68	0.45–1.02	
>=2.6	0.62	0.36–1.06	p for trend 0.33
Foods with tomato sauce (servings/week)			
<=1.5	1.0		
1.6–2.1	0.70	0.46–1.09	
2.2–3.0	0.59*	0.39–0.88	
>=3.1	0.30*	0.17–0.52	p for trend <0.001
All foods with Tomato (servings/week)			
<=2.0	1.0		
2.1–3.6	0.72	0.47–1.12	
3.7–5.5	0.44*	0.28–0.68	
>=5.6	0.34*	0.21–0.53	p for trend <0.001

Adjusted by age, residence, urban/rural status, family history of BC in 1° relatives, body mass index, age at menarche, parity, menopausal status and total calories consumption
* = statistically significant

Food groups and dietary items were adjusted by total energy intake using the residual method [10]. The regression model adjusted by age, years of urban status, educational level, body mass index, age at menarche, menopausal status, family history of BC, number of live births, total energy and total fruits.

The ORs of BC for dairy products are shown in Table 11.6. Several items displayed an association with increased risk of BC: milk (OR = 2.84), chocolate milk (OR = 2.85), total milk (OR = 1.99), quartirolo cheese (OR = 1.66), gruyere cheese (OR = 1.93) and ice cream (OR = 1.98). Of them, only quartirolo cheese was not significantly associated in the highest tertile. Furthermore, most products displayed a risk increase with dose-response pattern except for chocolate milk. In addition, an inverse and significant association is shown with the skimmed yoghurt intake (OR = 0.29), total yoghurt (OR = 0.41) and ricotta cheese (OR = 0.45), also having a dose-response pattern. Other items showed an absence of association for the highest tertiles of consumption. Besides, both intakes at the age of 18 displayed similar results that in adult age: whereas the milk intake was positively associated with the risk of BC (OR = 2.66, p for trend = 0.002), the butter intake did not show association (OR = 0.49, p for trend = 0.18), even tending to an apparently protective direction. The items having significant associations are shown in Fig. 11.2, in descendent order.

Our results support the existence of opposite associations of different dairy products and the risk of BC. On one hand, high intakes certain products recognized as low-fat such as skimmed yoghurt and ricotta cheese were inversely associated with the risk

Table 11.6 Relative risks of breast cancer for intake of dairy products

Variable	Tertils I	II	III	p-value for trend
Whole milk	**1.0**	**2.47***	**2.84***	0.007
Skimmed milk	1.0	0.63	0.89	0.72
Chocolate milk	1.0	**3.22***	**2.85***	0.06
Total milk	1.0	1.41	**1.99***	0.04
Whole yoghurt	1.0	1.41	1.03	0.97
Skimmed yoghurt	1.0	1.00	**0.29***	<0.001
Total yoghurt	1.0	0.73	**0.41***	0.008
Total milk + yoghurt	1.0	1.22	0.87	0.68
Ricotta cheese	1.0	0.60	**0.45***	0.01
Mozzarella cheese	1.0	0.63	1.12	0.71
Quartirolo cheese	1.0	**1.96***	1.66	0.15
Parmesan cheese	1.0	1.36	1.17	0.63
Gruyere cheese	1.0	1.40	**1.93***	0.03
Total cheese	1.0	0.61	0.83	0.53
Butter	1.0	0.92	0.92	0.80
Ice cream	1.0	1.02	**1.98***	0.02
Chantilly cream	1.0	0.80	1.18	0.68
Total dairy	1.0	1.08	1.16	0.65
Milk at age 18	1.0	1.26	**2.66***	0.002
Butter at age 18	1.0	1.29	0.49	0.18

Adjusted by: age, years of urban status, education, age at menarche, family history of BC, number of live births, BMI, menopausal status, total energy and total fruits. In bold, the statistically significant risks

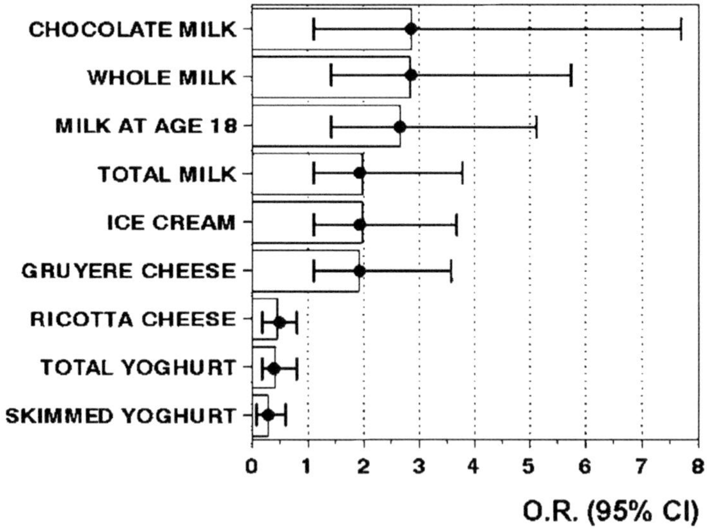

Fig. 11.2 Dairy foods with statistical significant relative risks

of BC. On the other hand, high intake of fatty products such as whole milk, chocolate milk, gruyere cheese and ice cream were clearly associated with the risk of BC. Nevertheless, we found that other fat-rich products as butter and Chantilly cream did not show a risk association (OR = 0.92 and OR = 1.18 respectively). Some total items as milk + yoghurt (OR = 0.87), cheese (OR = 0.83) and dairy (OR = 1.16) showed neither any association: this fact suggested us that perhaps when some studies analyzed items as "milk", "cheese" and "yoghurt", possible hidden differences coming from their varieties could have led results to null. In addition, we must recognize that certain particular preferences among individuals or populations could lead to findings oriented towards opposite directions.

We have found no association for skimmed milk and a positive association for whole and chocolate milk, as well as for total milk. In addition, the analysis of cheese revealed opposite associations with the risk of BC for high intakes of those varieties located at the extreme of the range: whereas the cheese having the lowest fat content (ricotta) tended to show a significant inverse association (OR = 0.45), the one with the highest fat content (gruyere) displayed a significant positive association (OR = 1.93). Besides, yoghurt tended to be protective, both the skimmed one (OR = 0.29) as well as the total one (OR = 0.41). Our results agreed to those obtained in a study performed in Dutch women [11], where a negative association (OR = 0.33) was reported for the combination of low fat intake + high intake of fermented milk and fibre, which was the best performance among 6 types of assessed combinations.

Regarding the analysis of possible mechanisms which could explain the results, we accept that fat content can be related with some risks (inverse association of skimmed yoghurt and ricotta cheese, positive association of whole and chocolate milk, gruyere cheese and ice cream), but there were non significant differences related to the intake of butter and chantilly cream, which have the highest fat levels. We could cautiously accept that fat level plays some role, but it would not be determinant by itself only.

Moreover, the levels of protective substances like vitamin D and conjugated linoleic acid (CLA) depend on the actual fat level. In this sense, the liquid skimmed products (milk and yoghurt) lack of adequate levels of vitamin D, at least. Fortified products were not introduced in the Uruguayan market until the late 90's, hence, it can not be considered as likely an exposure of partially skimmed milk plus extra vitamin D and/or calcium.

Other components deserve to be taken into account, for example carbohydrates like lactose and galactose (linked to ovarian cancer [12]) and proteins such as IGF-I (Insulin simil growth factor I), which seem to increase the risk of BC [13, 14]. Both combined, lactose inducing a sustained insulin response and IGF-I reproducing the action of the latter, derive in the upstream of immune and metabolic steps which are linked to pro-inflammatory events. These facts are described and commented in chapter on Insulin resistance and BC.

Comments on fermented products usually refer to yoghurts, but some cheeses require also fermentation in their production process, based on whey. It is interesting to remark that whey proteins have a considerable amount of three amino-acids that are common to one of the most powerful antioxidant and anticarcinogenic substances found in foods: glutathione. Whey protein is also the richest known source of naturally occurring branched chain amino acids (leucine, isoleucine and valine) and also of glutamic acid and cysteine. These amino acids are also present in the human maternal milk. The fermentation process, besides, guarantees at the same time a strong reduction of the lactose levels, something that could contribute with a protection against the development of a metabolic syndrome.

The observed negative association of ricotta cheese as well as of skimmed yoghurt with the risk of BC enabled us to think that perhaps both conditions (fermentation and skim) and not only one of them – whichever it were – could be necessary to provide a risk reduction. In fact, whole yoghurt (which is not low-fat) showed no association; skimmed milk (which is not fermented) did not showed any association either; other cheese types that are not low-fat showed lack of association or a positive association. Finally, whole milk, chocolate milk, ice cream, chantilly cream or butter are neither low-fat nor fermented products and they tended to have no association or to be positively associated. These facts suggest that beneficial effects of vitamin D and CLA can be overwhelmed in both senses: on one hand, skim and fermentation seemed to have better protective effect if both were present even though the levels of vitamin D and CLA were reduced; on the other hand, high fat levels and no fermentation seemed to have a higher risk if they were present, even though vitamin D and CLA were increased.

There is a potential protective effect of bacteria found in fermented milk on the health risks that aromatic heterocyclic amines (HCAs) involve. A study suggested that the detoxifying mechanism would be through a direct binding of HCAs to the cell walls of certain bacterial strands present in fermented foods [15]. Besides, we have reported in our studies [1, 2] evidence of links between BC and the intake of HCAs, mostly derived from cooking methods of red meats. Therefore, a protective effect of yoghurt and ricotta cheese could be expected to occur in the Uruguayan population, which has the highest beef intake in the world [16]. In addition, a beneficial effect on cholesterol metabolism was also suggested by other studies [17, 18] and the potential protection expected from prebiotics and probiotics due to their contribution in lactobacillus and phytosterols deserves to be taken into account [19].

Bioavailability of calcium and other minerals as magnesium and zinc is enhanced by fermented dairy foods [20–22]. Taking into account that: (a) diets with high saturated fat contents could produce deleterious effects in the absorption of dietary calcium [23]; and (b) this latter implies a protective action against BC and other tumour sites such as colon [24–26], it seems logic to think that both features (low-fat and fermentation) are required to optimize calcium bioavailability.

The concentration of folate-bounded proteins in different dairy products is closely related to the folate absorption [27, 28] and it can play a role in its bioavailability, not only for the own folates of dairy foods but also for those present in foods of vegetable sources, which have been shown as powerful protective factors against BC [29, 30].

White Meat

In 2003 another paper whose results came from population affiliated to the private healthcare system was published [31] and it analyzed possible associations of white meat consumption and the risk of BC. As it has been mentioned in the corresponding chapter, the general trend of the analyses on white meat consumption has been to consider it not associated with BC as well as a slight reduction of risk of the disease.

In this work we queried about the intake of: skinless chicken, chicken with skin, fried fish, not fried fish. As a consequence, new variables emerged after their combination: total chicken (skinless chicken + chicken with skin), total fish (fried fish + not fried fish), lean white meat (skinless chicken + not fried fish), fatty white meat (chicken with skin + fried fish), and total white meat (sum of the four original variables). Other food groups were created to be assessed: total vegetables, total fruits, red meat, total dairy, total oil, grains, desserts.

Table 11.7 presents the results of the analyses, following a similar methodology to the one applied for the study of dairy foods. Crude and adjusted odds ratios are presented.

(a) Logistic regression model adjusted by: years of urban status, age at first birth, age at menarche, number of live births, months of breastfeeding, body mass index, family history of BC, total dietary energy, total vegetables and fruits, total dairy, total oil and oil reutilization.

A significant increase of risk for high intake of fried fish was observed (OR = 1.99). On the other hand, the intake of not fried fish had a significant inverse association with the risk of BC (OR = 0.48), the same as with skinless skin intake (OR = 0.42) and both items combined (OR = 0.34). Total white meat showed a risk reduction of almost a half, borderly significant (OR = 0.55). Besides, the other fatty products displayed a trend towards the risk increase, although they did not reach a statistical significance probably due to the sample size: chicken with skin (OR = 1.54) and fatty white meat (OR = 1.62). The fact that both total consumptions of chicken and fish showed lack of association (OR = 0.78 and OR = 0.79 respectively) is not negligible. It remarks once again the problem faced by research focused on dietary items simply labelled as "chicken", "fish" or others: if each of them is composed by products which have opposite associations, these possible hidden differences could lead results to the null (Fig. 11.3).

The performed analyses could explain the still not very consistent findings on white meat consumption that the specialized literature cites [4]. Although these limitations are recognized based on previous studies, the intake of white meat has been recommended as a part of what is known as a "prudent" diet. Nevertheless, extreme caution should be present about this recommendation since chicken is the food belonging to the white meat group that has the highest concentration of heterocyclic amines among all meats. In addition, the feeding conditions for animals might represent another reason for the inconsistencies reported in the specialized literature. Currently, poultry are usually exposed to special methods in order to enhance their growing process and development, which include supplements of corn seeds and

Table 11.7 Crude and adjusted relative risks of breast cancer for white meat intake levels

Variable	Tertiles	Cases/ Controls n	p-value	OR Crude	(95% CI)	OR Adjusted	(95% CI)
Chicken with skin	Low	42/74		1.00	–	1.00	–
	Mid	21/74		0.50	(0.27–0.92)	1.07	(0.49–2.32)
	High	48/74	0.020	1.14	(0.68–1.93)	1.54	(0.86–2.77)
Skinless chicken	Low	53/74		1.00	–	1.00	–
	Mid	28/74		0.53	(0.30–1.52)	0.62	(0.34–1.15)
	High	30/74	0.038	0.57	(0.33–1.13)	0.42	(0.23–0.79)
Total chicken	Low	52/74		1.00	–	1.00	–
	Mid	30/74		0.58	(0.33–1.00)	0.85	(0.46–1.56)
	High	29/74	0.056	0.56	(0.32–0.97)	0.78	(0.42–1.47)
Fried fish	Low	35/74		1.00	–	1.00	–
	Mid	41/74		1.17	(0.67–2.04)	1.35	(0.72–2.54)
	High	35/74	0.81	1.00	(0.57–1.77)	1.99	(1.02–3.88)
Not fried fish	Low	44/74		1.00	–	1.00	–
	Mid	39/74		0.88	(0.52–1.52)	1.46	(0.76–2.79)
	High	28/74	0.29	0.64	(0.36–1.13)	0.48	(0.24–0.93)
Total Fish	Low	53/74		1.00	–	1.00	–
	Mid	17/74		0.32	(0.17–0.60)	0.52	(0.26–1.05)
	High	41/74	0.001	0.77	(0.46–1.30)	0.79	(0.44–1.42)
Lean white meat	Low	53/74		1.00	–	1.00	–
	Mid	31/74		0.58	(0.33–1.01)	0.61	(0.33–1.14)
	High	27/74	0.035	0.51	(0.29–0.90)	0.34	(0.18–0.65)
Fatty white meat	Low	29/74		1.00	–	1.00	–
	Mid	44/74		1.52	(0.86–2.68)	1.91	(1.02–3.58)
	High	38/74	0.35	1.31	(0.73–2.34)	1.62	(0.85–3.11)
Total white meat	Low	55/74		1.00	–	1.00	–
	Mid	30/74		0.55	(0.31–0.94)	0.59	(0.33–1.09)
	High	26/74	0.015	0.47	(0.27–0.83)	0.55	(0.29–1.02)

other products while they are confined to reduced spaces. Consequently, their flesh and fat accumulate high contents of Ω-6 PUFAs instead of the natural Ω-3 PUFAs that would derive from eating a variety of their animal and vegetable sources if they could grow free in farms. In conclusion, it has still not been defined whether diets high in poultry have any association with BC. Preparation forms, hence, could be related to the disease. We think that these facts deserve considerable attention because recommendations probably should be expanded to promote the consumption of these white meats, but after having preparation modalities which do not imply the intake of high levels of some fats or the production of HCAs during cooking.

Fruit Consumption

The results of this research were published in 2006 and in 2008 in different books [32, 33]. With similar criteria to our previous studies, the following items were analyzed looking for possible associations with the risk of BC: orange, orange juice,

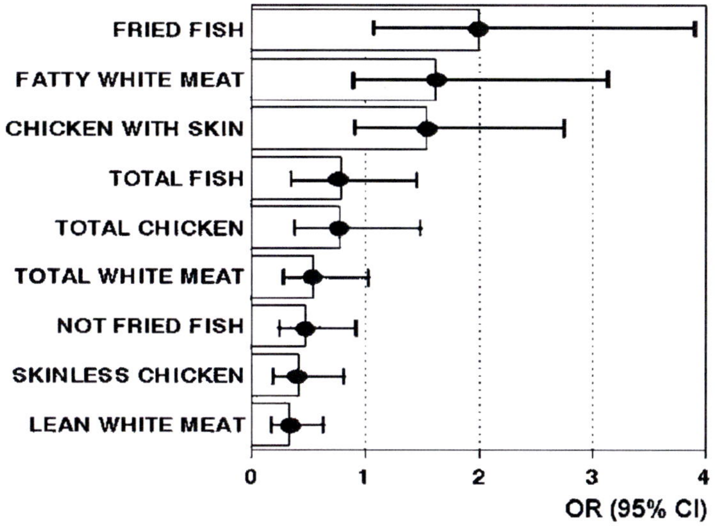

Fig. 11.3 Bar graphics derived from the original data of highest tertiles of intake for each dietary item, with their corresponding odds ratios and confidence intervals

tangerines, red apples, green apples, plums, watermelon, Moscatel grapes, common grapes, bananas, peaches, pears, fruit salad, citrus fruits, non citrus fruits, total fruits and dietary vitamin C. The regression model controlled for: age, age at menarche, menopausal status, menstruation duration, number of live births, dietary energy, family history of BC, smoking status, total vegetables, total meat, total dairy and exercise frequency. The main findings were a protective effect of total fruits, oranges, orange juice and citrus fruits. Besides, when the regression model included a term for vitamin C the negative association improved in all of them, in particular for orange and citrus fruits, suggesting a probable co-responsibility of other substances in the protection. The main results are shown in Table 11.8 and in Fig. 11.4, as follows:

It is interesting to remark the differences generated by citrus and non citrus fruits: only the latter displayed a protective effect (Fig. 11.5). The intake of green apples (Granny Smith type) was associated with a borderline risk reduction but with a significant trend (p=0.025), whereas red apples did not show an association with the risk of the disease (Fig. 11.6).

Although a high intake of both foods was associated with a risk reduction (with a dose-response trend), the reduction effect appeared to be stronger for orange juice. Anyway, after adjusting by vitamin C, each one of both foods reduced the risk around 77–78%, as it shows Table 11.9.

The protective effect of citrus fruits together (OR=0.27) and even more controlling for vitamin C (OR=0.13) was high. In nutritional epidemiology of cancer, a significant reduction of 87%, such as in the latter, is very strong and deserves to be remarked.

Table 11.8 Crude and adjusted relative risks for each analyzed variable

Variable	Tertiles	Intake*	Controls/ Cases n	p-value (trend)	Crude OR	Crude (95% CI)	Adjusted** OR	Adjusted** (95% CI)
Oranges	Low	0–52	73/46		1.00	–	1.00	–
	Mid	53–364	74/44		0.94	(0.56–1.59)	0.62	(0.33–1.16)
	High	>=365	75/21	0.012	0.44	(0.24–0.82)	**0.51**	(0.26–0.98)
Orange juice	Low	0–156	73/77		1.00	–	1.00	–
	Mid	157–364	74/18		0.23	(0.13–0.42)	0.16	(0.08–0.32)
	High	>=365	75/16	<0.0001	0.20	(0.11–0.38)	**0.26**	(0.13–0.54)
Tangerines	Low	0	73/28		1.00	–	1.00	–
	Mid	1–52	74/46		1.62	(0.92–2.87)	1.03	(0.54–1.99)
	High	>=53	75/37	0.439	1.28	(0.71–2.31)	1.20	(0.64–2.26)
Red apples	Low	0–104	73/39		1.00	–	1.00	–
	Mid	105–260	74/33		0.83	(0.47–1.47)	0.92	(0.49–1.73)
	High	>=261	75/39	0.925	0.97	(0.56–1.68)	1.31	(0.71–2.43)
Green apples	Low	0–104	73/52		1.00	–	1.00	–
	Mid	105–208	74/30		0.57	(0.33–0.99)	0.66	(0.36–1.21)
	High	>=209	75/29	0.025	0.54	(0.31–0.95)	0.55	(0.31–1.01)
Grapes –moscatel type	Low	0	73/23		1.00	–	1.00	–
	Mid	1–52	74/67		2.87	(1.62–5.10)	2.61	(1.37–4.98)
	High	>=53	75/21	0.760	0.89	(0.45–1.74)	0.96	(0.46–1.99)
Grapes –common type	Low	0	73/42		1.00	–	1.00	–
	Mid	1–12	74/21		0.49	(0.27–0.91)	0.93	(0.45–1.94)
	High	>=13	75/48	0.647	1.11	(0.66–1.88)	1.48	(0.82–2.65)
Bananas	Low	0–104	73/45		1.00	–	1.00	–
	Mid	105–156	75/19		0.41	(0.22–0.77)	0.44	(0.23–0.87)
	High	>=157	74/47	0.891	1.03	(0.61–1.74)	1.14	(0.64–2.03)
Plums	Low	0–12	74/50		1.00	–	1.00	–
	Mid	13–24	74/21		0.42	(0.23–0.77)	0.59	(0.30–1.15)
	High	>=25	74/40	0.360	0.80	(0.47–1.35)	0.62	(0.34–1.11)
Peaches	Low	0–24	73/30		1.00	–	1.00	–
	Mid	25–48	75/38		1.23	(0.69–2.19)	1.56	(0.82–2.96)
	High	>=49	74/43	0.233	1.41	(0.80–2.49)	1.29	(0.68–2.43)
Watermelon	Low	0	73/47		1.00	–	1.00	–
	Mid	1–12	74/24		0.50	(0.28–0.91)	0.98	(0.48–2.00)
	High	>=13	75/40	0.461	0.83	(0.49–1.41)	0.79	(0.45–1.40)
Pears	Low	0–5	73/29		1.00	–	1.00	–
	Mid	6–24	74/31		1.05	(0.58–1.92)	0.65	(0.33–1.27)
	High	>=25	75/51	0.049	1.71	(0.98–2.99)	1.35	(0.72–2.54)
Fruit salad	Low	0	73/34		1.00	–	1.00	–
	Mid	1–24	74/49		1.42	(0.83–2.45)	0.99	(0.54–1.82)
	High	>=25	75/28	0.495	0.80	(0.44–1.45)	0.86	(0.45–1.64)
Citrus fruits	Low	0–348	73/71		1.00	–	1.00	–
	Mid	349–663	74/25		0.35	(0.20–0.61)	**0.32**	(0.18–0.60)
	High	>=664	75/15	0.0001	0.21	(0.11–0.39)	**0.27**	(0.13–0.55)
Non citrus fruits	Low	0–554	74/33		1.00	–	1.00	–
	Mid	555–867	73/35		1.08	(0.60–1.91)	0.99	(0.53–1.87)
	High	>=868	75/43	0.371	1.29	(0.74–2.24)	1.07	(0.58–1.97)
Total fruits	Low	<=1019	74/46		1.00	–	1.00	–
	Mid	1020–1436	73/40		0.88	(0.52–1.50)	0.86	(0.48–1.55)
	High	>=1437	75/25	0.040	0.54	(0.30–0.96)	**0.44**	(0.23–0.86)

* = Times or units/year

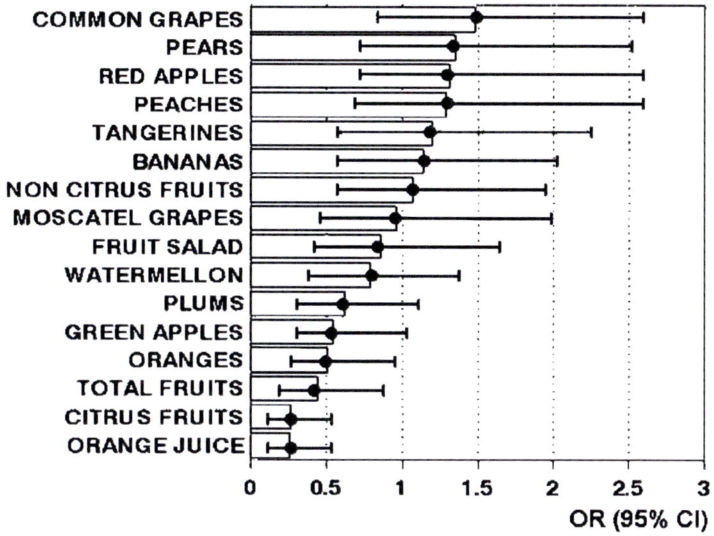

Fig. 11.4 Bar graphics derived from the original data of highest tertiles of intake for each fruit item, with their corresponding odds ratios and confidence intervals

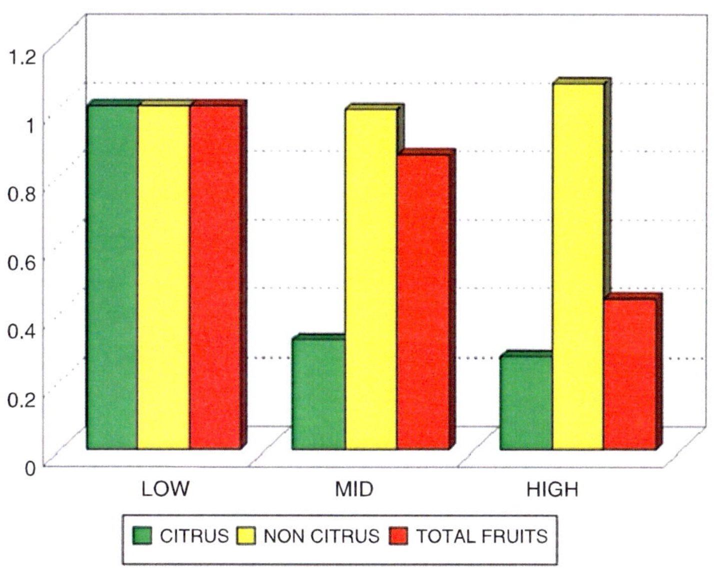

Fig. 11.5 Odds ratios for fruit intakes, categorized into tertiles

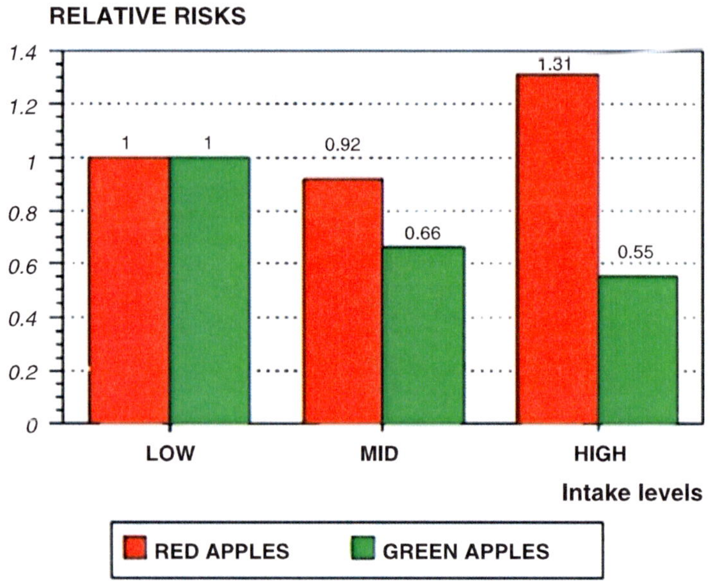

Fig. 11.6 Odds ratios for apple intakes, categorized into tertiles

Table 11.9 Adjusted relative risks after including vitamin C in the regression model

	RR	RR	
		Including vitamin C	
Variable	Without vitamin C	Mid tertile	High tertile
Orange	0.51 (0.26–0.98)	0.44 (0.19–1.03)	0.22 (0.08–0.64)
Orange juice	0.26 (0.13–0.54)	0.16 (0.08–0.31)	0.23 (0.11–0.48)
Citrus fruits	0.27 (0.13–0.55)	0.23 (0.11–0.46)	**0.13** (0.05–0.33)
Total fruits	0.44 (0.23–0.86)	0.81 (0.43–1.55)	0.35 (0.16–0.76)

We reproduce here some preliminary and still unpublished results about the orange consumption and the risk of BC among women in Uruguayan public hospitals. As a result of the combination of two databases, an old one with 773 patients and a new one with 1596, the final database (n=2369) was divided into quintiles to be statistically analyzed. A crosstabulation and an estimation of relative risks through unconditional logistic regression were performed. The regression model controlled by: age, education, age at menarche, menopausal status, number of live births, age at first delivery, months of breastfeeding, family history of BC in degree relatives and body mass index. These results are shown in the following Figs. 11.7 and 11.8.

Breast cancer cases are more frequent among the low intakes of oranges. An additional detail: category I (the lowest quintile) represents those women who are no consumers of oranges, that is, near 20% of the Uruguayan female population (assisted at public hospital system) do not consume oranges at all.

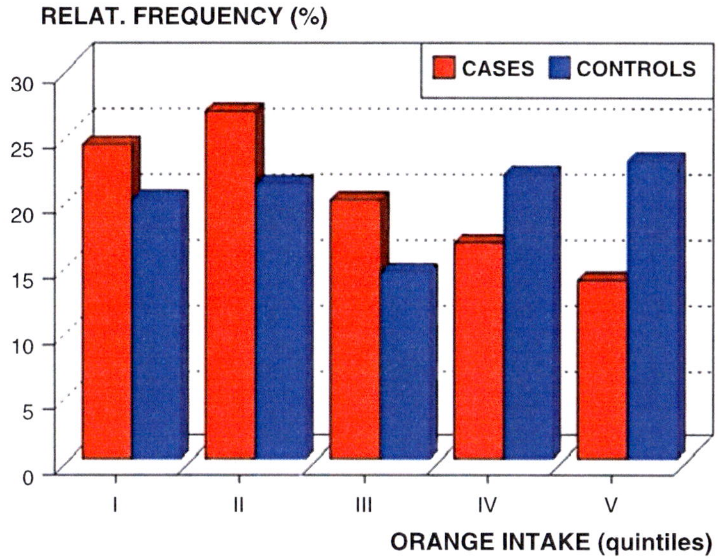

Fig. 11.7 Orange consumption

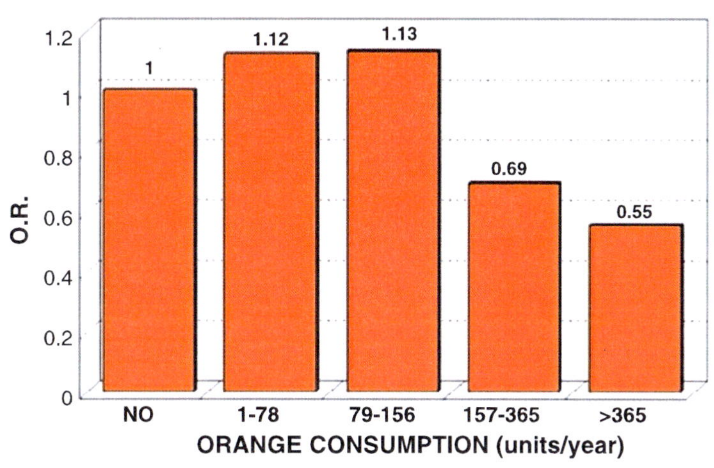

Fig. 11.8 Relative risks for orange intake

The most important change is seen between the third and fourth quintiles. This latter represents an intake of more than three and up to seven oranges/week (up to a mean of one unit per day). The highest quintile is composed by those women who have an intake over one orange per day.

The multivariate analysis showed that the Relative Risk of BC for eating more than three oranges/week is 0.69 (that is, 31% of protection), compared to those non-eaters. Furthermore, when consuming more than a unit per day, the risk decreases up to 0.55 (a 45% of protection). Both estimates were statistically significant.

This reduction was more evident for postmenopausal women (RR = 0.45) than for premenopausal ones (RR = 0.70). This fact – which is rather common in dietary studies – suggests that the time of action is very important, regarding the putative protective role of this food. More important than the hormonal status could be the time of action, could be assumed after the facts, since the analyses performed by age groups found the same proportions.

As it was possible to observe for the reader, the risk for the group with highest orange intake found among the private healthsystem (in tertiles) was 0.51 and the risk for those belonging to public healthsystem was 0.55 (in quintiles). Despite that the adjustment terms for the regression model were not exactly the same but shared some variables, the coincidence between both estimations – and in addition, the displayed pattern – suggests that we are facing a strong protective factor for BC in the studied population.

As a conclusion, we have observed that the studies involving patients coming from the public as well as from the private healthcare system, from all social strata, have demonstrated that women with absence of BC tend to be frequent consumers of citrus fruits and those women afflicted with BC tend to be unfrequent or no consumers of citrus fruits. Albeit fruits have been subject of numerous analyses and there is no complete universal coincidence on their protective role, the evidence is pointing to define this latter as likely. We have confirmed a very clear and definited population trend in Uruguay: Women with BC usually have low citrus consumption and women without BC are frequent citrus consumers.

References

1. Ronco AL, De Stéfani E, Mendilaharsu M et al (1996) Meat, fat and the risk of breast cancer: a case-control study from Uruguay. Int J Cancer 65(3):328–331
2. De Stéfani E, Ronco AL, Mendilaharsu M et al (1997) Meat intake, heterocyclic amines, and risk of breast cancer: a case-control study in Uruguay. Cancer Epidemiol Biomarkers Prev 6:573–581
3. World Cancer Research Fund (1997) Food, nutrition and the prevention of cancer: a global perspective. American Institute for Cancer Research, Washington DC, pp 252–287
4. World Cancer Research Fund/American Institute for Cancer Research (2007) Food, nutrition, physical activity, and the prevention of cancer: a global perspective. American Institute for Cancer Research, Washington DC
5. Steinmetz KA, Potter JD (1991) Vegetables, fruit and cancer. I. Epidemiology. Cancer Causes Control 2(5):325–357
6. Steinmetz KA, Potter JD (1991) Vegetables, fruit and cancer. II. Mechanisms. Cancer Causes Control 2(6):427–442
7. Ronco AL, De Stéfani E, Boffetta P et al (1999) Vegetables, fruits, and related nutrients and risk of breast cancer: a case control study in Uruguay. Nutr Cancer 35(2):111–119
8. Giovannucci E, Ascherio A, Rimm EB et al (1995) Intake of carotenoids and retinol in relation to risk of prostate cancer. J Natl Cancer Inst 87:1767–1776
9. Ronco AL, De Stéfani E, Dáttoli R (2002) Dairy foods and risk of breast cancer: a case-control study in Montevideo, Uruguay. Eur J Cancer Prev 11(5):457–463

10. Willett WC, Stampfer MJ (1986) Total energy intake: implications for epidemiologic analyses. Am J Epidemiol 124:17–27
11. Van't Veer P, Van Leer EM, Rietdijk A et al (1991) Combination of dietary factors in relation to breast cancer occurrence. Int J Cancer 47(5):649–653
12. Webb PM, Bain CJ, Purdie DM et al (1998) Milk consumption, galactose metabolism and ovarian cancer (Australia). Cancer Causes Control 9(6):637–644
13. He Y (1999) Comment on the association between Insulin-like Growth Factor-I (IGF-I) and bone mineral density: further evidence linking IGF-I to breast cancer risk. J Cell Endocrinol Metab 84:1760
14. Outwater JL, Nicholson A, Barnard N (1997) Dairy products and breast cancer: the IGF-I, estrogen and bGH hypothesis. Med Hypotheses 48(6):453–461
15. Knasmuller S, Steinkellner H, Hirschl AM et al (2001) Impact of bacteria in dairy products and of the intestinal microflora on the genotoxic and carcinogenic effects of heterocyclic aromatic amines. Mutat Res 1:129–138
16. Matos E, Brandani A (2002) Review on meat consumption and cancer in South America. Mutat Res 506–507:243–249
17. Ashar MN, Prajapati JB (2000) Verification of hypocholesterolemic effect of fermented milk on human subjects with different cholesterol levels. Folia Microbiol (Praha) 45(3):263–268
18. Rizkalla SW, Luo J, Kabir M et al (2000) Chronic consumption of fresh but not heated yogurt improves breath-hydrogen status and short-chain fatty acid profiles: a controlled study in healthy men with or without lactose maldigestion. Am J Clin Nutr 72(6):1474–1479
19. St-Onge MP, Farnworth ER, Jones PJ (2000) Consumption of fermented and nonfermented dairy products: effects on cholesterol concentrations and metabolism. Am J Clin Nutr 71(3):674–681
20. Ghanem KZ, Hussein L (1999) Calcium bioavailability of selected Egyptian foods with emphasis on the impact of fermentation and germination. Int J Food Sci Nutr 50(5):351–356
21. Scholz-Ahrens KE, Schaafsma G, van den Heuvel EG et al (2001) Effects of prebiotics on mineral metabolism. Am J Clin Nutr 73(2 Suppl):459S–464S
22. Van't Veer P, Dekker JM, Lamers JW et al (1989) Consumption of fermented milk products and breast cancer: a case-control study in The Netherlands. Cancer Res 49(14):4020–4023
23. Wohl GR, Loehrke L, Watkins BA et al (1998) Effects of high-fat diet on mature bone mineral content, structure and mechanical properties. Calcif Tissue Int 63(1):74–79
24. Garland CF, Garland FC, Gorham ED (1999) Calcium and vitamin D. Their potential roles in colon and breast cancer prevention. Ann N Y Acad Sci 889:107–119
25. Lipkin M, Newmark HL (1999) Vitamin D, calcium, and prevention of breast cancer: a review. J Am Coll Nutr 18:392s–397s
26. Xue L, Lipkin M, Newmark H et al (1999) Influence on dietary calcium and vitamin D on diet-induced epithelial cell hyperproliferation in mice. J Natl Cancer Inst 91:176–181
27. Forssen KM, Jagerstad MI, Wigertz K et al (2000) Folates and dairy products: a critical update. J Am Coll Nutr 19(2 Suppl):100S–110S
28. Wigertz K, Svensson UK, Jagerstad M (1997) Folate and folate-binding protein content in dairy products. J Dairy Res 64(2):239–252
29. Prinz-Langenohl R, Fohr I, Pietrzik K (2001) Beneficial role for folate in the prevention of colorectal and breast cancer. Eur J Nutr 40(3):98–105
30. Shrubsole MJ, Jin F, Dai Q et al (2001) Dietary folate intake and breast cancer risk: results from the Shanghai breast cancer study. Cancer Res 61(19):7136–7141
31. Ronco AL, De Stéfani E, Fabra A (2003) White meat intake and the risk of breast cancer: a case-control study in Montevideo, Uruguay. Nutr Res 23(2):151–162
32. Ronco AL, De Stefani E, Deneo-Pellegrini H (2006) Fruit consumption and risk of breast cancer: a case-control study. In: Flaps P (ed) New developments in nutrition research. Nova, New York, NY
33. Ronco AL, De Stéfani E, Deneo-Pellegrini H (2008) Fruit intake and risk of breast cancer: a case-control study. In: Fortugno LP (ed) Frontiers in breast cancer research. Nova, New York, NY, pp 175–186

Chapter 12
The Role of Nutrients and Other Substances

Fats

The RRs of BC for intake of dietary lipids [1] are shown in next place (Table 12.1). The intake of total fat was associated with a moderate increase of risk (RR = 1.5) in the highest quartile, after adjusting for the main confounding factors.

Saturated fats, which have shown RR up to 1.9 in other regression models, disappeared as a risk factor (RR = 0.84) after adjusting by other fat types. A moderate although non significant increase of risk was observed for monounsaturated fat (RR = 1.50). On the contrary, polyunsaturated fats were associated with an inverse and significant relationship with the risk of BC. More precisely, the group of higher consumption displayed a significant protective effect (RR = 0.38), which is equivalent to a risk reduction of 62%.

Linoleic acid, besides, was associated with a significant risk reduction of BC (RR = 0.24). Conversely, the other essential fatty acid, the α-linolenic was significantly associated with an important risk increase (RR = 2.76). Regarding the latter, it is of interest to explain that although it is a Ω-3 polyunsaturated fatty acid, it proceeds from several animal and vegetable sources. There have been studies which recognize in it an indicator of a high intake of red meat, for example. There is not a countersense when a high intake of this Ω-3 polyunsaturated fatty acid (PUFA) was associated with the risk of BC.

Finally, cholesterol was shown also as a statistically significant risk factor, with the highest RR observed in these groups (RR = 4.31) for the highest consumers.

Dietary Fibre

The adjusted RR of BC associated with dietary fibre intake in Uruguayan women [2] are shown in Table 12.2. An inverse relationship with a significant risk reduction of 49% for the group with the highest consumption (highest quartile) is evident.

A.L. Ronco and E. De Stéfani, *Nutritional Epidemiology of Breast Cancer*,
DOI 10.1007/978-94-007-2397-9_12, © Springer Science+Business Media B.V. 2012

Table 12.1 Relative risks of breast cancer for dietary fat

	Quartils of consumption				
Dietary item	I	II	III	IV	p-value (trend)
Total fat					
g/day	<57.5	57.6–73.8	73.9–88.7	88.8+	
RR	1.0	0.68	1.57	1.53	0.01
Saturated fats					
g/day	<20.9	21.0–28.8	28.9–37.7	37.8+	
RR	1.0	1.55	1.33	0.84	0.56
Monounsaturated fats					
g/day	<14.5	14.6–21.1	21.2–26.8	26.9+	
RR	1.0	1.23	1.16	1.50	0.55
Polyunsaturated fats					
g/day	<13.1	13.2–14.0	14.1 15.2	15.3+	
RR	1.0	0.67	0.67	0.38*	0.005
Linoleic acid					
g/day	<13.0	13.1–13.9	14.0–15.0	15.1+	
RR	1.0	0.66	0.44*	0.24*	<0.001
α-linolenic acid					
g/day	<0.8	0.9–1.0	1.1–1.2	1.3+	
RR	1.0	0.94	1.24	2.76*	0.02
Cholesterol					
mg/day	<314.9	315.0–427.7	427.8–538.1	538.2+	
RR	1.0	1.57	2.13*	4.31*	<0.001

Adjusted by age, residence, urban/rural status, family history of BC in 1° degree relatives, body mass index, age at menarche, parity, alcohol consumption, total calories consumption, dietary fibre, folate intake and quartiles of the other dietary fats

* = statistically significant

Table 12.2 Relative risks of breast cancer associated with fibre intake

	Quartils of consumption				
Dietary item	I	II	III	IV	p-value (trend)
Total fibre	1.0	1.15	0.69	0.51*	<0.001
Grain fibre	1.0	0.89	0.54*	0.65	0.02
Vegetable fibre	1.0	0.92	0.59*	0.56*	0.005
Fruit fibre	1.0	1.13	0.89	0.77	0.18

* = statistically significant

Also the p-value for trend was highly significant ($p<0.001$). When fibre consumption was analyzed according to its original source, fibre from cereals were associated with a RR = 0.65 for the quartil of highest consumption. Fibre from fruits was not associated with a significant risk reduction. Other adjustments performed in the regression model, by vitamin C, α-tocopherol, folate and lignans did not modify the estimations.

Table 12.3 Relative risks of breast cancer associated with non-starchy polysaccharides

	Quartils of consumption				
Dietary item	I	II	III	IV	p-value (trend)
Total NSP	1.0	1.26	0.50*	0.50*	<0.001
Soluble NSP	1.0	0.94	0.41*	0.49*	<0.001
Insoluble NSP	1.0	0.97	0.52*	0.45*	<0.001
Cellulose	1.0	0.85	0.72	0.68	0.11

Adjusted by age, residence, family history of BC in 1° degree relatives, previous history of benign breast diseases, total dietary calories, red meat, lutein, quercetin and menopausal status
* = statistically significant

We examined the risk of BC associated with the intake of Non-starch polysaccharides (NSP) in Table 12.3. The effect of a high intake of these polysaccharides was associated with a strong reduction of risk (RR = 0.50). When NSP were separately analyzed according to their solubility condition, the RRs were similar. Both types of fibre did not display major risk differences between pre- and postmenopausal women (results not shown here), but both were associated with a strong risk reduction. Finally, the intake of cellulose was associated with a protective effect, although statistically non significant (RR = 0.68 for the highest intake quartile).

The combined effect of fibre, fat, quercetin and lutein/zeaxanthin is displayed in Table 12.4. We showed in a multivariate model including total energy intake how a high total fat consumption and a low fibre consumption were associated with a significant increase of BC risk (RR = 3.30). High intake levels of quercetin and fibre were associated with a significant risk reduction of 64% (RR = 0.36), whereas the combined effect of lutein and fibre showed a reduction of 67% (RR = 0.33), which was also significant.

It has been suggested that the risk reduction of BC associated with a high fibre intake could be a marker of the effect of other substances which are present in plants, or even of phytoestrogens. Since information of lignans and other phytoestrogens in foods was limited it was difficult to adjust by these substances, however, we included lignans and flavonoids in our regression models. Whereas lignans did not show themselves as confounding factors of the relationship to be studied, quercetin (the most important flavonoid) was strongly associated with dietary fibre and the risk of BC.

Anyway, although our results should be interpreted with caution, we accept that the combined effect of quercetin and dietary fibre derived into a strong reduction in risk for the studied disease.

Heterocyclic Amines

As it was already mentioned in the corresponding section of international literature, aromatic heterocyclic amines, or simply heterocyclic amines (HCA) are produced as a consequence of pyrolysis of meat aminoacids during the cooking process at

Table 12.4 Relative risks of breast cancer for the combined effects of dietary fibre and other nutrient and non nutrient substances

	Cases/Controls	RR	(95% IC)
Fats			
High fibre intake			
Low fat intake	64/113	1.0	
High fat intake	78/98	1.44	(0.93–2.25)
Low fibre intake			
Low fat intake	93/84	2.01*	(1.30–3.10)
High fat intake	116/61	3.30*	(2.11–5.16)
Quercetin			
High fibre intake			
Low quercetin intake	117/79	1.0	
High quercetin intake	92/66	0.89	(0.57–1.37)
Low fibre intake			
Low quercetin intake	73/85	0.58*	(0.38–0.90)
High quercetin intake	69/126	0.36*	(0.24–0.55)
Lutein			
High fibre intake			
Low lutein intake	95/57	1.0	
High lutein intake	114/88	0.72	(0.46–1.12)
Low fibre intake			
Low lutein intake	51/53	0.58*	(0.35–0.98)
High lutein intake	91/158	0.33*	(0.21–0.50)

Adjusted by age, residence, family history of BC in 1° relatives, previous history benign breast disease, total energy, red meat and menopausal status
* = statistically significant

high temperatures. HCA are highly mutagenic and induce the formation of tumours in several sites, including the breast and this was seen in different animal species. HCA are the following:

IQ = 2-amino-3-methylimidazo (4,5-f) quinoline (imidazoquinoline)
PHiP = 2-amino-1-methyl-6- phenylimidazo (4,5 f) piridin (phenylimidazopiridin)
MeIQx = 2-amino-3,8 dimethylimidazo (4,5 f) quinoxalin (methylimidazoquinoxalin)

The food composition table for HCA concentration which is shown below (Table 12.5) was based on data of the existing literature cited in our respective work [3]. Contents were calculated as continuous variables in ng/g of each food.

The Relative Risks of BC for the exposure to HCA, taking into account the cooking methods assessed and the values communicated in the literature, are shown in Table 12.6. All HCA were associated to significant risk increases and the IQ showed a threefold risk increase for all women, despite their menopausal status. The PHiP was associated with a positive gradient of risk and a significant dose-response effect. In particular, postmenopausal women were associated with a threefold increased risk for the highest estimated PHiP quartile.

Table 12.5 HCA Concentration in foods (in ng/g)

Food	IQ	MeIQx	PHiP
Fried cow meat	3.79	2.35	13.19
Barbecued cow meat	0.50	2.11	15.70
Barbecued lamb	n/a	1.01	42.50
Grilled chicken	n/a	2.33	38.10
Fried fish	0.61	6.44	19.60
Grilled fish	1.80	2.20	37.50

n/a = not available

Table 12.6 Relative risks of breast cancer associated with exposure to HCA (ng/g)

	Quartils of consumption				
HCA menopausal status	I	II	III	IV	p-value (trend)
IQ	<=0.42	0.43–0.66	0.67–1.01	>=1.02	
All	1.0	1.22	1.87*	3.34*	<0.001
Pre	1.0	1.89	2.70*	2.15	0.24
Post	1.0	1.11	1.75	3.80*	<0.001
MeIQx	<=2.50	2.51–3.42	3.43–4.52	>=4.53	
All	1.0	1.12	1.60	2.13*	0.002
Pre	1.0	2.03	2.53	1.97	0.23
Post	1.0	0.92	1.49	2.14*	0.006
PHiP	<=11.07	11.08–15.26	15.27–20.14	>=20.15	
All	1.0	1.06	1.81*	2.59*	<0.001
Pre	1.0	1.19	1.24	1.16	0.84
Post	1.0	1.02	1.85	3.31*	<0.001

All risks were adjusted by age, residence, family history in 1° relatives, age at menarche, parity, previous history of benign breast disease, total energy, vegetable intake and fats intake
* = statistically significant

Most of the described fat types and HCAs combined emerged as a risk nutrient pattern in a recent factor analysis study performed by our group [4]. We reported an increase of risk (OR = 3.50, 95% CI 1.94–6.30) for the highest quartile of intake.

Bioactive Compounds

Our research had the goal of assessing whether the protective effect for BC of some vegetables and fruits could be explained by nutrients and bioactive substances which were present in those foods: carotenoids, phytosterols, vitamins, antioxidants and fibre [5]. Results are shown in Table 12.7.

Inverse associations (protective effects) were observed for dietary fibre, vitamin C, lycopene, vitamin E, folate and phytosterol intake. A strong risk reduction was observed for dietary fibre (RR = 0.41). Among carotenoids, lycopene, α-carotene and lutein showed a significant risk reduction (highest intake of lycopene RR = 0.30).

Table 12.7 Relative risk of breast cancer for nutrients and bioactive substances present in plant-origined foods

	Quartils of consumption				
Dietary item	I	II	III	IV	p-value (trend)
Total dietary fibre	1.0	0.68	0.63*	0.41*	0.001
Cereals fibre	1.0	0.87	0.86	0.58*	0.01
Vegetal fibre	1.0	0.89	0.55*	0.43*	<0.001
Fruit fibre	1.0	0.88	0.76	0.58*	0.05
β-carotene	1.0	0.92	0.72	0.72	0.19
α-carotene	1.0	0.61*	0.62*	0.52*	0.08
Lutein/Zeaxanthin	1.0	0.87	0.67	0.66	0.06
Lycopene	1.0	0.47*	0.42*	0.30*	<0.001
β-cryptoxantin	1.0	0.61*	0.62*	0.52*	0.08
Vitamin C	1.0	0.67	0.61*	0.45*	<0.001
Vitamin E	1.0	0.53*	0.50*	0.40*	<0.001
Folate	1.0	0.98	0.56*	0.70	0.01
Phytosterols	1.0	0.79	0.85	0.37*	<0.001
Glutathione	1.0	1.04	1.35	1.09	0.16

Adjusted by age, residence, urban/rural status, family history of BC in 1° degree relatives, total dietary calories, body mass index, age at menarche, parity and menopausal status
* = statistically significant

Also folate, vitamin E and phytosterols were significantly associated with a reduction of BC risk.

The previous risks are presented now as a bar graphics, ordered from major to minor values (Fig. 12.1).

The factor analysis study on nutrient patterns and risk of BC performed by our group [4] reported a risk reduction for the high intake of the so-called "antioxidants" pattern (OR = 0.44, 95% CI 0.27–0.74). It was significant only among all postmenopausal women (OR = 0.63, 95% CI 0.51–0.79) and even more among those ones who have a family history of BC (OR = 0.17, 95% CI 0.06–0.48). Such antioxidants pattern showed high loadings for the intake of: vitamin C, vitamin E, carotenoids, flavonoids, phytosterols, glucose and fructose, remarking the protective role for the whole combination of bioactive substances.

As another example of the complex interrelationships among dietary elements, in this particular case of vitamins, the 3-D graphics of Fig. 12.2 indicates how the intakes of vitamin C, vitamin E and lycopene are related. It can be seen that controls have a dark red zone corresponding to high intakes of the three components and the dark green (low consumers) area is relatively small. On the contrary, BC cases showed no more than an intermediate level of vitamin C together with a high intake of the other two elements. In other words, the consumption pattern of certain selected antioxidant substances keep some differences between cases and controls.

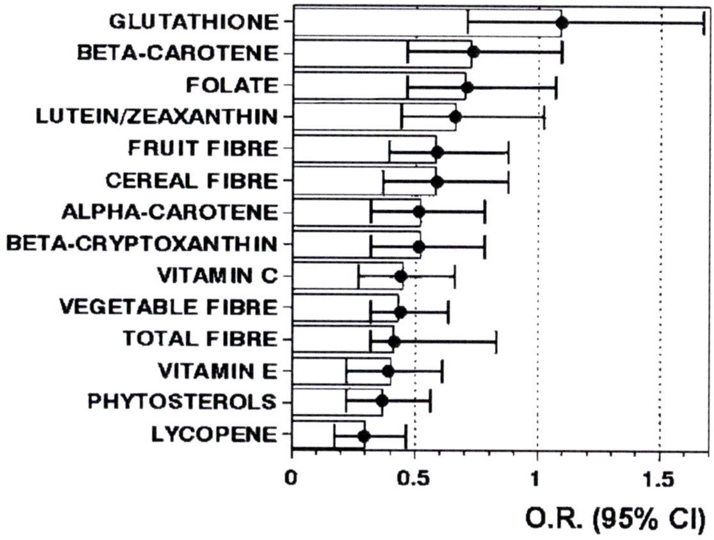

Fig. 12.1 Relative risks of BC for the studied nutrients and bioactive substances

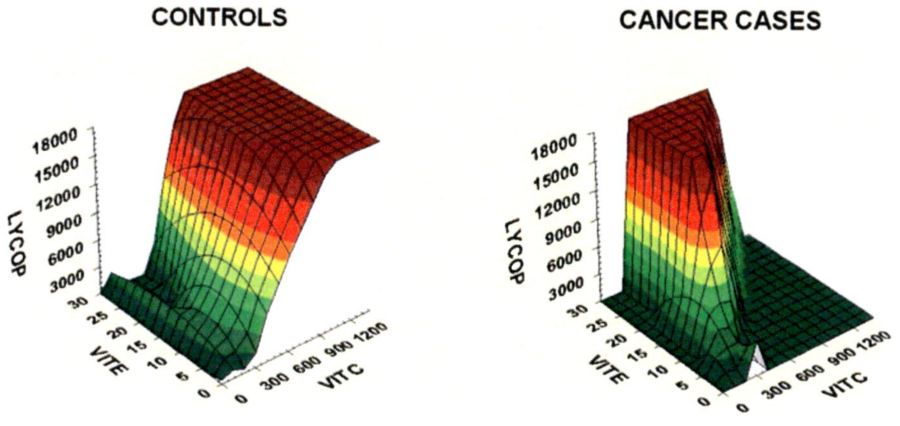

Fig. 12.2 3-D Graphics comparing the intake of selected antioxidants between controls and BC cases

Phytoestrogens

Given the need of counting on effective substances for the primary prevention of BC, the authors have considered years ago [6] that attempting to estimate the resulting effects of phytoestrogen intake constituted a priority in a community like the Uruguayan, with recognized high BC rates. Based on the data of Thompson et al.

Table 12.8 Principal foods sources of phytoestrogens (category = lignans), expressed in μg/100 g of each food

Food	Enterolactone	Enterodiol
Oat	265	386
Corn	168	480
Wheat	269	298
Rice	134	47
Sorghum	199	56
Garlic	81	326
Squash	271	110
Carrot	284	62
Sweet potato	240	55
Cauliflower	68	77
Lettuce	58	63
Potato	33	50
Cabbage	30	34
Tomato	11	10
Lentils	789	998
Kidney beans	329	232
Pear	112	69
Banana	55	14
Orange	27	12
Apple	34	1

[7], we present the Table 12.8, in which the main foods that are sources of enterolactone and enterodiol (lignans) are cited.

The Relative Risks of BC for foods or food groups which constitute an important source of phytoestrogens are shown in Table 12.9. The intake of cereals displayed a strong inverse (protective) association with a RR = 0.27 for the highest level of consumption. The intake of vegetables also was associated with a significant risk reduction (RR = 0.47), whereas tubers did not display a protective trend. Legumes intake, besides, was associated with a significant reduction of BC risk next to 47%. Finally, dietary fibre showed again a significant risk reduction (RR = 0.29) and a high intake of fruits also displayed a reduction (RR = 0.70), although it was not statistically significant.

Relative Risks of BC for phytoestrogen intake are presented in Table 12.10. A high consumption of enterodiol was associated with a significant protective effect of 57% (RR = 0.43). Also enterolactone and total lignans showed a significant risk reduction, which was lignans similar to that estimated for enterodiol.

In the following figure (Fig. 12.3), we present the graphic translation of the ORs of both phytoestrogens and their main sources, ordered in a descendent way. It is interesting to remark that on one hand, foods like tubers and total fruits tended to be protective or not associated with the risk of BC. Despite their content of phytoestrogens, items like carbohydrates such as sucrose and fructose could represent an opposite trend, because they can be included into the list of high-glycemic load foods, which involve potential risks through the upstream of insulin and cytokines

Table 12.9 Relative risks of breast cancer for foods which are source of phytoestrogens

	Quartils of consumption				
Dietary item	I	II	III	IV	p-value (trend)
Cereals					
intake	<=494	495–651	652–885	>=886	
RR	1.0	0.44*	0.36*	0.27*	0.002
Vegetables					
Intake	<=298	299–454	455–656	>=657	
RR	1.0	0.59*	0.54*	0.47*	<0.001
Tubers					
Intake	<=128	129–182	183–234	>=235	
RR	1.0	0.94	0.85	0.91	0.64
Legumes					
Intake	<=12	13–24	25–96	>=97	
RR	1.0	0.96	0.92	0.53*	0.004
Dietary fibre					
Intake	<=11,0	11,1–14,5	14,6–18,5	>=18,6	
RR	1.0	0.53*	0.36*	0.29*	<0.001
Fruits					
Intake	<=182	183–262	263–390	>=391	
RR	1.0	1.04	0.93	0.70	0.11

The values correspond to servings/year except fibre (grams/year). The model includes adjustment by age, residence, urban/rural status, education, age at menarche, parity, menopausal status, alcohol intake and total energy
* = statistically significant

pathways. On the other hand, items like fibre and cereals, overcome the own protection of phytoestrogens, suggesting that they provide something else than these latter. In the case of fibres, it is probable that their mechanical work in the bowel helping to remove estrogens, cholesterol, heterocyclic amines and several other substances from re-entering the circulation could explain partially this protective effect.

Polyunsaturated Ω-6 and Ω-3 Fatty Acids

This study [8, 9] emphasized the analysis of the sources of polyunsaturated fatty acids (PUFA) such as oils, meats, fried foods and bakery products. After adjusting by age, years of urban status, education, age at menarche, menopausal status, number of live births, breastfeeding, use of oral contraceptives, use of hormonal replacement therapy, current body mass index and at age 18, dietary energy, intake of oranges and tomatoes and dietary cholesterol, a multivariate analysis found that high intakes of Ω-6 PUFA were positively associated with the risk of BC (OR = 4.20 for the highest tertile). The ratio Ω-6/Ω-3 was also positively associated (OR = 2.88

Table 12.10 Relative risks of breast cancer for phytoestrogens. Discriminated by menopausal status

	Quartiles of consumption				
	I	II	III	IV	p-value (trend)
Enterolactone					
Intake	<=922	923–1,154	1,155–1,461	>=1,462	
All	1.0	0.87	0.53*	0.55*	0.001
Pre	1.0	0.84	0.58	0.74	
Post	1.0	0.96	0.54*	0.55*	
Enterodiol					
Intake	<=748	749–942	943–1,166	>=1,167	
All	1.0	0.53*	0.48*	0.43*	<0.001
Pre	1.0	0.87	0.42	0.61	
Post	1.0	0.53*	0.51*	0.40*	
Total lignans					
intake	<=1,656	1,657–2,136	2,137–2,645	>=2,646	
All	1.0	0.61*	0.56*	0.43*	<0.001
Pre	1.0	1.18	0.45	0.91	
Post	1.0	0.57*	0.64*	0.38*	
Isoflavones					
Intake	<=13	14–62	63–114	>=115	
All	1.0	1.15	1.23	0.62*	0.07
Pre	1.0	1.79	1.57	1.12	
Post	1.0	1.04	1.11	0.51*	

Intake in μg/100 g of foods, except in Isoflavones (mg/100 g)
* = statistically significant

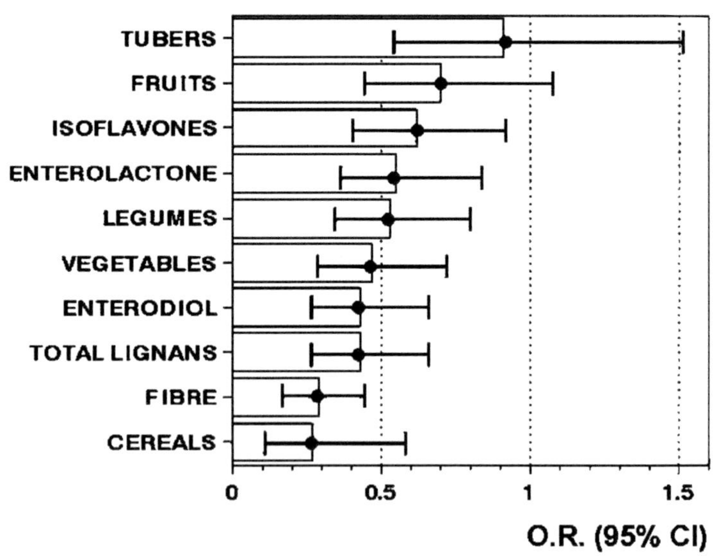

Fig. 12.3 Relative risks of breast cancer for the highest quartiles of phytoestrogens intakes and their main sources

Table 12.11 Estimated risks for dietary Ω-6 and Ω-3 PUFA according ages

		Age<=54		Age>=55	
	Tertiles	OR	(95% CI)	OR	(95% CI)
Ω-6	I	1.00	–	1.00	–
	II	1.26	(0.21–7.49)	2.81	(1.17–6.75)
	III	**7.20**	(1.45–35.7)	**4.05**	(1.65–9.94)
Ω-3	I	1.00	–	1.00	–
	II	0.26	(0.06–1.11)	1.65	(0.72–3.78)
	III	**0.20**	(0.04–0.96)	0.67	(0.26–1.76)
Ω-6/Ω-3	I	1.00	–	1.00	–
	II	1.84	(0.52–6.60)	0.98	(0.51–1.89)
	III	**5.51**	(1.77–17.2)	1.09	(0.55–2.13)

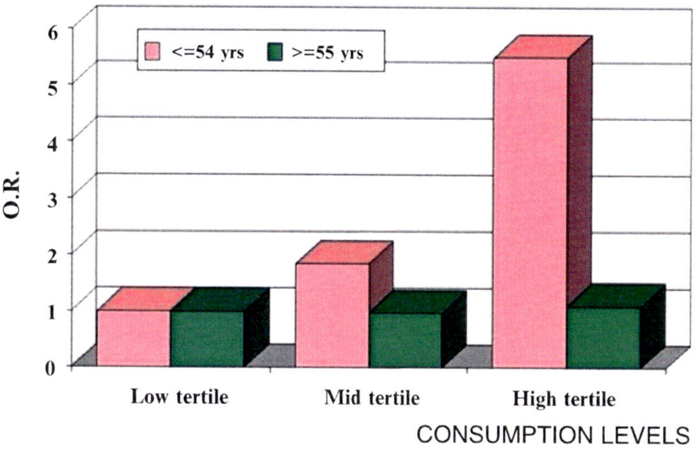

Fig. 12.4 Risk associations of dietary Ω6/Ω3 ratio stratified by age groups

for the highest tertile). The intake of Ω-3 was negatively associated (OR = 0.57 for the highest tertile). Although results come from a small sample of patients belonging to the subset with highest risk in Montevideo, the evidence reinforces the preventive potential of dietary recommendations with the aim of reducing the impact of the disease.

When the analysis was stratified by age (cutpoint in the sample median, 55 years), interesting results derived, as it can be seen in Table 12.11. Among premenopausal women the associations were stronger, in the risk increase of Ω-6 PUFA as well as the risk reduction of Ω-3 PUFA. These facts are reflected in the Table also for the ratio Ω-6/Ω-3. The risk increase for the sample (OR = 2.88) is explained mainly by the risk in the premenopausal subset (OR = 5.51), since there was no risk association among postmenopausal women (OR = 1.09). These results are expressed graphically in Fig. 12.4.

Apparently the protective effect of Ω-3 PUFA is stronger among younger women (mostly presumably premenopausal) and the risk increase of Ω-6 PUFA is also stronger than among the older ones (mostly presumably postmenopausal). Undoubtedly, if these results are confirmed by new analyses the possibilities of having basic recommendations for primary prevention of BC are encouraging since young women are a subgroup which is difficult to protect through nutritional guidelines. In fact, contrary to what happens to postmenopausal women, there are a few items suggesting a role of risk association or a protective association among young, premenopausal women. The rationale and numerous advantages for recommending a frequent intake of fishes that are rich sources of Ω-3 PUFA (tuna, sardines, salmon, cod, among others) as well as the supplementation through the intake of oil fish are commented in the Chapter on PUFA and BC.

References

1. De Stéfani E, Deneo-Pellegrini H, Mendilaharsu M et al (1998) Essential fatty acids and breast cancer: a case-control study in Uruguay. Int J Cancer 76:491–494
2. De Stéfani E, Correa P, Ronco A et al (1997) Dietary fiber and risk of breast cancer. Nutr Cancer 28:14–19
3. De Stéfani E, Ronco AL, Mendilaharsu M et al (1997) Meat intake, heterocyclic amines, and risk of breast cancer: a case-control study in Uruguay. Cancer Epidemol Biomarkers Prev 6:573–581
4. Ronco AL, De Stéfani E, Aune D et al (2010) Nutrient patterns and risk of breast cancer in Uruguay. Asian Pac J Cancer Prev 11(2):519–524
5. Ronco AL, De Stéfani E, Boffetta P et al (1999) Vegetables, fruits, and related nutrients and risk of breast cancer: a case control study in Uruguay. Nutr Cancer 35(2):111–119
6. Ronco AL, De Stéfani E (1999) Fitoestrógenos y riesgo de cáncer mamario: un estudio caso control. Rev Med Uruguay 15(2):94–102
7. Thompson LU, Robb P, Serraino M et al (1991) Mammalian lignan production from various foods. Nutr Cancer 16:43–52
8. Ronco A, De Stéfani E, Deneo-Pellegrini H et al (2005) Consumo de grasas poliinsaturadas y riesgo de cáncer de mama: un estudio caso-control. Rev Bras Nutr Clin 20(Suppl 1):S1–SS8, p 12
9. Ronco A, De Stéfani E, Deneo-Pellegrini H (2006) Polyunsaturated fatty acids intake and risk of breast cancer: a case-control study. XIV world congress on breast diseases, Zagreb, 18–21 May 2006

Chapter 13
Anthropometry

Body Composition

Body composition is a division or fractioning of the total body weight into its components, in order to perform its quantification and further analyses with targets related with nutrition, health, sport performance, among others. Aside from technicalities that exceed the boundaries of this book, we are interested in remarking the major components: fat mass, muscle mass, skeletal mass and residual mass. These correspond respectively to the adipose tissue, the muscular tissue, the bones and the rest of elements grouped (skin, inner organs, vessels, etc.). Occasionally, when body composition is classified in fatty fraction and lean fraction, this latter includes the other components together.

The inconvenience of assessing with the simple body weight or with the body mass index (BMI) is that they do not distinguish between fat mass and lean mass. Although BMI keeps a high correlation with fat mass (r=.60–.70), we have also observed that it correlates well with muscle mass [1]. According to their BMI some athletes could be correctly classified as having overweight or even obese, due to having a large muscle mass and at the same time low fat mass. Conversely, it can happen that a fat excess covers hides a muscle mass deficit without reflecting it in the total weight, such as it happens in sedentary people. These aspects should be taken into account when they are linked to our findings after having studied body composition in women with and without BC.

According to Latin American authors who have thoroughly revised the issue [2, 3], studies about body composition have been during long time focused on determination of body fat. Nevertheless, the interest in muscular mass began to increase in recent years due to its relationship with numerous aspects of human health, such as protein reserve of the body [4], functional capabilities and thermal regulation [5] and immune capability [6].

Historically, it was accepted that muscles represent the most abundant tissue in human organism, being in average 30% of total weight in a woman and 40% in a man. It is possible that these percentages are higher, indeed. In the last decades, new

A.L. Ronco and E. De Stéfani, *Nutritional Epidemiology of Breast Cancer*,
DOI 10.1007/978-94-007-2397-9_13, © Springer Science+Business Media B.V. 2012

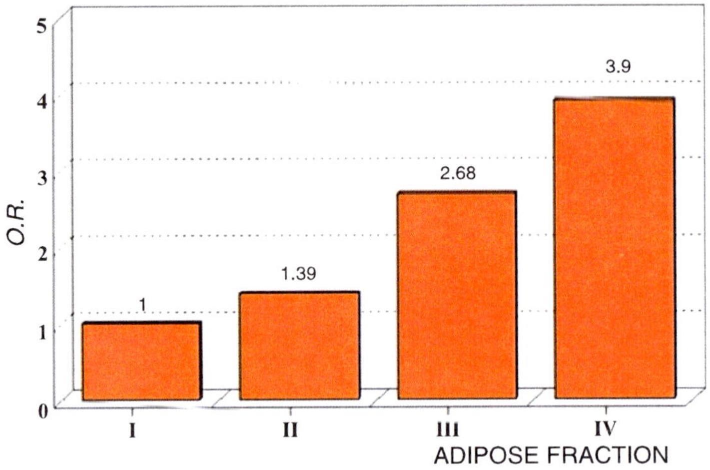

Fig. 13.1 Relative risks of the adipose fraction, expressed in quartiles

scientific evidence about the detrimental effects on health caused by the loss of muscular mass has been generated [7]. Since muscle mass is the main protein reserve of human body, its decrease has been also associated to reduced immune capabilities and of thermal regulation. The reduction of muscle mass is a phenomenon observed with aging, but it is enhanced in the sedentary lifestyles and even in those subjects who do not handle adequately the stressor factors, because these latter release hormones such as corticoids, who lead to a loss of muscle.

In our epidemiologic case-control studies which explored body composition and its possible associations with BC in a sample of almost 1.400 women [1, 8] we reported that the higher the fat fraction was, higher was the risk of the disease (Fig. 13.1). At the same time, the lower the muscle fraction was, also higher was the risk of BC (Fig. 13.2).

When fat mass increased, the muscle mass decreased. Having observed these facts, we created a simple Fat/Muscle Ratio, which additionally enhanced the quoted concept. The low level of risk involved similar proportions of both fat and muscle fraction, or even when fat mass was lower than muscle (FMR<=1). We observed intermediate levels with FMR from 1 to around 1.5, and the high-risk level corresponded to FMR values higher than 1.5 (Fig. 13.3).

In Fig. 13.4 are shown the relative risks for the FMR, regarding the whole sample. Significant differences of distribution and a strong linear trend were found in this analysis.

We observed that this ratio reflected apparently higher risk among premenopausal than postmenopausal women, but there was no statistical heterogeneity between both subsets.

Perhaps the most interesting finding was that the risk was increased in women with overweight (OR=4.83, 95% CI 2.22–10.5) and obesity (OR=7.13, 94% CI

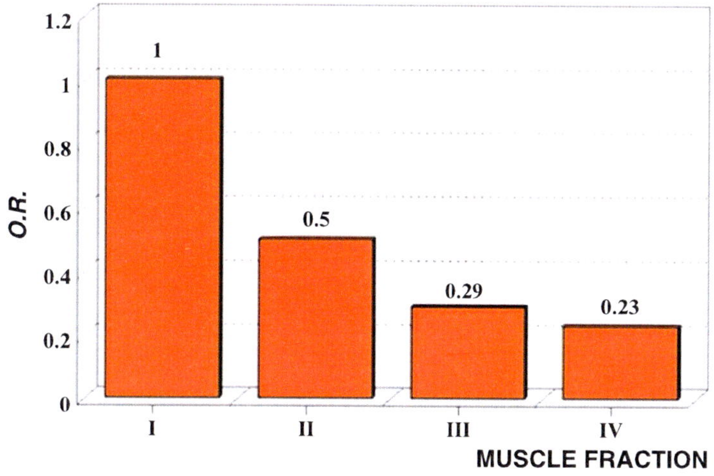

Fig. 13.2 Relative risks of the muscle fraction, expressed in quartiles

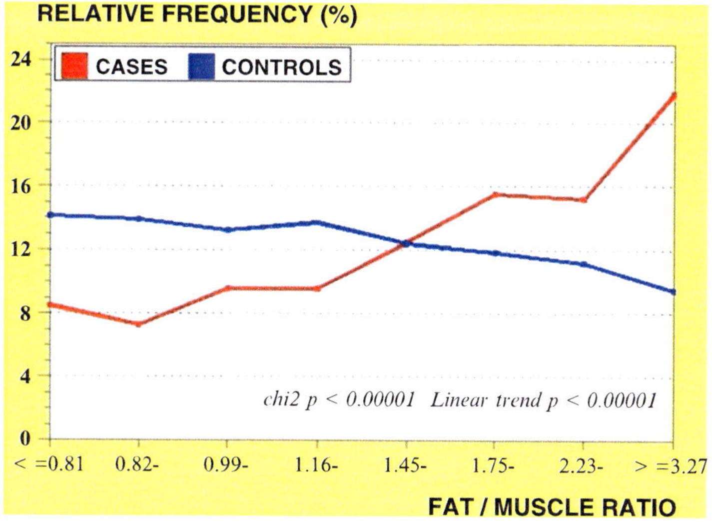

Fig. 13.3 Distribution of cases and controls according to the FMR (divided into octiles)

3.18–15.9) but also in women with normal BMI (OR=3.56, 95% CI 1.95–6.51). Those results mean that **in all women a high FMR implied a risk increase.** If the estimated FMR was high, the body mass index seemed to be not so important. The Fig. 13.5 displays the risks calculated for BMI strata.

We began then to understand how did things worked in those patients afflicted with BC who have a thin, slender body type. In these women without a visible overweight,

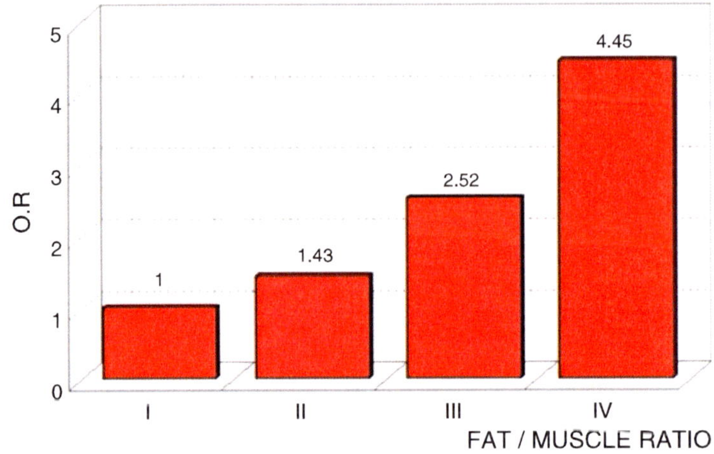

Fig. 13.4 Relative risks for the FMR, expressed in quartiles

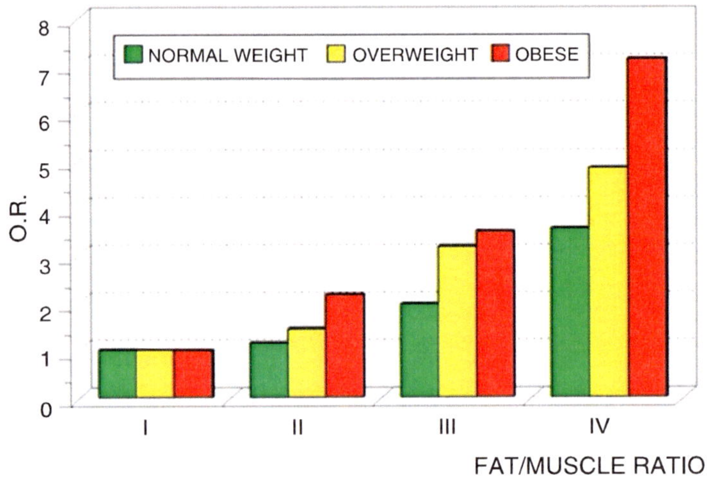

Fig. 13.5 Calculated relative risks for FMR stratified by BMI level

there was not actually any fat excess in terms of absolute weight. They lack of an adequate muscle mass and the current fat represents a **relative** very high fraction.

Hence, the problem could be double: the fat mass is excessive in relative terms for the existing body structure and the muscle mass is insufficient. Such women would be probably facing an excessive androgen aromatization, a high synthesis of cytokines, an excessive metabolization to "bad" estrogens (16-α-OHestrogens) and at the same time an insufficient immune system parallel to a poor muscular mass. The fat produces elements which limit the muscular development and in addition if

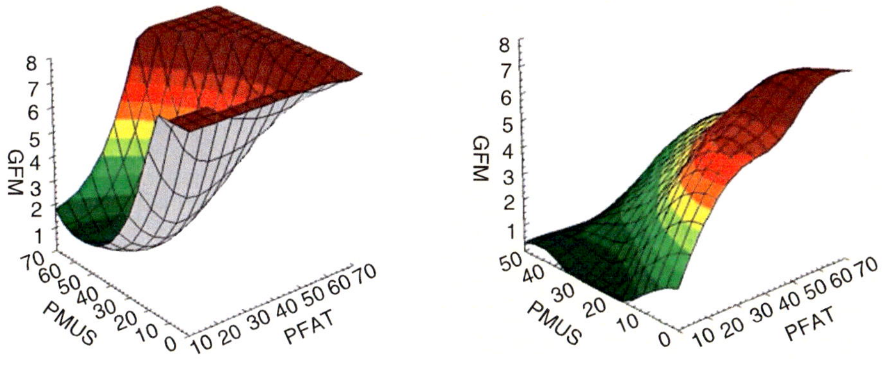

Fig. 13.6 3-D graphic representing the interaction of fat/muscle ratio with its components muscle percentage and fat percentage in healthy controls (*left*) and in cancer cases (*right*). Abbreviations: *GFM* (Fat/muscle ratio grouped in octiles), *PMUS* (muscular fraction) and *PFAT* (fat fraction)

the woman is sedentary there would not be a compensation in order to avoid the muscular loss, reaching for the latter inadequate levels.

Figure 13.6 displays a 3-D graphics, corresponding to the interaction of Fat fraction, muscle fraction and FMR. Cases (right side) show a concentration of high FMR (dark red zone) mainly located with extremely high Fat fraction together with extremely low Muscle fraction. Differently, healthy controls display wide strips of high FMR (dark red zone) but not restricted to low muscle fraction. Instead, controls have subjects with high FMR having low and high muscle fraction and having also low and high fat fraction. It appears to more likely to have high fat and high muscle combined together. The differences suggest different trends of anthropometric patterns for each condition.

We should need to know how the body composition is and not only to remain basing our criterium on what the weighscale displays, because there could be high differences among women with the same BMI and with rather similar body shapes (Fig. 13.7). Some cases of physical thinness or slenderness can belong to what is known as sarcopenia (a muscle mass deficit). Also some situations determine the so called "sarcopenic obesity" (fat excess with muscle deficit), opposed to other cases such as the "muscular obesity", where both components are abundant. In our research we were able to confirm that a certain proportion of large-size women (obese ones from the viewpoint of BMI) keep a FMR close to the unit.

Undoubtedly, factors like hormonal status, ethnical features and age can play a considerable role and they must be taken into account before thinking about a generalization to other populations. This research is brand new and we should analyze the evidence from other studies performed in different ethnic groups and countries to confirm or not the validity of the findings.

Some investigations have examined the interrelationships between skeletal muscle and the adipose tissue, in health as well as in disease. For example, some studies

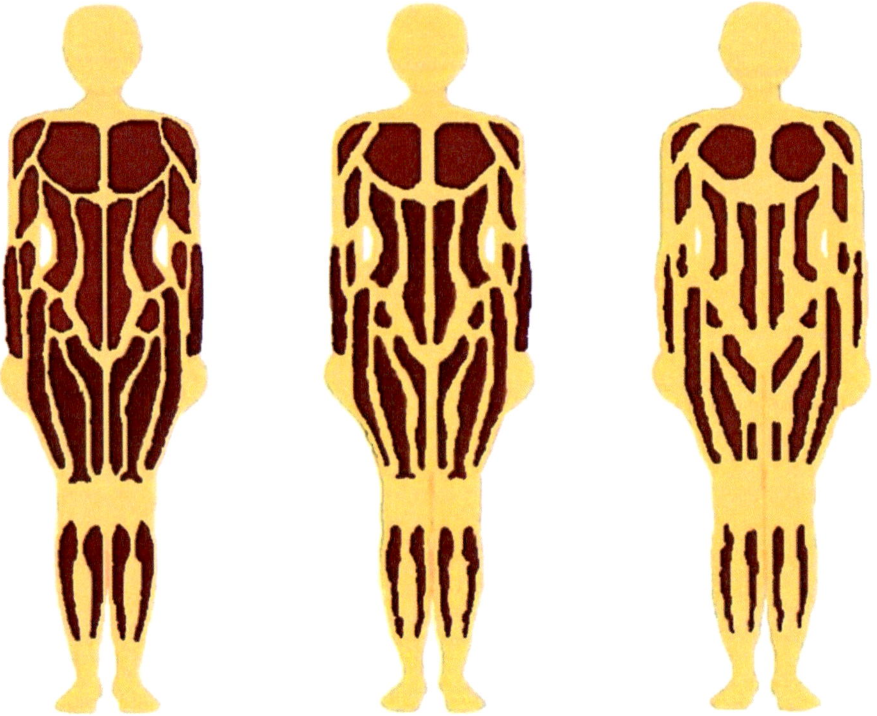

Fig. 13.7 Possible differences underlying similar external physical shapes. A woman can vary from having a good muscle mass and reduced adiposity (*left*) up to having a poor muscle mass with plenty of adiposity (*right*), without experiencing important weight or morphologic changes. This remarks the insufficiency of BMI

have found direct relationships among muscle mass, activity and adipose mass, suggesting that resistance training aside from preventing insulin resistance in humans, can influence in both muscle and adipose tissues in normal as well as in obese humans and animals [9–11].

The adipose tissue releases pro-inflammatory cytokines, such as TNF-α (tumoral necrosis factor alpha) which induces degradation of proteins and apoptosis in miofibres [12, 13]. Leptin, besides, has the ability to reduce the protein synthesis in skeletal muscle [14]. Experimental research has shown that there is a reduced protein content in the muscles of obese animals [15]. The administration of several cytokines (TNF-α, Interleukin-6, among others) leads to an increase of serum triglycerides and of fats production in the liver [16, 17]. During an infection the cytokines production is triggered and these latter take the organism towards an alteration of lipid metabolism. Due to these reasons, two decades ago the quoted lipid changes triggered by cytokines were postulated as a defense mechanism against invasive stimuli just as bacterial infections or tumour growth [18].

Conversely, muscular hypertrophy leads to a reduction of the adipose tissue [19–21], thanks to some other cytokines produced by the former. One of them, the

Interleukin-15 (IL-15) stimulates the muscular fibres to accumulate large amounts of proteins [22]. This represents the chance of reducing the cachexia produced by a tumour [23]. As it were not enough to, IL-15 is beneficial for the immune system: it induces proliferation of T-lymphocytes [24], increases cytotoxicity of Natural Killers [25] and protects these and other leukocytes from cell death [26, 27].

The interrelationship between muscular and adipose tissue, thoroughly studied by Spanish authors [28], leads to the concept of reciprocal regulation of both tissues, not restricted to the action of cytokines and hormones but also of nutrients as circulating fats and carbohydrates. Whether it is faced from the viewpoint of homeostasis or from the newer and complex field of cybernetics, everything points to recognize a feedback system that works under healthy and under pathologic conditions. According to Argilés, "This new vision of an adipose-muscular axis could contribute to the future design of new therapeutical approaches to face the therapy of diseases related with the control of body weight, such as obesity or cachexia".

What was previously exposed indicates that the presence of the muscular mass is important for its own maintenance, as well as for the regulation of fat synthesis and deposition and for the support of immune system. Probably appears now as more clear why could be an increase of risk in slender women with a low BMI: they tended to have a high FMR, which was not due to a fat excess but to a reduced muscle mass (usually notably under a recommendable 40% of whole body weight). Under these conditions, everything points to assume that the most probably recommendable physical exercise would not be one of aerobic type (to burn fats) but one of anaerobic, muscle-building type, in order to increase the muscular mass.

AN ADEQUATE BODY COMPOSITION COULD BE PROTECTIVE AGAINST BREAST CANCER. ON THE CONTRARY, ADIPOSE EXCESS, MUSCULAR DEFICIT OR BOTH COULD BE A RISK FACTOR.

The Somatotype

As we have already seen, some studies examined the localized adiposity and the risk of BC. It has been described a central adiposity (in abdomen and trunk, the classical apple-shaped) associated to a risk increase in postmenopausal women, whereas only a weak increase has been reported in premenopausal ones [29–33]. Women having this pattern of fat distribution experience hormonal and metabolic changes such as insulin resistance, hyperinsulinemia, hyperandrogenemia and higher aromatization of these latter to estrogens within the adipose tissue [34], hence, such distribution pattern is linked to higher risks of diabetes and cardiovascular diseases would have higher risks of BC than women whose fat depots prevail in hips, buttocks and lower limbs.

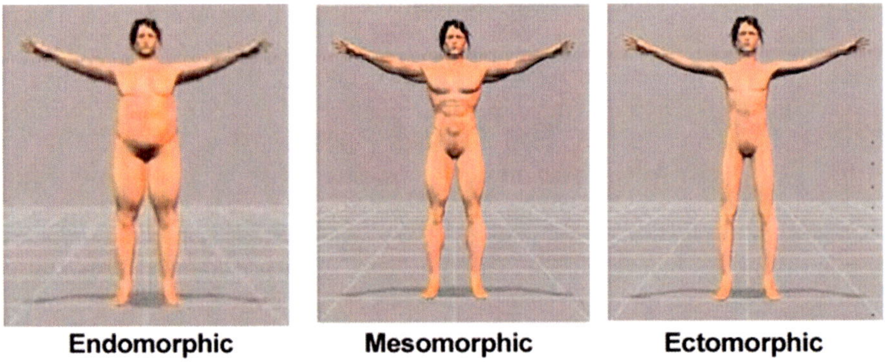

Fig. 13.8 Physical appearance of somatotype's components

According to the literature, the role of body shape as a measure of fat and muscle distribution is still not well defined. Recent reviews on body shape and size indicated that there was a need of new and better assessments [35]. Most studies have been performed on Anglosaxon populations. Therefore, this lack of information coming from other ethnical groups, the high incidence of BC in Uruguay, the easy access to patients and the low need of available resources led us to carry out a research within the public hospital frame. This research would allow to reach two objectives: To know the role (if any) of physical shape in a high-risk population like the Uruguayan, and at the same time to apply a methodology which was not previously used in the area of BC.

We investigated the possible role of physical shape in the risk of BC in a local population of 1.254 women, using an innovative methodology which was well known in the fitness world and athletic assessment: the somatotype [36]. It is defined as "a quantitative description of the present shape and composition of the human body" [37], a method developed by W.H. Sheldon in the first half of the past century [38]. This method describes three body components: (1) Endomorphy, which features the relative adiposity; (2) Mesomorphy, which features the muscular size; and (3) Ectomorphy, which features the linearity or slenderness derived from the ponderal index (height in cm divided by the cube root of weight in kg). These components differ among populations according to age, sex and origins. For example, an extreme endomorphism has a pear-shape, with wide hips and narrow shoulders. An extreme mesomorphism is featured by wide shoulders and relatively narrow hips (edge-shaped), more typical of men than of women. And an extreme ectomorphism has narrow shoulders, chest and hips, together with thin arms and legs and reduced amount of muscle or fat (Fig. 13.8).

Somatotype methodology has been scarcely used in the medical field, with examples related to cardiovascular risk [39–43], obesity [44, 45] and rarely in cancer research [46, 47]. The changes that occur in a somatotype happen during childhood to maturity and they can be modified through physical training and/or nutrition.

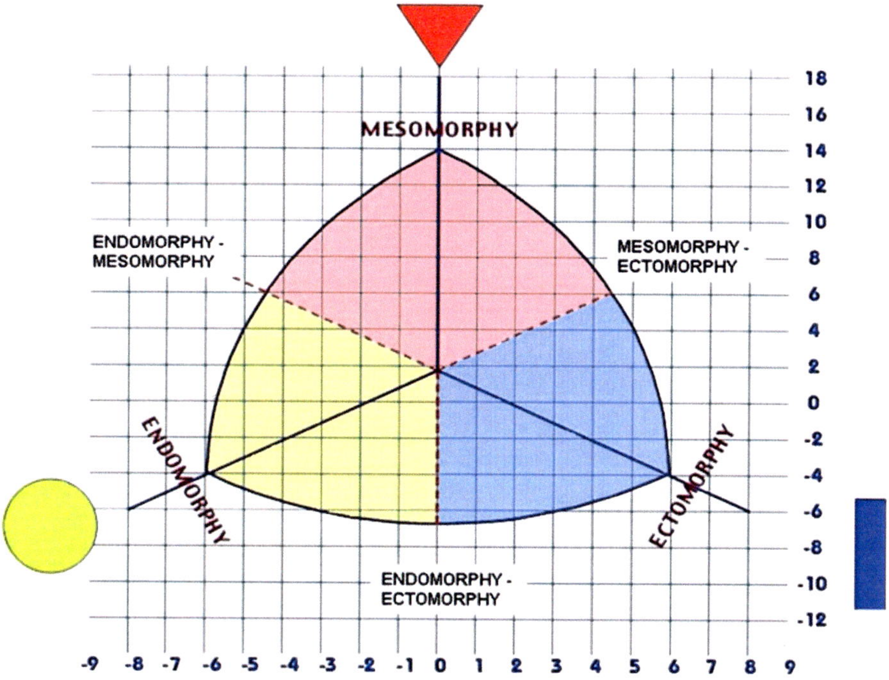

Fig. 13.9 Somatochart

The somatotype is expressed by a score produced by the three components, calculated from certain body measurements and specific formulas.

The somatochart is the graphic representation (Fig. 13.9) of a person through a point located within the references coordinates. Such point corresponds to the score previously calculated.

The study of the somatotype allowed us to quantify the proportions and shapes of the studied women. Women with BC displayed higher endomorphism than healthy controls. In other words, we have observed in our sample that patients with BC tended to be more "pear-shaped", regardless of their slender, medium or obese external appearance. Besides, we did not find differences in the mesomorphism and ectomorphism. Endomorphism exhibited a dose-effect pattern, which is a strength when being a possible risk factor. Results were also slightly more strong among premenopausal women and in women with normal weight (BMI<25 kg/m2), although they were not statistically heterogeneous [36].

From the viewpoint of somatotype, the color dots in the next somatochart (Fig. 13.10) translate the findings and represent the mean values of each subgroup. Postmenopausal women had almost the same values for BC cases and healthy controls (green and black dots). Healthy premenopausal women (blue dot) are less endo- and mesomorphic than postmenopausal ones. And premenopausal cases of BC (red dot) are somehow in the way between the normal premenopausal and the

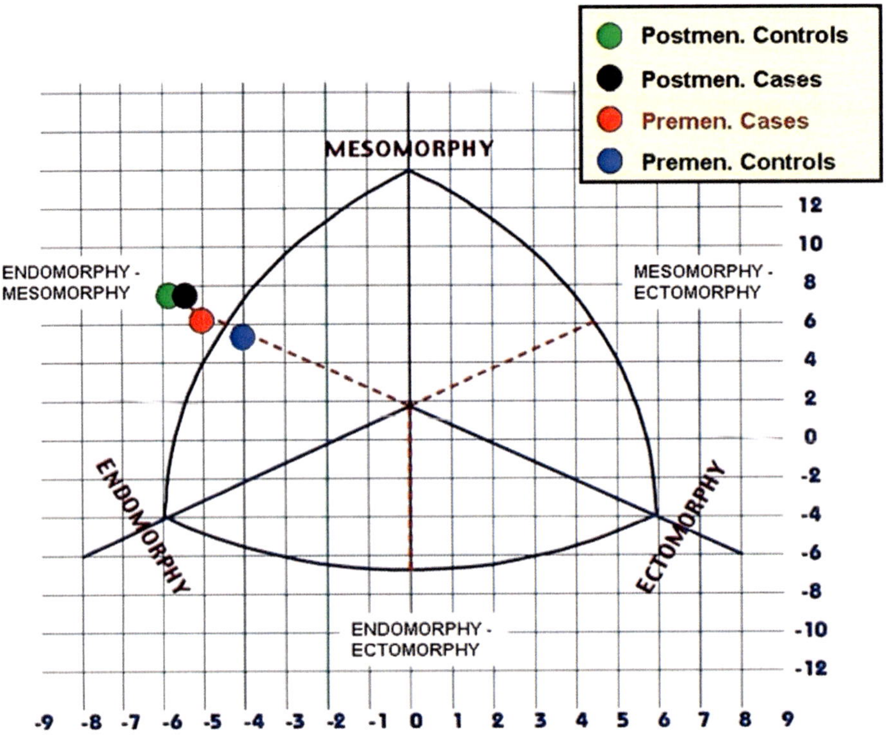

Fig. 13.10 Somatochart of the study in Uruguayan women (Ref. [36])

postmenopausal ones. It seems as if younger women with BC had acquired a body morphology which would be directed towards the one of older ones. In other words, the body shape of the former ones appears as if it were advanced in time getting closer to those of these latter.

As it can be appreciated in the corresponding Figure (Fig. 13.11), healthy controls showed a top surface of their FMR which was relatively constant (the red stripe), with a slight inclination. This top area corresponds to a endomorphic mid-to-high stripe, independently from the mesomorphism (from very low to high). Cases with BC, on the contrary, showed 2 areas grouping a very high FMR: one of them displayed a high endomorphism and low mesomorphism; the other one displayed high mesomorphism and low endomorphism. We might be witnessing the presence of two anthropometric clusters, something which deserves additional studies and having higher samples.

A recent study [48] performed in 1,537 patients showed that when the regression model included all terms of body composition and somatotype, involving mutual adjustments, there were changes in the estimates (mostly as an attenuation) of risk for fat weight (from OR = 4.57 to OR = 3.17), fat fraction (from OR = 3.43 to OR = 2.73) and for endomorphism (from OR = 5.45 to 3.27). In all cases the risks

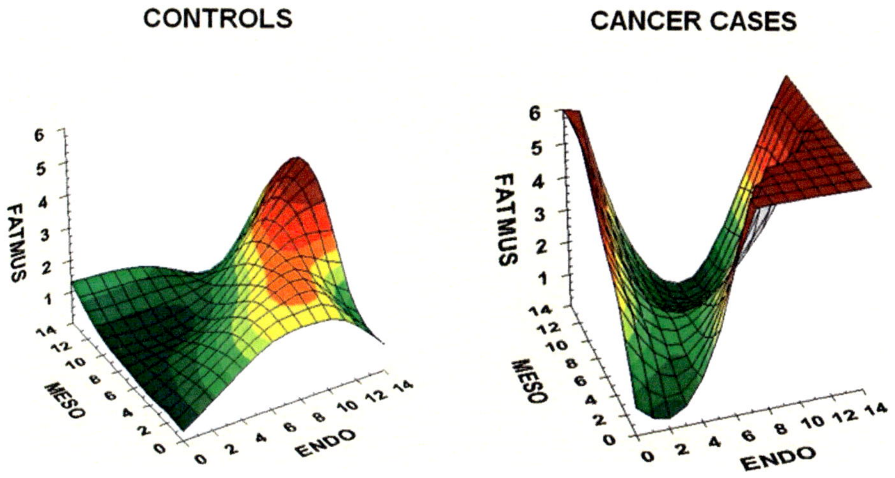

Fig. 13.11 Graphic comparison between BC cases and healthy controls, according to FMR, endomorphism and mesomorphism. Abbreviations: *FATMUS* (Fat/muscle ratio grouped in octiles), *MESO* (mesomorphism) and *ENDO* (endomorphism)

were statistically significant. Results suggest that these items have a certain value by themselves: the fat amount and fraction remained positively and significantly associated to the risk of BC despite the inclusion of body shape in the model, and viceversa.

Our studies have shown results that are different to the major part of the literature, because the gynoid-type obesity (expressed by a high endomorphism) has not been considered of high risk in the research performed in the first World. Nevertheless, it should be taken into account that more than two decades ago a higher aromatization in the body regions of endomorphism (hips, buttocks, thighs) [49] was already described, and that could be a plausible explanation for our findings.

Besides, the waist-to-hip ratio was similar for women with BC and healthy controls. The somehow unexpected findings, led us to consider that there are ethnic factors which should be taken into account, in view of the different origins of Uruguayan women (mainly an admixture of 80% Latin European and Hispanic ancestors with 20% of Amerindian and African ethnias), when compared with North American, Anglosaxon, Scandinavian or others coming from developed countries.

Hence, within a population in which a meso-endomorphic pattern prevails together with high occurrence of overweight and obesity, a pure central-type obesity is not suggested as a difference between both groups.

IN THE STUDIED POPULATION, A PHYSICAL SHAPE WITH MARKED ENDOMORPHISM SUGGESTED A RISK INCREASE, BUT MORE EVIDENCE FROM OTHER ETHNIC GROUPS IS NEEDED.

References

1. Ronco AL, Boeing H, De Stéfani E et al (2009) A case-control study on fat to muscle ratio and risk of breast cancer. Nutr Cancer 61(4):466–474
2. De Girolami DH (ed) (2003) Fundamentos de evaluación nutricional y composición corporal. El Ateneo, Buenos Aires
3. Fernández Vieitez JA. Estimaciones antropométricas del músculo esquelético en seres humanos. www.siicsalud.com/des/des042/05311002.htm. Accessed 17 Oct 2006
4. Hébuterne X, Berman S, Schneider SM (2001) Aging and muscle: the effects of malnutrition, renutrition, and physical exercise. Curr Opin Clin Nutr Metab Care 4:295–300
5. Anderson GS (1999) Human morphology and temperature regulating. Int J Biometeorol 43:99–109
6. Mariani E, Ravaglia G, Forti P et al (1999) Vitamin D, thyroid hormones and muscle mass influence natural killer (NK) innate immunity in healthy nonagenarians and centenarians. Clin Exp Immunol 116:19–27
7. Marcell TJ (2003) Sarcopenia: causes, consequences, and preventions. J Gerontol Med Sci 58A:911–916
8. Ronco AL, Varas X, Febles G et al (2006) Body composition and breast cancer: the role of menopausal status. XIV world congress on breast diseases, Zagreb, 18–21 May 2006
9. Fiebig RG, Hollander JM, Ney D et al (2002) Training down-regulates fatty acid synthase and body fat in obese Zucker rats. Med Sci Sports Exerc 200:153–160
10. Christ CY, Hunt D, Hancock J et al (2002) Exercise training improves muscle insulin resistance but not insulin receptor signaling in obese Zucker rats. J Appl Physiol 92:736–744
11. Knowler WC, Barrett-Connor E, Fowler SE et al (2002) Diabetes prevention program research group, reduction in the incidence of type-2 diabetes with lifestyle intervention or metformin. N Engl J Med 346:393–403
12. Fong Y, Moldawer LL, Morano M et al (1989) Cachectin/TNF or IL-1 alpha induces cachexia with redistribution of body proteins. Am J Physiol 256:R659–R665
13. Meadows KA, Holly JM, Stewart CE (2000) Tumor necrosis factor-alpha-induced apoptosis is associated with suppression of insulin-like growth factor binding protein-5 secretion in differentiating murine skeletal myoblasts. J Cell Physiol 183:330–337
14. Carbó N, Ribas V, Busquets S et al (2000) Short-term effects of leptin on skeletal muscle protein metabolism in the rat. J Nutr Biochem 11:431–435
15. Lanza-Jacoby S, Kaplan ML (1984) Alterations in skeletal muscle proteins in obese and nonobese rats. Int J Obes 8:451–456
16. Grunfeld C, Soued M, Adi S et al (1990) Evidence for two classes of cytokines that stimulate hepatic lipogenesis: relationships among tumor necrosis factor, interleukin-1 and interpheron alpha. Endocrinology 127:46–54
17. Grunfeld C, Adi S, Soued M et al (1990) Search for mediators of the lipogenic effects of tumor necrosis factor: potential role for interleukin-6. Cancer Res 50:4233–4238
18. Grunfeld C, Feingold KR (1992) Tumor necrosis factor, interleukin and interferon induced changes in lipid metabolism as part of host defense. Proc Soc Exp Biol Med 200:224–227
19. McPherron AC, Lee SJ (2002) Suppression of body fat accumulation in myostatin-deficient mice. J Clin Invest 109:595–601
20. Sutrave P, Hughes SH (1991) The ski oncogene. Oncogene 109:353–356
21. Costelli P, Carbó N, Busquets S et al (2003) Reduced protein degradation rates and low expression of proteolytic systems support skeletal muscle hypertrophy in transgenic mice overexpressing the c-ski oncogene. Cancer Lett 200:153–160
22. Quinn LS, Andreson BG, Drivdahl RH et al (2002) Overexpression of interleukin-15 induces skeletal muscle hypertrophy in vitro: implications for treatment of muscle wasting disorders. Exp Cell Res 280:55–63
23. Carbó N, López-soriano J, Costelli P, Busquets S et al (2000) Interleukin-15 antagonizes muscle protein waste in tumour-bearing rats. Br J Cancer 83:526–531

24. Burton JD, Bamford RN, Peters C et al (1994) A lymphokine, provisionally designated interleukin T and produced by a human adult T cell leukemia line, stimulates T cell proliferation and the induction of lymphokine-activated killer cells. Proc Natl Acad Sci USA 91:4935–4939
25. Carson WE, Giri JG, Lindemann MJ et al (1994) Interleukin(IL) 15 is a novel cytokine that activates human natural killer cells via components of the IL-2 receptor. J Exp Med 180:1395–1403
26. Akbar AN, Borthwick NJ, Wickremasinghe RG et al (1996) IL-2 receptor common gamma-chain signaling cytokines regulate activated T-cell apoptosis in response to growth factor withdrawal: selective induction of anti-apoptotic (bcl-2, bcl-xL) but not pro-apoptotic (bax, bcl-xS) gene expression. Eur J Immunol 26:294–299
27. Girard D, Paquet ME, Paquin R et al (1996) Differential effects of interleukin-15 (IL-15) and IL-2 on human neutrophils: modulation of phagocytosis, cytoskeleton rearrangement, gene expression and apoptosis by IL-15. Blood 88:3176–3184
28. Argiles JM, López-Soriano J, Almendro V et al (2005) Cross-talk between skeletal muscle and adipose tissue: a link with obesity? Med Res Rev 25(1):49–65
29. Kumar NB, Lyman GH, Allen K et al (1995) Timing of weight gain and breast cancer risk. Cancer 76:243–249
30. Männistö S, Pietinen P, Pyy M et al (1996) Body size indicators and risk of breast cancer according to menopause and estrogen-receptor status. Int J Cancer 68:8–13
31. Ng E-H, Gao F, Ji C-H et al (1997) Risk factors for breast carcinoma in Singaporean Chinese women. Cancer 80:725–731
32. Magnusson C, Baron J, Persson I et al (1998) Body size in different periods of life and breast cancer risk in postmenopausal women. Int J Cancer 76:29–34
33. Sonnenschein E, Toniolo P, Terry MB et al (1999) Body fat distribution and obesity in pre- and postmenopausal breast cancer. Int J Epidemiol 28:1026–1031
34. Bruning PF (1987) Endogenous estrogens and breast cancer a possible relationship between body fat distribution and estrogen availability. J Steroid Biochem 27:487–492
35. Friedenreich CM (2001) Review of anthropometric factors and breast cancer risk. Eur J Cancer Prev 10:15–32
36. Ronco AL, Mendoza B, Varas X et al (2008) Somatotype and risk of breast cancer: a case-control study in Uruguay. Braz J Epidemiol 11(2):215–227
37. Carter JEL, Heath BH (1990) Somatotyping: development and applications. Cambridge University Press, Cambridge
38. Sheldon WH (1951) The somatotype, the morphophenotype, and the morphogenotype. Cold Spring Harb Symp Quant Biol 15:373–382
39. Garn SM, Gertler MM, Sprague HB (1950) Somatotype and serum-cholesterol. Circulation 2:380–391
40. Gordon E, Tobias PV, Mendelsohn D et al (1987) The relationship between somatotype and serum lipids in male and female young adults. Hum Biol 59:459–465
41. Morris RW, Jacobs ML (1950) On the application of somatotyping to the study of constitution in disease. S Afr J Clin Sci 1:347–370
42. Valkov J, Matev T, Hristov I (1996) Relationship between somatotype and some risk factors for ischemic heart disease. Folia Med (Plovdiv) 38:17–21
43. Malina RM, Katzmarzyk PT, Song TMK et al (1997) Somatotype and cardiovascular risk factors in healthy adults. Am J Hum Biol 9:11–19
44. Seltzer CC, Mayer J (1969) Body build (somatotype) distinctiveness in obese women. J Am Diet Assoc 55:454–458
45. Koleva M, Nacheva A, Boev M (2000) Somatotype, nutrition, and obesity. Rev Environ Health 15:389–398
46. Kolodchenko VP (2000) Body build and soft tissue malignancies. Vopr Onkol 29:56–60
47. Eiben OG, Buday J, Bosze P (2004) Physique of patients with carcinoma of the female genital tract. Eur J Gynaecol Oncol 25:683–688

48. Ronco AL, De Stéfani E (2010) Interrelationships between body composition and somatotype and the risk of breast cancer. Proceedings of the XVI world congress of the senologic international society Valencia, 20–22 Oct 2010
49. Killinger DW, Perel E, Daniilescu D et al (1987) The relationship between aromatase activity and body fat distribution. Steroids 50(1–3):61–72

Chapter 14
Foods and Nutrients for Secondary Prevention: Risk Classification with Artificial Intelligence

Risk assessment related to breast cancer (BC) has been something necessary for the application of preventive and therapeutic strategies. Conventional risk analyses have shown certain limitations, mainly in relation to the cost/benefits ratio, taking into account the low detection rates of cancer cases the screening programmes achieved. The authors present herein an innovative proposal for estimating high- and low-risk condition using artificial neural networks models, based on an analysis of a database already used in a series of case-control studies. The inclusion of a large number of multifactorial variables made possible to achieve predictive values around 95%, a discriminant power which suggested the feasibility of BC selective screenings and primary prevention programmes on individual basis and with notably reduced costs.

Optimizing the definition of population at risk of BC constituted for one of the authors (A.R.) perhaps the most important target to reach during several years of his epidemiologic research, in view of how essential it was in order to impact on the disease from several angles, from the primary prevention up to the therapeutic strategies. With the aim of adequately documenting this objective, the present chapter exposes the rationale, the background, the prior experiences, the analyses, the findings and the resulting proposals about this issue.

Introduction

As it has already been mentioned, BC is the most frequent malignancy in women worldwide [1], prevailing previously in developed countries but currently also in developing ones. Several kinds of risk factors for the disease have been identified: menstrual and reproductive factors [2–4], family history of cancer [5, 6], alcohol consumption [7, 8], history of benign breast diseases [9, 10] and use of hormones [11–13] have been studied and found associated with the risk of BC. Besides, diet has been recognized as a very important environmental factor – within lifestyle, together with physical exercise – related to BC genesis and development [14].

A.L. Ronco and E. De Stéfani, *Nutritional Epidemiology of Breast Cancer*,
DOI 10.1007/978-94-007-2397-9_14,

Different strategies have been considered for the control of BC: primary prevention, secondary prevention or screening, and tertiary prevention or therapy optimization. Primary prevention involves all those interventions which intend to reduce the exposure to known risk factors, eventually also to enhance the exposure to known protective factors, something that aims to reduce the incidence of the disease. Secondary prevention refers to all means that can achieve an early diagnosis of the malignancy, if possible prior to the onset of symptoms. This is feasible within certain limits, and it is usually related to well-structured healthcare systems. For certain diseases like BC, an efficient screening system makes possible the reduction of the magnitude of this cancer. In a recent review, we have summarized the epidemiologic evidence generated in Uruguay which led us to propose a series of country-specific recommendations with that aim [15].

According to researchers, mammography-based breast screenings appear to be a necessary step in the control of the disease, and they have shown a considerable reduction of BC mortality [16–18], usually within ranges between 20% and 50%. There are two basic screening types: mass screenings and selective screenings. Mass screenings are directed to examine a population as much as possible, e.g., all adult women from 40 to 50 years old on. These procedures make no differentiation (or almost no one) between the real risk population and the rest of it. Concerning BC, there have been attempts of mass screening based on mammography, on breast clinical examination and on combination of both methodologies. In these programmes age factor has been the only one used as a classifier. Selective screenings have tried to reduce the risk population based on variables which were considered risk factors, or at least, that have had some discriminant value between populations afflicted with BC and other women not afflicted with it. Through this reduction of the sample it was expected to obtain a higher proportion of selected women who actually had a BC (true positives), whereas in the not selected group it was expected to avoid to find cancer cases as much as possible (false negatives).

Nevertheless, most of those conventional mass programmes have achieved detection rates around 10 cancers per 1.000 mammographies [17], and the inclusion of the age group under 50 years old has been controversial [17, 19] because of its even lower detection rate (about 3 or less per 1.000) [17], something that means an unsatisfactory cost/benefits ratio. Although BC could be cited as a model of a multifactorial disease, age is still considered as the main risk factor. Taking into account current detection rates of screening programmes as the above quoted, age factor should be recognized as an insufficient classifier, despite of the considerations about the initial age for being screened.

Due to the high costs of conventional screening programmes [20], we agree with the opinion about the potential convenience of selective BC screenings, an operative modality supported by scientific rational basis [21–23]. Estimating an increased risk through discriminant functions is something not new: in the late 60's Dunn [24] tried to identify a high-risk group of BC. Afterwards, other authors attempted to improve the performance of certain selected factors, anamnestic or not [25–28]. The analysis of Soini and Hakama [29] considering up to 20 combined variables, as well as the one of Seidman et al. [30] led them to recognize, however, the respective failure of such types of classification systems in order to be applied in the public health.

In the early 80's Toti et al. [31] attempted to calculate a discriminant value for women, based initially on 15 biologic variables from their medical history (furtherly they found four that were enough to discriminate cases from controls within some degree of uncertainty). Interesting studies in America [32] as well in Europe [33, 34] on surveillance of women at increased risk for BC confirmed that it is worthy to detect this tumour at early stages. A study with the same objective was proposed by us, in which a score was created based on socio-demographic, gyneco-obstetric, dietary and family factors [35]. The results, however, also led us to conclude the same as many of the authors did: although the high-risk group concentrated a high proportion of cancers, the group classified as low-risk one also included many cases of cancer (false negatives), who could have been wrongly excluded a priori if we had assumed the criteria as valid. Due to the complex, non-linear associations among factors related with BC, we considered as more appropriate the use of Artificial Neural Networks (ANN) to evaluate their discriminant capabilities, in order to classify subsets of women selected as of potentially high and low-risk of BC, to be further screened or not and also to be considered for primary prevention.

A limited number of previously published epidemiologic papers [36–39] and also only one targeting specifically high-risk cancer subjects [37] indicate, in our opinion, that epidemiology had not taken advantage of the potential usefulness of ANN until some years ago. In 1998 one of the authors of this book (A.R.) communicated the results of a pilot study based on a sample of 556 patients. The study was specifically designed to identify BC high-risk populations using ANN [40] and a new study in 1999 based on a 30% larger sample replicated the prior results [41]. Complementary communications on these points were made also further [42, 43]. Afterwards, we attempted to evaluate the different discriminant values of the data groups (gyneco-obstetric, socio-demographic, family history of cancer, selected food items and nutrients) after having expanded the dietary information by addition of several nutrients and a total number of 59 predictors to be analyzed with models of ANNs [44]. To our knowledge, this was the first time in the medical literature that foods and nutrients were considered as good discriminant factors of BC risk, according to the results.

Methodology

Data derived from a database used in part of a series of case-control studies about diet and BC already cited in this book, which were carried out in Uruguay between 1994 and 1999 [45–50]. Seven hundred and twenty interviewed women – patients coming from all regions of Uruguay and admitted to the six major hospitals in Montevideo – whose records were complete were considered eligible and included in the study from which 364 were afflicted with a histologically diagnosed incident BC and 356 were used as control population, not afflicted with oncologic, gynecologic, hormonal nor nutritional diseases. Controls were frequency-matched to cases on age and residence county. The database had 252 variables, including the original 66 food items asked in the questionnaire form and a number of macro- and micronutrients, calculated from the first ones. Basic statistical analyses were performed with an available statistical package [51] to almost all numerical variables of the database, considering a cutoff point a p-value of 0.10, in an attempt of maximizing discrimination even though some variables did not reach statistical significance. A total number of 60 variables entered the model comprising 59 independent variables or predictors (input layer) and 1 dependent variable or outcome (output layer). These discriminant variables belong to the following groups: socio-demographic and familial, gyneco-obstetric and dietary variables (divided into food items and nutrients).

Concerning the family history of cancer, it included a variable which was itself a score, applying for different combinations the same criteria we communicated more than a decade ago [40–44], discriminating between pre- and postmenopausal women. The presence of 1 familial case of BC represented respectively 4 and 3 points, the absence of any type of familial cases meant 1 and 0 point, for example. The outcome of interest was cancer, a binary variable, labeled as 1 = yes and 0 = no.

Logistic regressions were also performed in order to make comparisons between this procedure and the ANN, using the same number of variables and applying the same criteria for grouping these variables into gynecoobstetric, familial + sociodemographic, food items, nutrients and all together. Regressions were consecutively performed for each one of these groups of variables and for all of them together. Backward and forward step methods were used and the best results were registered when the predictive values were the highest possible, even though some of these models did not include all the variables of each group. Variables were introduced into the different models as they were originally collected, part of them continuous and part binary.

Neural Networks Features

ANNs are computational programs inspired in the functionality of biological neurons (Fig. siguiente), based on complex mathematical algorithms, which are composed by several layers of intelligent nodes called Neurons and which have the capability to find relationships between the input layers (containing the independent variables or predictors) and the output layer (containing the dependent variable or result) through the management of their respective numeric signals.

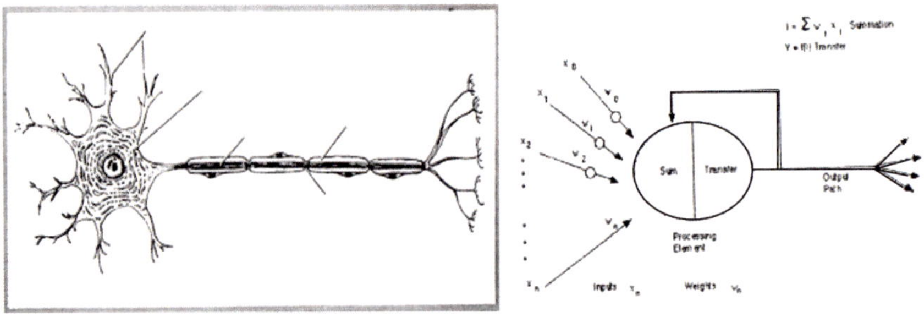

BIOLOGICAL NEURON ARTIFICIAL NEURON

Neurons form "processing units", which are linked among themselves, adopting inner structures similar to a network. Information moves among layers through connections carrying different weights, and there is a training process which attempts to minimize the error between observed and predicted outcomes by modifying those weights. During this training process, the calculated error is back-propagated to the network and weights are conveniently adjusted in order to improve the prediction.

ANNs are techniques applied to pattern recognition through a training based on several different examples, which enables them to model and make predictions in very complex systems. These mathematical techniques are applied to problems classification and temporal series, and they offer the potential of identifying connections that other techniques are not able to perform, because: (1) They use linear and non-linear relationships among data; (2) They model any type of data distribution (not only normal distribution); and (3) They deal with redundant data and/or inconsistencies in the information, missing values, noise and also data constructed from contradictory examples. The capability of manipulating these inaccurate data turns ANNs very effective in the processing of not well regulated information. ANNs could fail in the attempt if: (a) there are no deterministic relationships between the predictors and the expected outcome; (b) if insufficient training has been performed; or (c) if not enough neurons have been used.

We evaluated several network models based on a back-propagation type optimized with genetic algorithms (GA) provided by a commercially available program [52]. This type of ANN selects continuously the best combinations of variables according to the displayed sensitivity among the input and the output one(s). The GA allow to evolve neural network structures while simultaneously searching for significant input variables to maximize the predictive accuracy of the resulting ANN models. Thus, the user does not need to spend too much time attempting to find the best networks, significant input variables and performing other neural network development efforts manually.

In particular, some features of the used software deserve to be mentioned. Through the main screen one has the ability to import data (which need to be previously adequately edited), run the optimization search (there is an option to use the standard back-propagation or the optimized one), view the system activity, trends, plots, and finally, one has also the ability to change genetic, neural and system configuration. During a run, the program provides the ability to view the status of what is happening, view the evolving population, see the configurations and statistics of the top ten network models found so far, observe learning curves and view reports on the specifics of the system setup and the resulting top networks.

In Fig. 14.1 the trend of neural learning is shown. The graph helps to observe the progress of training. By observing the nature of the curves created as training progresses, one can get an idea of the degree the ANN is able to learn the relationships between inputs and output. For example, a flat or highly jagged curve indicates difficulty in learning while a smooth asymptotic curve that ramps up (for accuracy) or down (for error) shows that the network is strongly able to learn. During a run, different types of curves are possible to be seen, as alternative network structures are being evaluated.

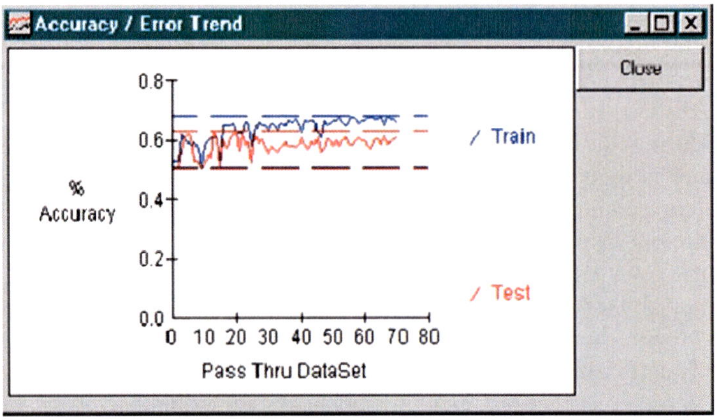

Fig. 14.1 Training and testing trends

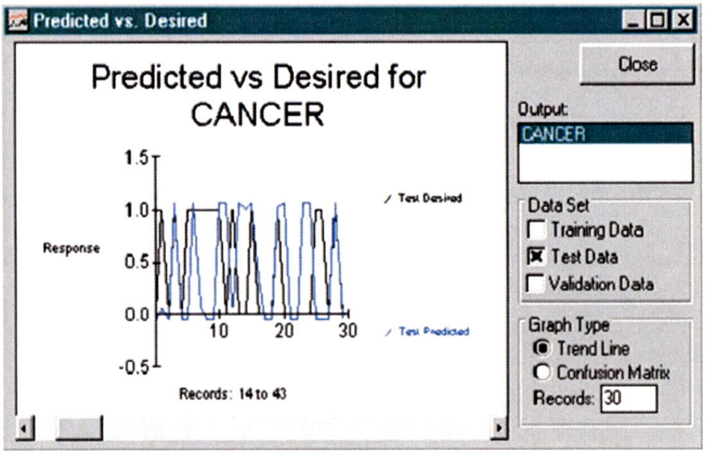

Fig. 14.2 Predicted vs. desired (expected) outputs

Figure 14.2 shows a graph of the window that enables one to view predicted (the actual network's output) vs. expected (the outputs as defined in the user's data) values of the currently training network's output. The option of "trend line" is herewith shown, where the X axis is the record number and the Y axis is the value in the original data range. There is also an option to select to view the values for the current training, testing and/or validation data sets, and another option to change the edit box from the total sample to a number or records that one considers as more appropriate to make the observations.

Network models worked with 16 up to 256 nodes in only one hidden layer. Logistic activation functions (sigmoid) are recognized as very adequate for a dichotomous outcome [53] (e.g. 0 = no and 1 = yes) and we used them for the recent studies.

As with logistic regressions, we ran different models of ANN which were consecutively performed for each group of variables. All networks were trained with a randomly selected subset of patients (from 50% to 84%), while the other subset (from 16% to 50%) was used to test each model. Taking into account this split, it represented acceptable ratios observations/variables in each step of training and testing [53]. A minimum number of 15 iterations and a maximum of 110 were established for each network. A training stop was set after 30 iterations without finding a new maximum accuracy. Besides, we also established the searching stop for a prespecified value of 100% for the overall accuracy (which has been never accomplished) and the cutpoint for classification of patients was 0.5, which means that values between 0 and 0.49 correspond to not cancer and values between 0.51 and 1 to cancer. Particular features of the procedure like learning rates were established with default values (0.1–0.8), as well as the momentum (0.1–0.6) whereas the mutations type and value were set by random exchange of 20%.

Some comments are needed to explain the preceding features. The speed of learning is governed by the learning rate. If this is increased too much, learning becomes unstable; the net oscillates back and forth across the error minimum. One way of overcoming the limitations thus imposed is to alter the training rule from "pure" gradient descent to include a term which includes a proportion of the last weight change. Thus, if the previous weight change was large, so will be the new one. That is, the weight change carries along some momentum to the next iteration. This has a tendency to smooth out small fluctuations in the error-weight space (it is a low-pass filter).

Besides, GA are used by the software to search for or "evolve" neural networks to maximize some objective function, such as accuracy. The ANNs that have been developed are evaluated and selected on their ability to predict based on data. GA are a cyclic process which consists of several steps: creating an initial population of "genotypes" (a genetic representation of ANN); building the neural networks ("phenotypes") based on genotypes; training and testing the ANN to determine how good they are; comparing the fitness of networks and keeping the top 10 (the best ones); selecting those networks in the population which are better (population is the name given to the "chromosomes", representing the input variables used and the network structures); refilling the population back to the defined size; pairing up the genotypes of the ANN; "mating" the genotypes by exchanging genes (features) of the networks; finally, "mutating" the genotypes in some random fashion. Afterwards, the process begins from the 2° step and is continued until some stopping criteria or a manual stop of it. Methodology and results are described in detail in the original paper [44], and the theoretical basis of the proposal was also mentioned in a previous paper [41].

Table 14.1 shows the list of selected input variables: food items, nutrients or related items, gynecological and socio-demographical variables with the corresponding p-values for differences between cancers and controls without cancer. Features are described in detail also in the original source [44]. Some variables that were not significant from a statistical viewpoint have been excluded from the original table: age of first live birth (p=0.10), educational level (p=0.08), carbohydrates

Table 14.1 Selected input variables used in the ANN models of risk analysis (For complete details see Ref. [41])

	P value
Gynecoobstetric variables	
Age at menarche	0.006
Number of live births	<0.001
Nulliparous (yes-no)	0.002
Benign breast diseases (yes-no)	0.040
Number of ovulatory cycles	0.006
Total breastfeeding (months)	0.006
Sociodemographic and familial variables	
Breast cancer in mother	<0.001
Breast cancer in aunts	0.001
Familial score	<0.001
Dietary variables	
Proteins	<0.001
Total fat	<0.001
Saturated fat	<0.001
Energy (kcal)	<0.001
Ratio energy/BMI	<0.001
Hard liquor (drinker status)	0.021
Wine (drinker status)	0.043
Alcohol (drinker status)	0.012
Tea	0.016
Linolenic acid	<0.001
Linoleic acid	<0.001
Ratio linoleic/linolenic	<0.001
Polenta	0.011
Beef consumption	<0.001
Fried meat	<0.001
Barbecue	<0.001
Lamb	0.008
Liver	<0.001
Mortadella sausage	<0.001
Cow meat	<0.001
Fried eggs	0.050
Boiled eggs	<0.001
Milk	0.001
Butter	<0.001
Lentils	0.050
Calabash	0.027
Spinach	0.023
Lettuce	0.013
Rice pudding	0.028
Bread	0.011
Cholesterol	0.005

Table 14.2 Best results obtained with ANNs and logistic regressions

Neural networks		
Variables	P.P.V. (%)	N.P.V.(%)
FAM	65.04	87.88
GYN	87.55	50.75
FAM+GYN	69.45	88.30
Nut	58.03	85.11
Food	87.55	83.95
All	93.14	97.64
Logistic regressions		
Variables	P.P.V. (%)	N.P.V. (%)
FAM	39.29	83.43
GYN	65.93	58.43
FAM+GYN	58.52	67.42
Nut	64.84	70.22
Food	70.88	72.75
All	73.90	75.00

(p=0.06), salt-cured meat (p=0.09), stew (p=0.10), bakery products (p=0.08), dulce de leche (caramel) (p=0.09), ice cream (p=0.09), soft drinks (p=0.11) and "mate" (a local herbal infusion) (p=0.08).

Results

In Table 14.2 the best models of ANN are shown, according to their positive predictive value (PPV) and negative predictive value (NPV) results and for each one of the groups of variables. Definitions of predictive values are as follows:

PPV is the probability that someone with a positive screening test result really has the disease, according to the formula PPV=True positives/true+false positives

NPV is the probability that someone with a negative screening test result really has not the disease, according to the formula NPV=True negatives/true+false negatives

The columns include the following information: variable groups, PPV and NPV. Best results were obtained with the proposed ANN using 50–52 input variables (initially all of them having included the 59 inputs): the best NPV (97.64%) and PPV (93.14%) were achieved using networks with logistic neurons for the output function. Other ANN models obtained around 90% for any of the predictive values

Table 14.2 also displays the best results obtained by logistic regressions for each group of variables. Results were improved when using all variables, though the best ones (PPV 73.90% and NPV 75.00%) were achieved including between 45 and 47 items.

Best results of ANN and logistic regressions are shown in Fig. 14.3, based on their respective best PPV and NPV. Both systems found the best predictive performance considering the inclusion (at least initially) of all variables, both displayed

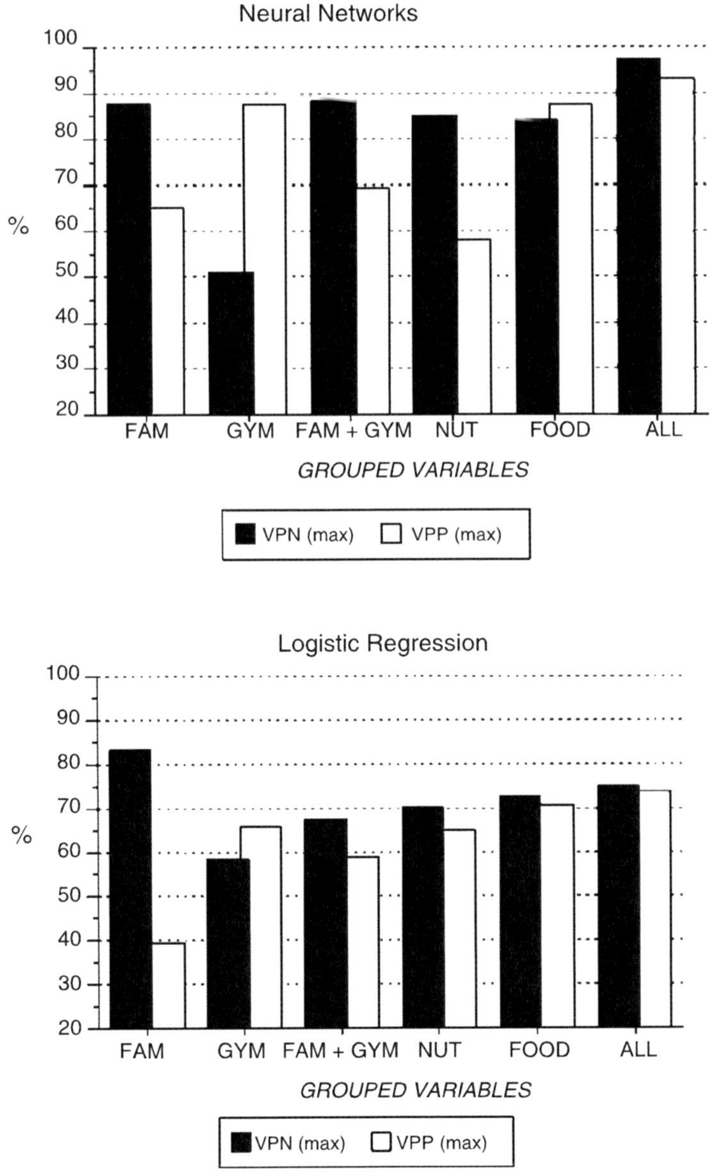

Fig. 14.3 Comparison of performances obtained with ANNs (*up*) and logistic regressions (*down*)

high discrimination using food items and both also achieved a narrow difference between predictive values. Nonetheless, results obtained by ANN were finally around 20% better than logistic regressions.

The inclusion of 31 food items, 15 nutrients or dietary constituents (total kilocalories, proteins, carbohydrates, saturated fat, cholesterol, fatty acids, among others), together with 13 items of gyneco-obstetric, socio-demographic and family cancer history allowed the achievement of a high-level prediction for the considered sample, showing the usefulness of some variables that may not be necessarily risk factors but play a role as discriminant ones. Results confirmed the findings of our previous reports [41, 44], the first one of which had included 39 dietary variables and 15 more belonging to the other groups. The current study showed a PPV of 93.14% and a NPV of 97.64% which evidences that high proportions of cases have fitted to the classification category in which the ANN located them.

Previous attempts to selective screenings were based on few variables [22–31], mainly gyneco-obstetric ones. We agree with those authors who say that family history cannot be used as risk classifier, because that would mean to be taking into account about 5–15% of the population and leaving out the other 85–95% [17]. Moreover, gyneco-obstetric factors were not able to overcome an average of 25% of population involved, thus, the same considerations can be stated: around 75% of women would be out of the system [17]. Finally, the inclusion of selected dietary factors was an unsuccessful attempt, perhaps due to the prevalence of some selected habits and consumptions like a high-fat diet [30], something that could have taken statistical differences to the null. These authors recognized that despite their efforts to determine risk factors for BC, they have not appreciably increased the ability to identify substantial numbers of truly high-risk women. Summarily, results were not so good as it was expected beforehand, suggesting us to believe that selection criteria perhaps should be based on a multifactorial basis, according to the principles of convergent and reciprocal causation [54].

A particular model of risk classification based mainly in gyneco-obstetric and familial variables has been created by Gail [55, 56], which is being taken into account as a way of predicting chances of developing a BC within certain time periods in the future. In our opinion, the model assumes that the risk estimates of those variables are the same for the American women and for women from anywhere, and that would mean a similar behaviour of BC in every population.

From this viewpoint, local or regional environmental factors (diet and lifestyle included) are not being taken into account for its prediction and such exclusion means to us having an uncomplete information. If environmental factors are considered important in the occurrence and evolution of BC, we think that they should not be excluded at least a priori from the different models of risk assessment.

Gynecoobstetric variables did not show remarkable results for the regression, and this should be taken into account as a possible explanation for what was mentioned above about selective screenings. On the contrary, ANN could reach rather good PPV (between 73.9% and 87.6%) only with this group of variables. Besides, food items, more than nutrients, seemed to be good discriminant in our sample: they overcame 70% of both predictive values in logistic regressions and more than 80% in ANN, narrowing the distance between the highest values in each analysis system. Data displayed on Fig. 14.3 allows us to have a graphical perspective of the predictive capabilities that ANN and logistic regressions showed. The analysis has taken advantage of the discriminant value of food items, showing that their inclusion in the different models improved substantially the final accuracy. Although the issues of fat, saturated fat, fatty foods and BC have not been already elucidated and it is still under controversy their eventual role as risk factors [57], we recognize the important value of these variables (as well as other ones) playing a discriminant role between cancer patients and controls. In other words, there are some elements which differentiate two profiles (mainly lifestyle, familial and dietary) from an apparently homogeneous population. Perhaps this applies mainly to Western populations, who are characterized by some particular nutritional styles, but it allows thinking on terms of classification tools to be utilized in an attempt of selection of risk population.

In our opinion, the key issue to be addressed in order to improve the efficiency of selective screenings is the number of considered variables. We still do not know how the increase of prediction accuracy does evolve through the increase of the amount of variables, if it is a linear function, or an asymptotic one, or some other type. Anyway, a sigmoid (linear) function was already described for some combinations of variables in one of the above quoted papers [29].

Figure 14.4 explains from a graphical viewpoint what we stated before. Being situated in the lower left corner, we are managing few variables and therefore achieving a low discriminant capability. On the upper right corner, examples managing high amount of variables allowed to achieve a high discriminant capability (examples of Djordjevic [33, 34] and ours [41, 44]). The corollary of working with different methodologies was that both studies led us to the idea of two levels of risk: a population level, achieved by using a few discriminant variables, and an individual level, achieved by using a high number of discriminant variables (Fig. 14.5). We also make ourselves the question if there is any critical mass of data over which the accuracy of classification is particularly improved.

Further questions arise from these observations. If BC is a multifactorial disease, why should one think that a unifactorial classifier (age) or an oligofactorial classifier (gynecoobstetrics, reproductive, family history, etc., considered individually) might be the best ones? Couldn't be wrong an excessively simplified focus, from a conceptual viewpoint? Couldn't be necessary to manage a multilevel classification? In this sense, the use of ANN has meant an adequate management of variables which are related in a complex form. Neural networks are recognized as capable to address complex factor relationships where linear models are not enough to define them [53]. We consider BC as an example of an outcome from such complex interactions of factors, in other words, of risk and protective factors.

Networks can express hidden patterns of associations of variables that perhaps are not statistically risk or protective factors (others which can be considered as indicators but are not risk factors by themselves, like for example educational level), but who are valuable discriminants. The comparison of results with ANN and a logistic regression is reassuring these facts and show that ANN could find combinations among variables that are finally more discriminant for both subpopulations involved. Logistic regressions are the commonest form of analysis used to compare to ANN, mainly due to the linearity of their algorithms. Indeed, they represent linear discriminant models which belong to orthodox statistics. Besides, the use of back-propagation ANN with logistic activation function allowed the authors to achieve

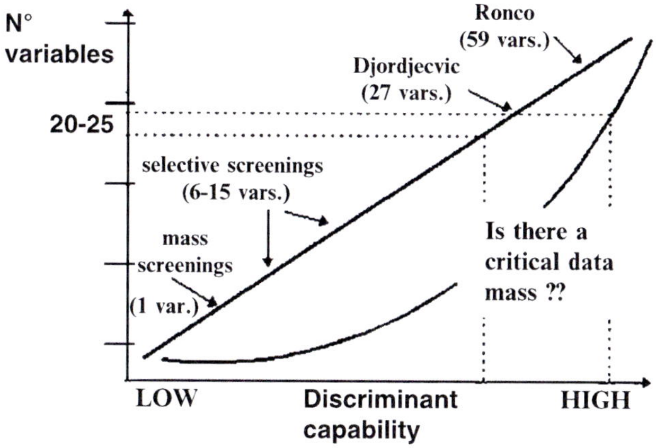

Fig. 14.4 A theoretical approach of the relationship between the amount of information used and the discriminant capability within screenings

Fig. 14.5 Interpretation of risk levels according to the amount of information used and the discriminant capability achieved

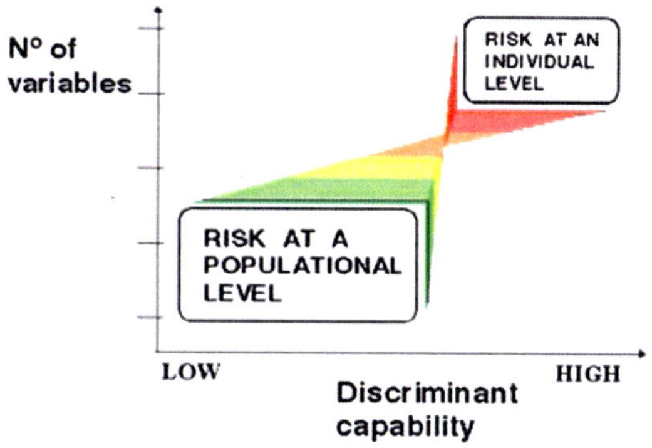

the best possible results for a dichotomized outcome, as we have already reported in the communications on BC [40–44, 58, 59] and in further studies on prostate cancer [60, 61], dementias [62] and osteoporosis [63].

Some limitations should be recognized to the proposed methodology. First, complexity and length of the questionnaire form requires the use of interviewers in order to reduce possible biases inherent to self-administered questionnaires. These latter ones are forms given to study subjects who are asked to complete them, they are one of the cheapest ways of collecting information, but also have the limitation that they can be used only in literate populations and the researcher has relatively little control on the data quality. Thus, this means that trained personnel is needed to perform the above quoted interviews and to process data in the computer, in order to avoid those limitations. Second, the database involved information from the low socio-economic-cultural strata who are admitted to public hospitals, a subset of Uruguayan women in which only about 20–25% of all incident BC cases occur. Therefore, the results should not be extrapolated to the pre-paid healthcare subpopulations, because dietary, socio-demographic and cultural patterns from the first ones might not correspond to these latter ones, who represent the other 75–80%. Furthermore, it would not be either adequate to extrapolate the patterns to other geographic regions or countries, something that emphasizes the relatively important role of environmental factors [15].

Taking into account the potential costs of implementing a screening programme, ANNs can be valuable tools with capabilities of classifying women with estimated high and low risks of BC. Network models including dietary information could operate as guidelines to select those asymptomatic women to be entered into a mammographic screening programme, as well as, for example, to receive adequate nutritional advice in those cases where dietary patterns imply a high risk, as well as to receive a chemoprevention as an attempt of simultaneous primary prevention. Another destination of the generated information could be the therapeutic optimization, that is, towards a tertiary prevention. In current days, maybe the best example of this latter could be the chance of selecting women in order to apply a strategy of double prevention, BC and osteoporosis, through the administration of raloxifene (a drug whose profile suggests that in the future could be more frequently taken into account).

A population-based pilot study to test the herewith proposed methodology would be required in order to demonstrate the feasibility of an intelligent selective BC screening programme, which was for the first time proposed, to our knowledge, by one of the authors [43]. The addition of new information, as anthropometry and serum levels of substances as vitamin D, lipids, insulin, among others, for example, could expand the possibilities for an ultra-selective methodology like the one herewith presented, and of course, it is reasonable to think that the accuracy in the risk classification could be even higher. All these points were taken into consideration as a previous step to the design of the Risk Profile Report, which is described in a separate chapter. These are tasks which could be developed in the future, if circumstances are appropriate.

References

1. Parkin DM, Whelan SL, Ferlay J et al (eds) (2002) Cancer incidence in five continents, vol VIII, IARC Scientific Publications No. 155. IARC, Lyon
2. Cole P, MacMahon B (1969) Oestrogen fractions during early reproductive life in the aetiology of breast cancer. Lancet 1:604–606
3. Layde PM, Webster LA, Baughman AL (1989) The independent associations of parity, age at first full term pregnancy, and duration of breast-feeding with the risk of breast cancer. J Clin Epidemiol 42:963–973
4. Trichopoulos D, MacMahon B, Cole P (1972) Menopause and breast cancer risk. J Natl Cancer Inst 48:605–613
5. Brinton LA, Hoover R, Fraumeni JF Jr (1982) Interaction of familial and hormonal risk factors for breast cancer. J Natl Cancer Inst 69:817–822
6. Newman B, Austin MA, Lee M, King MC (1988) Inheritance of human breast cancer. Evidence for autosomal dominant transmission in high-risk families. Proc Nat Acad Sci (Wash) 85:3044–3048
7. Longnecker MP, Berlin JA, Orza MJ (1988) A meta-analysis of alcohol consumption in relation to risk of breast cancer. JAMA 260:652–656

8. Willett WC, Stampfer MJ, Colditz GA (1987) Moderate alcohol consumption and the risk of breast cancer. N Engl J Med 316:1174–1179
9. Dupont WD, Page DL (1987) Breast cancer risk associated with proliferative disease, age at first birth, and a family history of breast cancer. Am J Epidemiol 125:769–779
10. Monson RR, Yen S, MacMahon B (1976) Chronic mastitis and carcinoma of the breast. Lancet 2:224–226
11. Colditz GA, Stampfer MJ, Willett WC (1990) Prospective study of estrogen replacement therapy and risk of breast cancer in postmenopausal women. JAMA 264:2648–2653
12. Meirik O, Lund E, Adami HO (1986) Oral contraceptive use and breast cancer in young women: a joint national case-control study in Norway and Sweden. Lancet 2:650–654
13. Miller DR, Rosenberg L, Kaufman DW (1989) Breast cancer before age 45 and oral contraceptive use: new findings. Am J Epidemiol 129:269–280
14. World Cancer Research Fund (1997) Food, nutrition and the prevention of cancer: a global perspective. American Institute for Cancer Research, Washington DC, pp 252–287
15. Ronco AL, De Stéfani E, Stoll M (2010) Hormonal and metabolic modulation through nutrition: towards a primary prevention of breast cancer. Breast 19:322–332
16. Day NE, Miller AB (1988) Screening for breast cancer. International union against cancer. Hans Huber Publishers, Stuttgart, pp 119–121
17. Jatoi I (1997) Breast cancer screening. Medical intelligence unit. Landes Bioscience, Austin, pp 9–34
18. Shapiro S (1994) Screening: assessment of current studies. Cancer 74:231–238
19. Kopans DB (1996) Mammography screening for women ages 40-49: the controversy and the facts. In: Proceedings of the 32nd annual meeting of the ASCO, educational book. Philadelphia, pp 142–145
20. Parkin DM, Day NE (1985) Evaluating and planning screening programmes. In: Parkin DM, Wagner G, Muir C (eds) The role of the registry in cancer control, IARC Scientific Publications N°66. International Agency for Research on Cancer, Lyon, pp 45–63
21. Mettlin C (1994) The relationship of breast cancer epidemiology to screening recommendations. Cancer 74:228–230
22. Schechter MT, Miller AB, Baines CJ et al (1986) Selection of women at high risk of breast cancer for initial screening. J Chron Dis 39(4):253–260
23. Torner J, Fernández Martínez I, Granell J et al (1996) Mass screening versus selective screening. Rev Senologia y Patol Mam 10(1):31–43, in Spanish
24. Dunn JE (1969) Epidemiology and possible identification of high-risk groups that could develop cancer of the breast. Cancer 23:775–780
25. Shapiro S, Goldberg J, Venet L et al (1973) Risk factors in breast cancer –a prospective study. In: Doll R, Vodopia J (eds) Host environment interactions in the etiology of cancer in man, IARC Scientific Publication N°7. IARC, Lyon, pp 169–182
26. Farewell VT (1977) The combined effect of breast cancer risk factors. Cancer 40:931–936
27. Wolfe JN (1976) Breast parenchymal patterns and their changes with age. Radiology 121:545–552
28. Fournier D, Kuttig H, Müller A et al (1977) Brustkrebsfrüherkennung: Kontrolle von Risikogruppen oder Massescreening –wer soll geröntgt werden? Med Welt 28:359–363
29. Soini I, Hakama M (1978) Failure of selective screening for breast cancer by combining risk factors. Int J Cancer 22:275–281
30. Seidman H, Stellman SD, Mushinski MH (1982) A different perspective on breast cancer risk factors: some implications of the non attributable risk. CA- Cancer J Clin 32(5):301–313
31. Toti A, Piffanelli A, Pavanelli CN et al (1980) Possible indication of breast cancer risk through discriminant functions. Cancer 46(5):1280–1285
32. Chart PL, Franssen E (1997) Management of women at increased risk for breast cancer: preliminary results from a new program. CMAJ 157(9):1235–1242
33. Djordjevic M, Vuletic L, Jovicevic-Bekic A et al (1994) Follow-up of risk groups for breast cancer 1990–2000. In: Sankaranarayanan R, Wahrendorf J, Demaret E (eds) Directory of ongoing research in cancer epidemiology 1994, IARC Scientific Publications N° 130. International Agency for Research on Cancer, Lyon, p 510, abstract 1242

34. Djordjevic M, Babic M, Drecun V et al (1999) Results of the questionnaired selective screening for the breast cancer. In: Proceedings of the I conference on screening and early detection of cancer, development of a European strategy, Viena, p.39, Abstract 9006
35. Ronco AL, Carámbula JA (1998) The breast cancer risk score: in search of high-risk premenopausal women for screening. X international congress on senology, Oporto. Breast J 4(Suppl 1): 17 (abstract N° 331)
36. Waschulzik T, Quandt K, Lewis M et al(1993) Evaluation of an epidemiological data set as an example of the application of neural networks to the analysis of large medical data sets. In: Andreassen S et al (eds) Artificial intelligence in medicine, proceedings of the fourth European conference on artificial intelligence in medicine Europe, IOS, Amsterdam, pp 466–476
37. Speight PM, Elliott AE, Jullien JA et al (1995) The use of artificial intelligence to identify people at risk of oral cancer and precancer. Br Dent J 179:382–387
38. Ioannidis JP, McQueen PG, Goedert JJ et al (1998) Use of neural networks to model complex immunogenetic associations of disease: human leukocyte antigen impact on the progression of human immunodeficiency virus infection. Am J Epidemiol 147:464–471
39. Hammad TA, Abdel Wahab MF, Declaris N et al (1996) Comparative evaluation of the use of artificial neural networks for modelling the epidemiology of schistosomiasis mansoni. Trans R Soc Trop Med Hyg 90(4):372–376
40. Ronco AL (1998) Evaluation of classificatory capabilities of an artificial neural network in search of breast cancer risk populations: a pilot study. X international congress on senology, Oporto. Breast J 4(Suppl 1): 22 (abstract N° 120)
41. Ronco AL (1999) Use of artificial neural networks in modeling associations of discriminant factors: towards an intelligent selective breast cancer screening. Artif Intell Med 16(3):299–309
42. Ronco AL (1999) Discriminating breast cancer high-risk individuals with artificial neural networks: a novel approach to selective screenings. In: Proceedings of the I conference on screening and early detection of cancer, development of a European strategy, Viena, p 51. Abstract 9030
43. Ronco AL (1999) Artificial intelligence-based screening for breast cancer: a pilot project. In: Proceedings of the I conference on screening and early detection of cancer, development of a European strategy, Viena, p 37. Abstract 9001
44. Ronco AL, De Stéfani E (1999) Role of classical and dietary discriminant factors for classification of breast cancer high-risk populations: a study with neural networks. Cancer Strategy 1:203–209
45. Ronco AL, De Stéfani E, Mendilaharsu M et al (1996) Meat, fat and the risk of breast cancer: a case-control study from Uruguay. Int J Cancer 65:328–331
46. De Stéfani E, Ronco AL, Mendilaharsu M et al (1997) Meat intake, heterocyclic amines, and risk of breast cancer: a case-control study in Uruguay. Cancer Epidemiol Biomarkers Prev 6:573–581
47. Ronco AL, De Stéfani E (1999) Phytoestrogens and risk of breast cancer: a case-control study. Rev Med Urug 15(2):94–102, in Spanish
48. De Stéfani E, Correa P, Ronco AL et al (1997) Dietary fiber and risk of breast cancer. A case-control study in Uruguay. Nutr Cancer 28(1):14–19
49. Ronco AL, De Stéfani E, Boffetta P et al (1999) Vegetables, fruits, and related nutrients and risk of breast cancer: a case control study in Uruguay. Nutr Cancer 35(2):111–119
50. De Stéfani E, Deneo-Pellegrini H, Mendilaharsu M et al (1998) Essencial fatty acids and breast cancer: a case-control study in Uruguay. Int J Cancer 76:491–494
51. Spss/PC+Version 5.0 for D.O.S (1992) SPSS Inc, Michigan
52. NeuroGenetic Optimizer Version 2.5 for Windows (1995) BioComp Systems Inc. Redmond
53. Tu JV (1996) Advantages and disadvantages of using artificial neural networks versus logistic regression for predicting medical outcomes. J Clin Epidemiol 49:1225–1231
54. Anderson NB (1998) Levels of analysis in health science: a framework for integrating sociobehavioral and biomedical research. In: McCann SM (ed) Neuroimmunomodulation: molecular aspects, integrative systems and clinical advances, vol 840, Annals of the New York Academy Science. New York Academy of Sciences, New York, pp 563–576

55. Gail MH, Brinton LA, Byar DP et al (1989) Projecting individualized probabilities of developing breast cancer for white females who are being examined annually. J Natl Cancer Inst 81:1879–1886
56. Constantino JP, Gail MH, Pee D et al (1999) Validation studies for models projecting the risk of invasive and total breast cancer incidence. J Natl Cancer Inst 91:1541–1548
57. Wu AH (2000) Diet and breast carcinoma in multiethnic populations. Cancer 88(S5):1239–1244
58. Ronco AL, Carámbula JA (1998) Classificatory improvement of a breast clinical screening programme by application of an artificial neural network: a pilot study. X international congress on senology, Oporto. Breast J, 4(Suppl 1): 21 (abstract N° 332)
59. Ronco AL, Quarneti A, Febles G et al (2010) Anthropometric variables as risk classificators of breast cancer: comparing neural networks and logistic regressions. XVI World congress on breast diseases, Valencia, 20–22 Oct 2010
60. Ronco AL, Fernández W, Aparicio D et al (1997) Diagnostic optimization of the transrectal ultrasonography by application of an artificial neural network: preliminary results. VIII congress of the world federation of ultrasound in medicine and biology, Buenos Aires, Ultrasound Med Biol, 23(Suppl 1): S58
61. Ronco AL, Fernández R (1999) Improving ultrasonographic diagnosis of prostate cancer with neural networks. Ultrasound Med Biol 25(5):729–733
62. Ronco AL, Sosa Alvarez A (2000) Uso de redes neurales artificiales en la orientación diagnóstica de las demencias: resultados preliminares. Publicación oficial del I Congreso Uruguayo de Neurología. Punta del Este, Uruguay, 10–12 Aug 2000, p 168
63. Ronco AL, Hernández J, Mendoza B (2001) Preselection of women with high risk of osteoporosis with artificial neural networks: a pilot study. Proceedings of the II international congress of bone and mineral metabolism, Rio de Janeiro, 25–27 Oct 2001

Part III
Future Perspectives

Chapter 15
Primary Prevention of Breast Cancer: A New Challenge

Many people still do not know or place obliquely the importance of other risk factors which are different from the classic ones (menstrual-reproductive history, family history of cancer). As a consequence, the former ones could appear as inexistent. Despite any kind of purpose of such attitude – a fact that we will not analyze here – we should remark that it has an important weight for the public opinion and also at an individual level, especially if comments proceed from specialists who can be considered as opinion leaders.

It is a positive fact to recognize and emphasize that BC is an essentially preventable tumour, through the different ways that prevention can be developed. Primary prevention attempts to reduce the incidence of the disease through a reduction in the exposure to risk factors and through a simultaneous increase in exposure to protective factors.

The main goal of this chapter is to consider within realistic terms what could be expected from primary prevention to be achieved in a close future. In this sense, we would recommend the readers to see a recent review performed by us, which was focused on the nutritional potential for modulating hormones and metabolism [1]. Posing certain futuristic scenarios as for example telomerase or apoptosis manipulation or some other types of molecular processes does not correspond to the focus of our present work, but also it would mean remaining in merely theoretical stages of the problem when we are actually interested in improving certain aspects from a practical viewpoint.

There are currently different strategies of primary prevention, which are handled for given cases of high risk, mainly of genetic background. There is the prophylactic mastectomy, a surgical procedure destined to remove both mammary glands and replacing them by internal synthetic prostheses. There is also chemoprevention, by the administration of substances which occupy the place of female hormones or that change the circumstances of their receptors. In addition, there are sophisticated therapies at a genetic-molecular level which are being projected to the future. All of the quoted strategies share a common goal, which is **stopping the initiation or promotion of the cancer process**. In the present work we are not

A.L. Ronco and E. De Stéfani, *Nutritional Epidemiology of Breast Cancer*,
DOI 10.1007/978-94-007-2397-9_15, © Springer Science+Business Media B.V. 2012

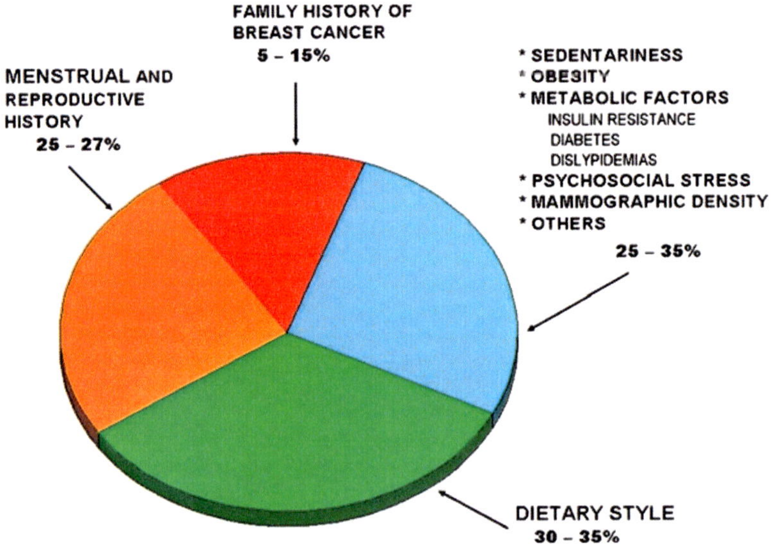

Fig. 15.1 Known risk factors of breast cancer

focusing these modalities – which have their respective specialists, like the surgeon or the oncologist – but on the impact on modifiable environmental factors.

In BC inherited elements linked to the family history are recognized as responsible of 5% and no more than 15% of cases. The group of menstrual and reproductive factors is attributed with around 25% of responsibility. Considered together, these classic risk factors – which could still be called not modifiable factors – explain between 30% and 40% of cases. Most of the rest are environmental modifiable factors, and they correspond to a 60–70%. Of these, diet is considered the most important one. It is accepted that a risk reduction through influencing dietary factors can reach a 30–35% of the whole risk. The rest of factors include: excess weight and obesity, metabolic factors (i.e. insulin resistance, low serum vitamin D level, dislypidemia, diabetes), sedentariness or low level of physical activity and psychosocial stress among other possible factors. The Figure summarizes the current risks that could be recognized for BC (Fig. 15.1).

Seven decades ago an experimental study found a higher incidence of BC in rats which were fed with a high-fat diet [2]. Over time, the scientific knowledge recognized that also high-energy diets tended to be associated with higher risks of the disease. Then some of the most powerful indicators relating diet to the etiology of BC emerged from ecologic and migrant studies, which demonstrated that migrants tended to acquire those cancer patterns belonging to the host countries [3]. The occurrence of the disease needed some time period to be modified: there were no substantial changes of BC incidence for the first-generation immigrants, but those expected changes would be probable found among the 2nd and 3rd generations [4].

Such time delay suggested a strong influence of factors linked to lifestyle, like nutrition, during the childhood period. This influence on the risk of BC enabled to consider the possible existence of long latency periods for the disease in which carcinogenic factors would exert their action. In the 90s two studies on migrants in Uruguay agreed with the existing literature, since they found that there were increased incidence risks for foreign Spanish and Italian residents in Uruguay compared to those ones of their home countries [5], and older mean ages – between 10 years and 15 years – were reported for cancer mortality among foreign women compared to the Uruguayan ones [6].

Nevertheless, large epidemiologic studies also reported that there was no association between fat intake and BC. Researchers observed later that the core of the problem was not centred in the total amount of fat but in the fat type, from the viewpoint of its chemical structure (saturated, monounsaturated, polyunsaturated).

In recent years, an international expert panel reported that nutritional features and their relationship with BC were not well established, with few exceptions like alcohol consumption and obesity among postmenopausal women [7]. The quoted report confirmed somehow certain points which had been posed a decade before [8], limiting the dietary recommendations only to general ones, which promoted reduced intake of red meats replacing them with white meats and also a frequent intake of plant foods (vegetables and fruits). This scheme would have two advantages: it can be easily understandable for everybody and it supposes a minimal strategy of primary prevention of cancer.

We had initially agreed in general terms with the quoted guidelines, however, more recently our concept about white meat white in replacement of red meat is rather different. In first place, any type of meat which is exposed to direct heat produces heterocyclic amines in its surface: it does not appear to be healthier the intake of white meat than the one of red meat. Second, if animals are fed with corn- or sorghum-enriched rations, their meat and fat will have an imbalance of Ω-6/Ω-3 PUFA. Hence, meat with source in poultry fed under these conditions would not be potentially healthier than cattle fed freely with green leaves and wild seeds.

Most specialized scientific studies on BC proceed from developed countries (e.g. North America, European Union, Oceania, Israel), understandable if we combine high incidences of the disease together with logistic resources for research. Anyway, this fact could be seen as a limitation by itself regarding the information derived from such studies. The main reason could be that environmental factors (diet included) are not the same in the developing world than in the developed one. Ethnic differences belong to local factors which could have influence in the process of developing a cancer. Beyond races, genomic research is constantly tending to wipe out the paradigm of the "average subject" who fits all situations. We should accept that some constitutive differences among individuals can make the difference: although menstrual and reproductive factors have reached a universal status, nutrition has not. In particular, remarkable differences might exist in the case of developing countries and as a consequence, perhaps a fraction of the information coming from the developed nations is not always applicable.

Besides, it is not mandatory to be a developing country to have low incidence rates: Japan has lower rates than Western countries from the Northern hemisphere. On the contrary, some Latin American countries as Uruguay, Argentina and Brazil stand out from the rest due to their higher rates. A continuous urbanization process combined together with improvements in the educational levels, higher industrialization and finally remarkable change of habits converge towards an increase of the occurrence of the disease. A sustained presence of women in the job market and higher educational levels are tightly linked to a reduction in the number of pregnancies and births, as well as a delay for having them at a first time and also for more reduced breastfeeding times. These environmental circumstances of urban life are linked to an increase in many outdoor job types which are low-active type when compared to rural ones. As a global consequence, psychosocial stress and high-caloric fast-foods become disruptors of metabolic and hormonal balances, leading to the development of pathologies such as overweight and obesity, insulin resistance and cancer.

Since several years Uruguay is located among those countries with the highest rates in the world [9] and Montevideo, its capital city, displays the highest age-adjusted incidence rate for a city [10]. This small Latin American country is featured by very particular indicators: First, it has a very high level of red meat consumption [11]. Second, it has a high human development index (50° in the world ranking of United Nations) [12]. And third, it has an aged population [13]. In view of these facts, we must accept that a developing country has shown a high occurrence of a disease which is typical of developed countries. Nevertheless, the quoted features describe a society profile that is not a typical one of developing countries. In these latter, the major impact of BC is on women belonging to mid-to-high socioeconomic and cultural classes, who accumulate menstrual- reproductive risk factors with some socio-economic and environmental ones. We have stated that such subpopulations constitute a "first world" within the third world [1]. Montevideo, whose surface reaches around 500 sq km, has a coastal strip of mid-to-high residential areas which in our opinion represents such "first world": its somehow privileged social fraction has a twice higher incidence than the rest of the city [14].

Furthermore, the region involving Uruguay, Argentina and specially Southern Brazil share some staple foods: there is a high consumption of red meat cooked by direct heat like barbecue, beefsteak and hamburgers. In this corner of Latin America meat – mainly red meat – is the axis food of the daily meal and it is a cheaper product than in North America or Europe because its price is lower despite the salaries are so. As an example, women belonging to the mid-to-low social strata who are admitted in the public hospital system in Montevideo have an average meat intake that is comparable to North American women (unpublished data). Conversely, low social classes of other Latin American nations have not developed high BC rates, presumably because while these population subgroups show protective reproductive factors, their dietary profiles have a higher proportion of plant foods, meat is not so accessible due to its high price.

From the perspective of nutrition, some cancers are generally associated to excesses or defects. Typical dietary patterns (Western, high-fat, high-dairy) include high meat intake, an excessive energy intake based on certain fats and refined sugars, as well as low intake of fish, vegetable and fruits. Such patterns, already found and analyzed in Uruguayan women [15, 16], converge along time towards several imbalances which build the proper biological environment to initiate and develop carcinogenesis in susceptible organisms.

Previous knowledge on classic risk factors (menstrual-reproductive history and family history of BC) has led to the idea that women who have been exposed for a longer time period or more intensely to endogenous estrogens will have an increased risk of BC. In fact, estrogens were recognized five decades ago as the main risk factor for developing BC [17]. Estrogens are known for their proliferative effects on estrogen-sensitive tissues resulting in tumorigenesis. Nevertheless, scientific research has shown that nutrition (through diet and body fat excess) together with a low level of physical activity can strongly affect their synthesis and bioavailability, independently from bearing any of the mentioned "classic" risk factors [18, 19].

As with other cancers and other modern, chronic diseases, scientific knowledge has given evidence of a multifactorial background interacting at different levels (biological, socio-cultural, environmental) during years, due to which in certain given conditions a BC will be initiated and promoted. Nowadays, the epidemiologic, clinical and experimental evidence is such that enables us to state that BC is a complex hormonal, metabolic and immune problem. Nevertheless, since the key hormones – the estrogens – were already recognized as the main risk factor for developing BC, it seems that most factors converge towards an inadequate exposure to some of them during an inadequate time period. This is our reason to believe that the ultimate goal of any strategy of primary prevention of BC should be to achieve a hormonal and metabolic modulation through nutritional factors, those which are playing a major role within lifestyle.

More than a decade ago [20] we showed that foods were so good discriminant – and also better- between women with BC and without it as other variables did (menstrual-reproductive, family history, socio-demographic ones), at least for the Uruguayan population. A sample of more than 700 women enabled us to state that the feeding profile had the potential of contributing to define a risk population. Once again we must take into account that even though every adult woman belongs theoretically to the risk population, there are subgroups which can be defined as high-risk, based on the relative importance of certain items in those subgroups. And if we have observed remarkable differences of given intakes between a subset which is afflicted by BC and other subset which has not developed the diseases, then such nutritional profile must be probably playing some role. Although our knowledge about such role is actually incomplete, there is some basis from which it would be possible to take profit. Therefore, we believe that a proposal of dietary changes pointing to a primary prevention of the disease could turn into an extremely useful tool to face an unavoidable need in the modern societies.

This area of research has some philosophical implications, which could be controversial but also deserving our attention: *if the cause is not an only one, it is not wrong to think that the solution is not only either.* The data on menstrual and reproductive factors have led to think that women who exposed themselves much time or more intensely to estrogens increased their risk of developing the disease. And it is so, indeed. However, what is going on with those women who have no menstrual or reproductive risk factors? Could they be also exposed to high levels of estrogens

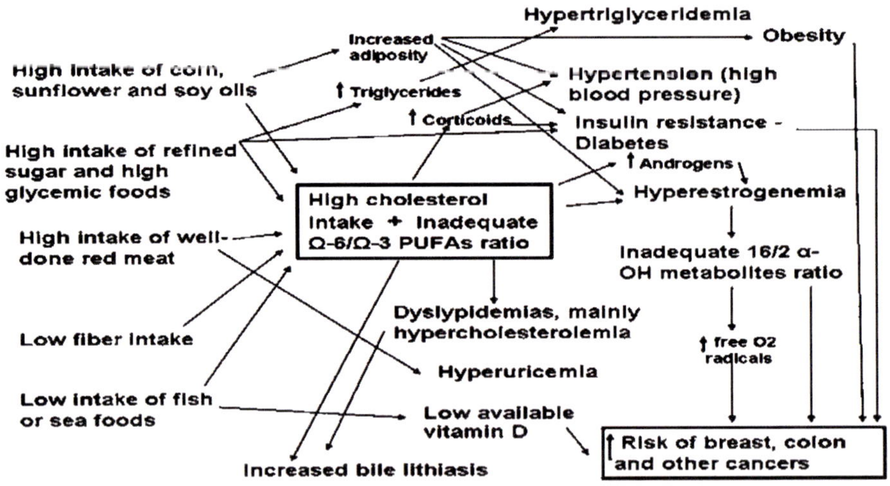

Fig. 15.2 Possible consequences of a Western diet

circulating in their bodies? The answer is yes, they could. The scientific research has evidenced that nutrition and the level of physical activity, as well as weight excess or adequacy can strongly condition the synthesis and availability of hormones.

The pie chart at the beginning of this chapter should be taken into account at this moment. If around 3 or 4 of each ten women with BC have reproductive of family risk factors, there are 6 or 7 that anyway developed the disease without such classical factors. These latter might have had hormonal and metabolic conditions derived from their lifestyle, from which resulted the development of a cancer.

These considerations about risk factors would make more understandable the reasons why Uruguayan women who belong to low socioeconomic strata could also be prone to developing cancer: albeit they have a more favourable reproductive history (several births beginning at early ages, long breastfeeding periods, i.e.) they tend to be overweight, have sedentary lifestyles and display dietary patterns which are more typical of Western developed societies: they have a very high intake of red meat exposed to direct heat (barbecued and grilled), high intake of fatty dairy foods, processed foods, fried foods, together with low intake of fish, fruits and vegetables. In addition, they tend to be obese or overweight, according to international standards. Should their reproductive history be protective, it seems insufficient to antagonize their environmental/lifestyle risk factors. It appears clearly why then those women belonging to low social strata in other Latin American countries have not so much BC, conversely: their diets have bigger proportions of fruits and vegetables, and red meat is not so accessible.

The following scheme (Fig. 15.2) displays in detail the probable consequences of the current Western nutritional style, which we have already described for Uruguayan women [1, 21]. In the central picture two key elements appear: excessive dietary cholesterol and an imbalance of Ω-6/Ω-3 PUFA ratio. The long sequence of metabolic and hormonal events resulting from these two excesses can

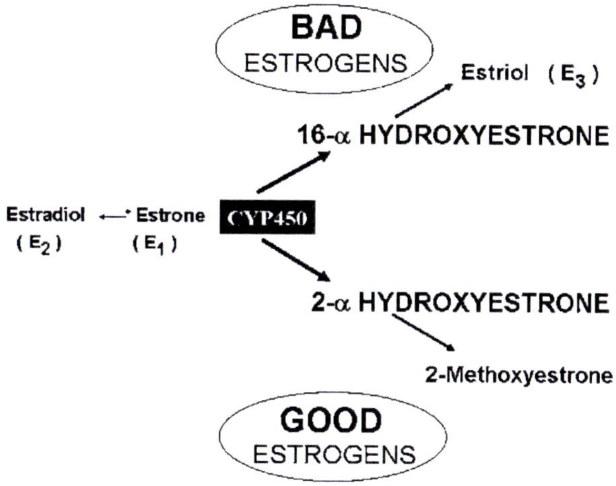

Fig. 15.3 Possible metabolic pathways of estrogens

finally facilitate the beginning and development of several cancers, among them BC, as well as several pathologic states involved in the metabolic syndrome.

The estrogens issue goes further. It is, in fact, a matter of excessive estrogenic "capital". This excess of estrogens represents a potential overnourishment of the mammary tissue. After some estrogens (estradiol and estrone) are synthesized, their life follows one of two possible pathways leading to catechol hormones [22]:

(a) They can derive into very active metabolites, the 16- and 4-α-hydroxy (OH) estrogens (the "bad" ones). Results of experimental research in over the last two decades have shown that a large part of the cancer-inducing effect of estrogen involves the formation of agonistic metabolites of estrogen, especially 16α-OHestrone.
(b) They can form low active compounds, the 2-α-OHestrogens (the "good" ones). These other metabolites, such as 2-α-OHestrone and 2-α-OHestradiol, offer protection against the estrogen-agonist effects of 16-α-OHestrone.

The phase I enzyme cytochrome P-450 (CYP450) – a kind of intracellular metabolic switch – derives the production of metabolites towards one or the other, depending on its state [23]. The initial findings [24] have led other authors to develop a theory [25], which has been supported by newer findings [26].

The following scheme (Fig. 15.3) illustrates better the process:

The "bad" estrogens are believed to have participation in the initiation process (they are genotoxic) as well in the promotion (enhancing cell proliferation). Altogether, having a dual role as substrate for phase I enzymes CYP450 (CYP 1A1 and 1B1) and as ligands for estrogen receptors they promote events that increase the risk of BC. On the contrary, "good" estrogens have also a weak anti-estrogenic capability [26] and this group of "good" estrogens is the one which can be modified. Furthermore, research has found that such CYP450 enzymes oxidize catechol estrogens to semiquinones and quinones, substances with common features of several chemical carcinogens [27, 28]. Especially 3, 4-quinones were postulated as a possible independent risk factor [29]. It has also been hypothesized that genotoxicity caused by the oxidative metabolism of estrogens can be reduced by reactions of metabolites with phase II enzymes, like catechol-o methyl-transferase (COMT) [30] and glutathione S-transferase P1 (GSTP1) [31]. As a consequence of these facts, women who metabolize a large proportion of their estrogens via the 16α-hydroxylation pathway might be at a higher risk of BC [32].

On the other hand, women with BC have an increased production of "bad" estrogens (16- and 4-α-OH metabolites), but conversely, healthy women produce them constantly. It is interesting to remark that the main conversion to 4-α-OHestrogens has been detected in uterine myometrium and benign myomas [33] and in benign and malignant mammary tumors [34]. The 16-α-OH metabolites have a higher affinity for the estrogen receptor (ER) than the 2-α-OH metabolites, while these latter may inhibit angiogenesis [35].

The ratio of 2/16-α-OH metabolites may be a marker for lifestyle influences on estrogen metabolism associated with westernization [36]. In addition, Parl et al. [29], having recognized that each of the phase I and II enzymes contains genetic polymorphisms [37, 38], remarked the possibility of developing better predictive models by integrating known reproductive and lifestyle factors with predicted exposure to estrogen-3,4 quinones determined by inherited variations in genes involved in estrogen metabolism. In our opinion, the 2/16-α-OH metabolites ratio is giving arguments to become an independent risk factor for BC [39]. According to the literature, there would be factors associated with the synthesis of 2-α-OHestrogens, but in opposite directions [40, 41], which exert some sort of actions on the CYP450 estrogenic "switch". On one hand, those factors which increase the risk of BC by reducing the 2/16-α-OH metabolites ratio, such as sedentariness, heritage, obesity, high-fat diet, human papilloma virus, dimethylbenzanthracene, polycyclic aromatic amines and high intake of Ω-6 fatty acids. And on the other hand, those factors which reduce BC risk by increasing the 2/16- α-OH estrogens ratio, such as physical exercise, muscularity, slenderness (low BMI), oil fish, cruciferous vegetables, indole-3-carbinol, diindolylmethane, high intake of Ω-3 fatty acids. Regarding cancers in estrogen-sensitive tissues such as the breast, Ω-6 fatty acids may have opposite effects to those of the Ω-3 series: a high intake of Ω-6 fatty acids linoleic acid and arachidonic acid inhibits the estrogens detoxification by 2-hydroxylation [42] and increases 16α-hydroxylation [43].

The estrogen synthesis occurs not only in the ovaries: after menopause, the suprarenal glands and the adipocytes are the major sources. Far from being an organ destined to be some kind of biological battery (an energy accumulating-releasing device), adipocytes constitute a giant gland which takes useful substances and also produces estrogens. An excess of body fatness is associated with an increased hormonal bioavailability. In addition, androgens which are catched from circulation are also converted into estrogens in the adipocytes through the action of the aromatase (also an enzyme of CYP450), in the process known as **androgen aromatization**. The point here is that an excess of estrogen synthesis means higher probability of producing more "bad" estrogens, which are metabolically very active. Regarding this, modern hormonal therapy through the administration of drugs such as letrozol or anastrozol is attempting to inhibit this process. In addition, obesity creates a doubly favourable environment for mammary carcinogenesis, since insulin requirements and androgen aromatization are stimulated and increased, the latter for producing more estrogens. Aromatization is stimulated bearing an excessive adipose mass, especially in the thighs, buttocks and abdominal-pelvic regions (what we accept as a gynoid-type of obesity), with a high intake of Ω-6 PUFA (mainly derived from common vegetable oils and margarines), and also having increased circulating glucocorticoids [44] (produced under sustained stress, also prescribed for the therapy of inflammatory pathologies). According to research, women require supplemental Indole-3-Carbinol (I3C) at 300–400 mg/day to significantly increase the 2/16- α-OHestrogens ratio [45]. Animal studies showed that diindolylmethane is the active promoter of greater 2-hydroxylation of estrogen associated with a cancer-resistant estrogen metabolism, more than the I3C [40].

As it has been exposed, the main problem for a woman is more complex than simply being highly exposed to hormones. The point is *to be exposed to high levels of some of them* in particular, in addition to the exposure time. It is an accumulative effect, in the sense of amount x time. Excessive and/or "bad" estrogens bind their receptors in those cells where they must take action and generate a cascade of molecular events which after years of influence might increase the risk of developing BC.

Furthermore, when there is an excess of estrogen, although it is eliminated through the bile duct to the intestines, part of it is captured by the liver and returns to the blood system (the enterohepatic circulation) and becomes available once again. The aforementioned situation is even more intense when a woman is afflicted by a slow intestinal transit: the more the stools remain in the bowel, the higher the opportunity of being reabsorbed and reutilized. Women should have some degree of certainty about the destination of such estrogens, attempting to actually eliminate what was thought to be eliminated. Among other reasons, the latter is useful to recognize the benefits of an adequate dietary fibre intake derived from fruits and vegetables.

Based on all the aforementioned concepts, we do not see as adequate to simply accept that a preventive strategy for BC is covered only by having periodical medical consultations and mammograms. We are convinced that achieving an impact on nutrition means doing something else for breast health than early detection. A primary prevention strategy added to secondary prevention will allow for even better results, not only in reducing mortality but also contributing to a reduction in incidence. With the knowledge of the effects of diet on estrogen metabolites, we assume that women may reduce their risk of an estrogen-associated tumour as BC.

After this insight on the influence of nutritional elements in the hormonal origin of BC (elements which could be absolutely modifiable), women who seem to be apparently healthy should be encouraged to make an attempt of changes in their nutritional style, in order to reduce their current risk. This is for us the current challenge of primary prevention of the disease. Moreover, perhaps there is no one only challenge, but actually there are several challenges (i.e. behavioural) to be faced in order to achieve the success of such nutritional prevention. What we are proposing to do in primary prevention of BC is mainly a quantitative and qualitative change in the bioavailability and exposure to the own estrogens, in other words, to manage fewer and better hormones.

References

1. Ronco AL, De Stéfani E, Stoll M (2010) Hormonal and metabolic modulation through nutrition: towards a primary prevention of breast cancer. Breast 19:322–332
2. Tannenbaum A (1942) Genesis and growth of tumors. III. Effects of a high-fat diet. Cancer Res 2:468–475
3. Nelson NJ (2006) Migrant studies aid the search for factors linked to breast cancer risk. J Natl Cancer Inst 98(7):436–438
4. Hemminki K (2003) Genetic and environmental factors in carcinogenesis. In: Vainio HU, Hietanen EK (eds) Mechanisms in carcinogenesis and cancer prevention. Springer, New York, pp 13–21
5. De Stéfani E, Parkin DM, Khlat M et al (1990) Cancer in migrants to Uruguay. Int J Cancer 46:233–237
6. Ronco A, Leibovici S, Vassallo JA (1994) Cancer mortality in migrants to Uruguay. Arch Med Int Urug 16:3107–3112, in Spanish
7. World Cancer Research Fund/American Institute for Cancer Research (2007) Food, nutrition, physical activity, and the prevention of cancer: a global perspective. American Institute for Cancer Research, Washington DC
8. World Cancer Research Fund (1997) Food, nutrition and the prevention of cancer: a global perspective. American Institute for Cancer Research, Washington DC, pp 252–287
9. Ferlay J, Bray F, Pisani P et al (2004) GLOBOCAN 2002: cancer incidence, mortality and prevalence worldwide IARC CancerBase No. 5. Version 2.0. IARC Press, Lyon
10. Parkin DM, Whelan SL, Ferlay J et al (eds) (2002) Cancer incidence in five continents, vol 8, IARC Scientific Publications No. 155. IARC, Lyon
11. Food and Agricultural Organization (2010) http://faostat.fao.org/site/610/Desktop Default.aspx?Page ID¼610#ancor. Accessed 30 Apr 2010
12. United Nations Organization, Program of Human Development (2009) Human development index rankings. Available at http://hdr.undp.org/en/statistics/; 2009. Accessed 27 Apr 10
13. U.S. Census Bureau (2010) International data base, http://www.census.gov/ipc/www/idb/country.php. Accessed 30 Apr 2010
14. Lafon L, Ronco AL (2002) Analysis of geographic distribution of cancer in Montevideo. Rev Med Uruguay 1:36–47, in Spanish
15. Ronco AL, De Stéfani E, Aune D et al (2010) Nutrient patterns and risk of breast cancer in Uruguay. Asian Pac J Cancer Prev 11(2):519–524
16. Ronco AL, De Stéfani E, Deneo-Pellegrini H et al (2010) Dietary patterns and risk of ductal carcinoma of the breast: a factor analysis in Uruguay. Asian Pac J Cancer Prev 11(5):1187–1193
17. MacMahon B, Feinleib M (1960) Breast cancer in relation to nursing and menopausal history. J Natl Cancer Inst 24:733–753
18. Hanf V, Gonder U (2005) Nutrition and primary prevention of breast cancer: foods, nutrients and breast cancer risk. Eur J Obstet Gynecol Reprod Biol 123:139–149
19. Duncan AM (2004) The role of nutrition in the prevention of breast cancer. AACN Clin Issues 15:119–135
20. Ronco AL, De Stéfani E (1999) Role of classic and dietary discriminant factors for classification of breast cancer high-risk populations: a study with neural networks. Cancer Strat 1:203–209
21. Ronco AL, De Stéfani E, Deneo-Pellegrini H et al (eds) (2008) Epidemiología nutricional del cáncer de mama. Ediciones De la Plaza, Montevideo
22. Sepkovic DW, Bradlow HL (2009) Estrogen hydroxylation e the good and the bad. Ann N Y Acad Sci 1155:57–67
23. Fishman J, Osborne MP, Telang NT (1995) The role of estrogen in mammary carcinogenesis. In: Bradlow HL, Osborne MP, Veronesi U (eds) Cancer prevention. Annals of the New York Academy Science, New York, pp 91–100
24. Fishman J, Boyar RM, Hellman L (1975) Influence of body weight on estradiol metabolism in young women. J Clin Endocrinol Metab 41:989–991

25. Bradlow HL, Hershcopf R, Fishman J (1986) Oestradiol 16 alpha-hydroxylase: a risk marker for breast cancer. Cancer Surv 5:573–583
26. Muti P, Bradlow HL, Micheli A et al (2000) Estrogen metabolism and risk of breast cancer: a prospective study of the 2:16 alpha-hydroxyestrone ratio in premenopausal and postmenopausal women. Epidemiology 11:635–640
27. Bolton JL, Trush MA, Penning TM et al (2000) Role of quinones in toxicology. Chem Res Toxicol 13:135–160
28. Li KM, Todorovic R, Devanesan P et al (2004) Metabolism and DNA binding studies of 4-hydroxyestradiol and estradiol-3, 4-quinone in vitro and in female ACI rat mammary gland in vivo. Carcinogenesis 25:289–297
29. Parl FF, Dawling S, Roodi N et al (2009) Estrogen metabolism and breast cancer. A risk model. Ann N Y Acad Sci 1155:68–75
30. Dawling S, Roodi N, Mernaugh RL et al (2001) Catechol-o-methyltransferase (COMT)-mediated metabolism of catechol estrogens: comparison of wild-type and variant COMT isoforms. Cancer Res 61:6716–6722
31. Hachey DL, Dawling S, Roodi N et al (2003) Sequential action of phase I and II enzymes cytochrome p450 1B1 and glutathione S-transferase P1 in mammary estrogen metabolism. Cancer Res 63:8492–8499
32. Cauley JA, Zmuda JM, Danielson ME et al (2003) Estrogen metabolites and the risk of breast cancer in older women. Epidemiology 14:740–744
33. Liehr JG, Ricci MJ, Jefcoate CR et al (1995) 4-Hydroxylation of estradiol by human uterine myometrium and myoma microsomes: implications for the mechanism of uterine tumorigenesis. Proc Natl Acad Sci USA 92:9220–9224
34. Liehr JG, Ricci MJ (1996) 4-Hydroxylation of estrogens as marker of human mammary tumors. Proc Natl Acad Sci USA 93:3294–3296
35. Fowke JH, Qi D, Bradlow HL et al (2003) Urinary estrogen metabolites and breast cancer: differential pattern of risk found with preversus post-treatment collection. Steroids 68:65–72
36. Falk RT, Fears T, Xu X et al (2005) Urinary estrogen metabolites and their ratio among Asian American women. Cancer Epidemiol Biomarkers Prev 14:221–226
37. Cascorbi I, Brockmöller J, Roots I (1996) A C4887A polymorphism in exon 7 of human CYP1A1: population frequency, mutation linkages, and impact on lung cancer susceptibility. Cancer Res 56:4965–4969
38. Hanna IH, Dawling S, Roodi N et al (2000) Cytochrome P450 1B1 (CYP1B1) pharmacogenetics: association of polymorphisms with functional differences in estrogen hydroxilation activity. Cancer Res 60:3440–3444
39. Lord RS, Bongiovanni B, Bralley JA (2002) Estrogen metabolism and the diet-cancer connection: rationale for assessing the ratio of urinary hydroxylated estrogen metabolites. Altern Med Rev 7(2):112–129
40. Jellinck PH, Forkert PG, Riddick DS et al (1993) Ah receptor binding properties of indole carbinols and induction of hepatic estradiol hydroxylation. Biochem Pharmacol 45:1129–1136
41. Bradlow HL, Sepkovic DW, Telang NT et al (1995) Indole-3-carbinol. A novel approach to breast cancer prevention. In: Bradlow HL, Osborne MP, Veronesi U (eds) cancer prevention, vol 768. Annals of the New York Academy Science, New York, pp 180–200
42. Davis DL, Bradlow HL, Wolff M et al (1993) Medical hypothesis: xenoestrogens as preventable causes of breast cancer. Environ Health Perspect 101:372–377
43. Bartsch H, Nair J, Owen RW (1999) Dietary polyunsaturated fatty acids and cancers of the breast and colorectum: emerging evidence for their role as risk modifiers. Carcinogenesis 20:2209–2218
44. McTernan PG, Anderson LA, Anwar AJ et al (2002) Glucocorticoid regulation of p450 aromatase activity in human adipose tissue: gender and site differences. J Clin Endocrinol Metab 87:1327–1336
45. Wong GY, Bradlow HL, Sepkovic D et al (1997) Dose ranging study of indole-3-carbinol for breast cancer prevention. J Cell Biochem Suppl 28–29:111–116

Chapter 16
Basic Nutritional Guidelines for Breast Health

The own dynamics of scientific knowledge makes us to rectify it in a continuous way. As a consequence, our knowledge becomes valid only temporarily. Only time and new research will say how many and which of our current statements are the most solid ones, but we account for a good evidence base. Within that frame and recognizing the difficulties to generalize information coming from heterogeneous populations, we summarize herewith a group of recommendations which emerged from a combination of international literature and the Uruguayan case-control studies on nutrition and BC. The background for these recommendations was thoroughly analyzed in a recent review [1].

Low Intake of Red Meat Prepared with Direct Heat

Those cooking methods as barbecue, grill or fried are not recommendable. In our studies, the low-risk subgroup had an intake up to once a week. It should be taken into account that Mediterranean diets deal with twice a month, for example. The stewed forms, which are accompanied by plenty of vegetables and legumes have defined a potentially protective style, on the contrary.

High Intake of White Meat Not Prepared with Direct Heat

Poultry like chicken prepared in barbecue or fried and with their skin are not a good choice. It is better without skin and also prepared in such way that the fat does not remain in the meat. Poultry which currently are fed with supplements of corn seeds and other products while they are confined to reduced spaces in order to enhance their growing process and development, accumulate high contents of Ω-6 PUFA instead of the natural Ω-3 PUFA that would derive from eating a variety of their

A.L. Ronco and E. De Stéfani, *Nutritional Epidemiology of Breast Cancer*,
DOI 10.1007/978-94-007-2397-9_16,

animal and vegetable sources if they could grow free in farms. We recommend a high intake of fish, and particularly not in fried form. The best fishes to achieve our goal are the fatty or "blue" fishes (sardines, tuna, salmon, herring, i.e.).

Preferential Intake of Extra Virgin Olive Oil

This oil should be exclusively consumed, instead of common vegetable oils (as corn, sunflower, soy, for example). Destinations like salad dressings as well as for preparation of several plates like pizzas and cakes. Fried foods should not be frequently consumed, however, using olive oil reduces the chance of producing *trans*-fatty acids (omega-6 fatty acids modified through heat). Olive oil is perhaps the main representative of Mediterranean diets.

High Intake of Citrus Fruits

In the populations studied by our group, a frequent intake of citrus fruits (in particular oranges, tangerines and orange juice) was a very powerful protective item. Apparently, a daily average of 1–2 units per day should be maintained. Also lemons, grapefruits, kiwi, strawberries should be taken into account. Vitamin C and flavonoids are elements whose contribution in the diet should be sustained.

Intake of Skimmed Dairy Foods

We find adequate to recommend the intake of skimmed milk fortified with calcium and vitamin D, and also skimmed yoghurt, among the fluid dairy foods. Regarding cheeses, ricotta and low-fat types are our recommendations, based on our studies. The intake of fatty cheeses – like the Gruyere, for example – as well as milk sour, Chantilly cream, ice cream and chocolate milk should be restricted.

Low Intake of High-Glycemic Load Foods

These foods, which after their ingestion request high insulin synthesis and peaks, should be reduced as much as possible. Bread and other derived from wheat, other cereals (especially refined ones), the pastry, sweets, marmalades, jams, among others, should be moderately consumed. The integral foods are more recommendable are more nutritive and determine a different metabolic behaviour. These foods should be combined with foods which are high in their protein content like dairy or meats, for example, in order to slow down the speed of raising blood glucose and the consequent insulin peaks.

Including Some Soy-Derived Foods

Currently, the availability of soy-derived products is something advantageous. There are soybeans, flour, sprouts and also prepared foods like hamburgers and others, which could be substitutes of foods like red meat, for example. Soy deserves to be present at least once a week in a meal, when thinking of proteins, phytoestrogens and their fat contribution.

Frequent Intake of Tomatoes

Tomatoes are foods which fortunately can be consumed in raw or cooked form, and whose characteristic protective elements – carotenoids – are better digested in an oily environment. These foods are closely linked to the Mediterranean dietary style and can be considered as an ally for mammary health.

Frequent Intake of Cruciferous Vegetables

Cruciferous is a vegetable group which includes cabbage, broccoli, cauliflower, Brussels sprouts, and it is recommendable to have some of them frequently in the meals. In addition to their anticarcinogenic capabilities, they enhance the synthesis of "good" oestrogens perhaps as no one else from the vegetable kingdom. Cabbage, for example, is perfectly adequate to any salad. The compatibility between taste and benefits should be achieved, looking for reasonable dressings to achieve it.

Supplementation with Ω-3

A frequent intake of certain types of fish is not feasible for everybody from a practical viewpoint. Hence, it is mandatory to include these fatty acids (DHA, EPA) which are almost not produced by human body. Due to: (1) Their antioxidant action; (2) Their enhancement of the immune system; (3) Their capability to help in the synthesis of "good" estrogens; and (4) Their contribution to balance the actions of Ω-6 PUFA, we consider that the supplementation of Ω-3 PUFA is a key point in current nutrition. This would be valid for cancer prevention as well as for optimizing treatments, helping to prevent the recurrence of tumours.

Supplementation with Vitamin D

Vitamin D has anti-tumour capabilities against breast, colon and probably prostate cancer. The intake of blue fishes is a good beginning, but receiving sunlight regularly would be the main source. Nevertheless, because of insufficient exposure or because the skin can respond under the necessary level to such stimulus, oral supplementation is recommendable, according to experts. Independently from drinking milk or other fortified foods, some hundreds of International Units could be an adequate daily amount. With that aim, consider a consultation with the Endocrinologist, since this specialist will prescribe the most adequate dose for each individual patient.

Achieving and/or Maintaining an Adequate Adipose Level

We have already commented how body weight and body mass index are insufficient to indicate us our actual adipose level. Body composition, through manual anthropometric measurements, through electric bioimpedance or through densitometry, lead us towards the reality. The fat/muscle ratio should not be higher than 1.5, according to what we have observed in Uruguayan women. The parity between both components would probably be fair. In the analyzed population, body fat fraction should be under 35% and muscle fraction over 27%.

We are trying to generate a new healthy nutritional pattern, combining 11 dietary items with an anthropometric one. Somehow, questioning the potential preventive efficacy of a proposal as the preceding one is something which deserves attention, because the necessary time to reduce risks cannot be still accurately estimated. Some prospective studies have suggested that a period under 10 years with certain nutritional styles did not mean a risk reduction. Probably 15 or more years of a given style will be needed to exert some effect. If near 15–20 years of smoking ceasing are needed to equal the risk of lung cancer among smokers to non smokers, it sounds logic to assume that at least such minimal amount of time will be needed the risk of BC, regarding something so complex as diet is.

What is a matter of high importance for us is not the possibility of achieving the same odds of those women who nourish themselves better, but that they set into motion into a style which is capable of reducing such odds, within better conditions of general health. **Up to our knowledge, there are no studies indicating that a prudent diet is pejorative for health.** Some studies show no differences and some of them suggest important reductions in the risk of developing the disease and of its recurrence. Hence, the balance of scientific evidence is beginning to incline itself towards a healthy style.

Which changes belong to this new proposed style? Those changes who determine an attenuation of excesses and deficits that the current modern Western diet has. In an extreme simplification, we attempt to reduce the volume of foods which increase the risk of developing the disease, and at the same time, to increase the volume of foods which reduce such risk. Instead of having a deficit of protective foods, we should achieve a deficit of risk foods. The schemes presented in Fig. 16.1 summarize the idea we want to communicate.

If we locate the components of each food group or component (protective, risk) of foods instead of the group itself, the previous scheme would acquire the appearance of a graphic equalizer, for example, suggesting an **inadequate** dietary pattern (Fig. 16.2).

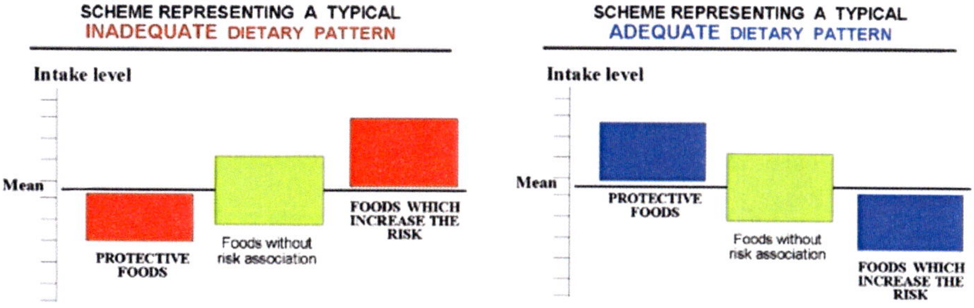

Fig. 16.1 General schemes of an inadequate nutritional pattern (*left*) and an adequate one (*right*) for preventing the disease

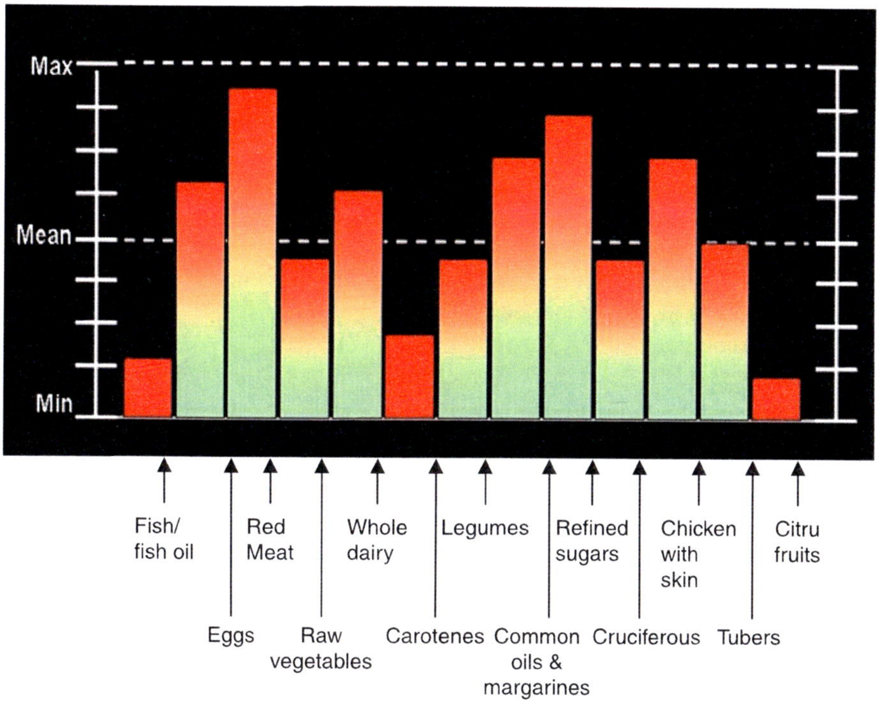

Fig. 16.2 An example of inadequate dietary pattern expressed by a graphic bar picture

The general idea implies modifying each selected term, upwards or downwards and according to the risk or protective nature of the term, towards the putative low-risk threshold or zone. The latter could be represented by the reference category of each dietary item for the case of risk factors, and the highest intake category for protective factors. For example, regarding the multivariate analysis of fried meat intake (which is a risk factor among Uruguayan women) and the risk of BC, the reference category comprises from none (0) up to 1 serving/week. This could be considered as the low-risk zone, therefore, recommendations should be oriented to reduce the intake no more than 1 serving/week. On the contrary, if we are speaking about a putative protective factor in the same population, like citrus fruits, the highest category of consumption includes >=8 units/week (oranges, orange juice servings, i.e.) and if it is possible, the woman should enter this low-risk category by means of increasing her daily citrus intake.

In fact, the proposal is next to make an equalization of food intakes: we would call it as ***nutriequalization***, a short form for nutritional equalization. While emphasizing the intake changes for each found risk or protective nutritional factor in a given population set, we are attempting to change its own dietary pattern. Therefore, if the dietary analysis is performed on a country-specific data series, the results apply to members of such population, since the lowest or highest categories of consumption might not coincide with the ones of other populations. This fact limits the generalization of results to other populations, indeed, unless coincident low-risk ranges among countries are found.

According to the current knowledge, we are limited only to propose a general scheme, mainly at a population level. But the possibilities of a tailored protective dietary style for a close future might exist, led by nutrigenomics of BC. Epidemiologic studies have communicated that certain genetic polymorphisms in several genes encoding biotransformation enzymes could be associated to increased risks of developing BC [2]. For example, the tissue composition of PUFA is important to health and depends on both dietary intake and metabolism controlled by genetic polymorphisms that should be taken into consideration in the determination of nutritional requirements [3].

Nevertheless, identifying those women who will or will not benefit from dietary intervention strategies is still not feasible. Adequate knowledge about how the responses depend on an individual's genetic background (nutrigenetic effects), as well as the cumulative effects of food components on genetic expression profiles through nutrigenomics, may assist in identifying responders and non-responders to such strategic changes. What to change, how much to change, for how long. That will be perhaps the time of individual *nutriequalization*.

It is important that the suggested changes involve not only the woman herself – we can not consider her always as a patient – but also the nucleus with whom she lives. This will make for her more tolerable and comfortable any type of modifications. And if that family core and her children are also involved, taking into account very specially the daughters, the potential risk reduction will be higher. This would happen since the time of exposure to an inadequate diet up to the present time would be reduced. Obviously, if a woman has been afflicted by a BC, the benefits are great, because the daughter with such family history is currently considered as with a statistically higher risk when compared to daughters of mothers without the disease. In the future it will not be the same a woman with high family risk following an adequate dietary style than a woman with high family risk whose nutrition is a combination of excesses and deficits. This is what could be called ***transgenerational prevention*** – or intergenerational, as Dr. Arnot says [4] –. In our opinion, it is an obligation as a citizen to think about the health of the next generation, taking profit of the created knowledge.

The exposure of a child or teenager to a protective dietary style will generate a risk reduction which is more important than the one achieved by an adult woman. The age differences between mother and daughter mean a benefit for the latter. Even there were no progress in the scientific knowledge in the next years (something highly unlikely), the women who belong to the next generation could locate themselves in a position which means lesser risk than their mothers. In this sense, a recent review recognized that overall, Ω-3 PUFA have promising cancer-preventive effects when introduced early in life, a time period when tissues are particularly sensitive to their environment [5].

An impact constituted by massive and sustained nutritional changes will be necessary to achieve some effect on the incidence of BC in many countries. Undoubtedly, an immediate change respect of the current situation of the disease cannot be expected, at least regarding what depends on this environmental factor. If a massive migration of dietary habits directed towards a healthy style does occur, we might be witnessing a reduction of incidence in rates in some countries perhaps during the next 30's decade. Nowadays it is not possible to propose a similar prognosis before, because the necessary process would take much time, from the viewpoint of the current knowledge. Mortality, besides, will surely go on downwards, but according to what is presented in this work, its reduction speed could accelerate even more. From our viewpoint, the following changes would be of utmost hierarchy: notably increasing Ω-3 PUFA and reducing Ω-6 PUFA and limiting the intake of barbecued and fried meat not beyond 2–3 times per month, as an average consumption like Mediterranean diets have.

Then, it will be mandatory to revise what does constitute a potential excess (to cut it down) and what does constitute a potential deficit (and compensate it). In this sense, a ***"far East"-type*** proposal (on a basis of increasing the intake of products derived from soy as beans, flour, tofu, miso) will remark important differences regarding the habits of the Western societies, albeit it could be excellent from the viewpoint of the theoretical protection against BC. We consider that including some products of the above quoted – as a partial substitution of beefsteak, processed meat and sausages, for example – is an excellent choice. Recent evidence, however, suggests that soy intake during early life may both reduce BC risk and risk of recurrence, in other words, the best time for including soy and soy-derived products appears to be no longer than the puberty [6]. However, a high intake of soy foods during adolescence was also associated with a reduced risk of premenopausal BC (OR = 0.57; 95% CI: 0.34–0.97) [7]. Lifetime soy intake at a moderate level could prevent BC recurrence through mechanisms that change the biology of tumors; e.g. women who consumed soy during childhood develop BC with significantly reduced Human epidermal growth factor receptor 2 levels [6]. Hence, this would limit somehow the perspective for such dietary style, if adult women make an attempt to change it radically, assuming that the consequences of this change would have some degree of uncertainty.

Anyway, it should be taken into account the ethnic and geographic origin from a large part of inhabitants of Latin America, part of the United States and Southern Europe itself, which is in particular Spain and Italy. In this sense, diets having a

"Mediterranean" orientation could be a solution which is at the grip of women in general, also taking into account that such diets *are not very much low-caloric ones*. It is of interest to remember that longevity observed in some Mediterranean populations (i.e. Cyprus, Greece, Malta, Italy, Spain) has been attributed, within a multifactorial spectrum, to the usual intake of fish, olive oil and tomatoes – the latter in raw form as well as cooked one –. The substitution of other common oils (corn, soybean, sunflower, as some of the most frequent consumption) by olive oil could constitute one of the most substantial advances towards the protection, in view of the results derived from research of the last years. And the protective elements of tomatoes, among which carotenoids prevail, were found as having a better absorption when foods are cooked in an oily environment. Therefore, foods like simple pizzas, sauces, some pasta dressed with tomato sauce could be a relatively frequent part of a healthy diet, when olive oil is included.

The preceding arguments and the existing literature has enabled the authors of this book to express the potential convenience of some recommendations that have similarities to the general ones suggested internationally [8] but that are also different from them, since the background of ours combines international with local evidences.

We are convinced that it is mandatory or at least convenient to recommend on this basis, if it is feasible to do so. It sounds as no very reasonable to wait still a decade or more to suggest recommendations, when probably some significant international studies will show positive results, especially if such recommendations are of high additional benefit to vessels, metabolism, joints and as protection against developing other cancers. The evidence for links among diet, chronic inflammation and cancer as well as with other high prevalent, chronic diseases must encourage to making the decision of recommending key changes in current dietary style. It would be convenient to consider that in the meantime, it is medically and ethically justified to recommend some nutritional changes to patients and to healthy women.

Although we have put particular emphasis on findings derived from local epidemiological studies, we have shown that the proposed changes would at least constitute an attempt at low cost intervention without adverse side effects, contrary to those one can expect from drug treatments. While there is no clear evidence that any specific dietary component can effectively reduce BC risk [9] the fact that several measures have convergence on the control of amount and quality of estrogens is something we can profit from. We have already something on which we can base our actions [1, 8, 10] and probably new studies which are ongoing probably will shed light to the question within some years, through confirmatory results.

References

1. Ronco AL, De Stéfani E, Stoll M (2010) Hormonal and metabolic modulation through nutrition: towards a primary prevention of breast cancer. Breast 19:322–332
2. Parl FF, Dawling S, Roodi N et al (2009) Estrogen metabolism and breast cancer. A risk model. Ann N Y Acad Sci 1155:68–75

3. Simopoulos AP (2010) Genetic variants in the metabolism of omega-6 and omega-3 fatty acids: their role in the determination of nutritional requirements and chronic disease risk. Exp Biol Med (Maywood) 235(7):785–795
4. Arnot R (ed) (1999) Dieta para la prevención del cáncer de mama. Urano, Barcelona
5. Maclennan M, Ma DW (2010) Role of dietary fatty acids in mammary gland development and breast cancer. Breast Cancer Res 12(5):211
6. Hilakivi-Clarke L, Andrade JE, Helferich W (2010) Is soy consumption good or bad for the breast? J Nutr 140(12):2326S–2334S
7. Lee SA, Shu XO, Li H et al (2009) Adolescent and adult soy food intake and breast cancer risk: results from the Shanghai Women's Health Study. Am J Clin Nutr 89(6):1920–1926
8. World Cancer Research Fund (1997) Food, nutrition and the prevention of cancer: a global perspective. American Institute for Cancer Research, Washington, DC, pp 252–287
9. Mahoney MC, Bevers T, Linos E et al (2008) Opportunities and strategies for breast cancer prevention through risk reduction. CA Cancer J Clin 58:347–371
10. World Cancer Research Fund/American Institute for Cancer Research (2007) Food, nutrition, physical activity, and the prevention of cancer: a global perspective. American Institute for Cancer Research, Washington, DC

Chapter 17
Prevention After Diagnosis

In a book on breast cancer (BC) published in Brazil more than a decade ago [1] there was a chapter on diet in which the gynecologist Dr. Menke made comments about dietary intervention in daily practice: *"There is no one single day in the medical office or in the outpatients area that patients bearing risk factors or patients who were already treated by a breast cancer make us the following questions: How should I care myself? What should I eat? And our answer flows fast with the scheme: self-examination, clinical examination and periodical mammogram. Regarding nutrition, we simply ignore it, or we give vague recommendations, considering the issue as a not very important one, which is time-consuming and frequently disobeyed by patients."*

It is so. Undoubtedly, it is not a Brazilian problem, of course. It is universal, according to a recent Finnish study [2], which found that there is a need of dietary and lifestyle counsel from Finnish and Australian women. The paper also states that "such need is poorly recognized currently by physicians."

Just in the last years have appeared results of scientific studies showing the advantages of an adequate diet for those women who were diagnosed with a BC regarding the disease-free survival and the overall survival. The survival has been increased in American postmenopausal women having a low fat intake and a high intake of fruits, vegetables and micronutrients derived from these latter [3, 4]. The intake of protective foods in Norwegian survivors of BC has been found similar to those of healthy women [5]. Women with high plasmatic levels of carotenoids (specially eating more tomatoes, carrot, red pepper) reduced significantly their recurrence risk compared to those ones with low levels [6]. Dietary styles ranging from macrobiotic to semivegetarian ones have been supported as coadjuvant with specific therapy of BC [7].

In addition, in the last years there were some communications that reported an improvement when some nutritional guidelines were followed focusing on the management of overweight and obesity [8–18]. In general terms, the evidence suggests that BC survival is reduced among women with general or abdominal obesity, as well as that obese women of all ages were more likely than non-obese women to have disease recurrence.

DOI 10.1007/978-94-007-2397-9_17,

Furthermore, large intervention studies are on-going in the developed World, probably enhanced by the great preventive potential this research area has, in which diet and exercise are being investigated in their capability of reducing the recurrence of BC, as the WHEL study in the USA [19] or others in the United Kingdom [20]. There are researchers who have already shown the efficacy of a multimodal approach to the problem, through telephone counsel, informative meetings, periodical bulletins and cooking classes [21]. There was feasible among them to achieve changes in the dietary habits of women who were previously treated by a BC. Undoubtedly, we are facing examples that can be followed, that should be developed from the own profile of each population, according to its culture, its customs and its way of thinking.

The main objective of therapies is **to avoid the reappearance of the disease**. Once the specific therapeutic has been applied in each situation, the therapies will point mainly to achieve the healing or the local control, regarding the situation of each patient. The reappearance can be called "recurrence" or "relapse", and medical treatments attempt to avoid its presence at a local, regional or systemic level. It has to do with several factors which belong to the tumour itself, and it is more likely to occur in younger women (under age 40) and within the first 2 years of the surgery, because the tumour aggressiveness is more frequent among them. Currently, some histopathologic factors aside from young age are known, and these factors have prognostic value for the recurrence of the disease. Specialists display the maximum efforts to avoid a loco-regional recurrence, since it increases around threefold the odds for distant metastases, which is a disadvantageous situation in the fight to control the disease.

The change of nutrition and lifestyle might probably allow achieving several goals, but we remark that such changes would give the possibility of optimizing the established therapies, what we can accept as tertiary prevention: they could help to delay a disease recurrence. When we talk about supporting the treatments for BC, we include them all: surgery, radiotherapy, chemotherapy, hormonal therapy and also immunotherapy. A mammary tumour is based on favourable hormonal and metabolic environments, but in addition, the immune system has at the same time failed. Besides, specific therapies imply higher or lower degree of aggression to the whole organism. Perhaps more localized or more generalized, there is an inevitable aggression for some organs which belong to the rest of the "healthy" body. If there were dietary elements at hand which could protect the healthy cells and empower the toxicity on tumour cells, we should recognize the advantage of using such elements.

Regarding BC patients, since several years are needed to modify the risks and currently there is lack of evidence in this sense, we cannot predict any given success for the patient at an individual level when a pure primary prevention is considered. In other words, we bring a rationale for adopting new nutritional and life styles, with the aim of helping the body to reject the possibility for the disease to come back again, working together with the conventional treatments. Albeit it is not possible to predict at an individual level, it is expected that under certain circumstances less cases of recurrence will appear within a subset of patients who make nutritional corrections.

When comparing the potential preventive action being in an apparent health status with having a diagnosed mammary pathology there is a difference of degree. Undoubtedly, there are also differences comparing benign pathologies (as a fibroadenoma), a pre-neoplastic lesion (as atypical lobular hyperplasia) and a cancer (intraductal, lobular, among others). Before classifying lesions, we should make more general considerations: the hormonal-metabolic-immune system is balanced or imbalanced. When a woman's breast has been any time studied – especially through puncture or biopsy, although there was a benign lesion – this fact is revealing her that there is a broken balance: the organ "breast" is giving signals about its tendency to get sick. And this was confirmed by epidemiologic research, indicating that the history of benign breast diseases increases modestly the likelihood of developing a cancer. The point is not a malignant transformation of the benign lesion, but a higher probability of having a malignancy in the future.

There are even stronger arguments for somebody whose lesion is precancerous: the patient has been advised that "if certain given circumstances do not change, it is highly likely that in the future you will develop a cancer". In the light of current knowledge, it does not seem good only to feel satisfied having made a consultation with the physician – perhaps more frequently than before- and continuing with the old scheme which indicates along time that "for the moment, there is no news about cancer". Let's analyze why.

We assume that the patient has been surgically operated and the tumour mass has been resected. Then, it is time to have an impact on cells that may have remained and perhaps have migrated by lymphatic vessels. Keep this concept in mind: **The main task is now done by the own body, therefore, help it.** Those possible remaining cancer cells should experience some cuts in their nourishment, avoiding for example the intake of high glycemic load foods such as common refined sugar, bread, desserts, soft drinks. The invading cells live more with low levels of oxygen and as a consequence the growth of new vessels (neo angiogenesis) is enhanced in order to continue growing. You must give them as much oxygen as possible – because it is harmful for cancer cells – through the intake of fish oil rich in Ω-3 fatty acids, extra virgin olive oil, and doing all the physical exercise that the patient is able to do, in order to oxygenize the whole body. If there were problems related to the arm at the operated side, walking is the last thing to be abandoned. But if the patient has the physical conditions and a medical authorization, she should gain some muscular mass – more than simply walking – since this will improve her immune system, among other consequences.

Let's put into consideration the time of radiotherapy. When a patient receives a radiation dose on the breast and on certain related lymphatic areas – as axillary, supraclavicular or internal mammary regions, i.e. – , the objective is to sterilize the tumour bed and the drainage regions. Although radiotherapy is a local and regional treatment, it implies a high likelihood of temporarily weakening the immune system. Radiotherapy produces free-radicals through peroxydation and the patient should help herself eliminating them more quickly. This therapy is aggressive with residual tumour cells, but also with healthy tissues. The patient should contribute to improving the oxygenation of those tissues in order to achieve that radiation affects more the tumour and less the healthy cells.

In these circumstances three types of substances are useful: antioxidants, substances which improve the tissue oxygenation and those which enhance the immune system. **All these can be found in two particular oils**: fish liver oil and extra virgin olive oil. Regarding this latter, it has a component, squalene, which does everything. It seems better to supplement with more concentrated oil, that is, the one extracted from the liver of sharks who live in deep waters, or purified from the olive [22, 23]. A recent experimental study reported that olive oil also inhibits the mutation of Her-2-neu oncogene (linked to BC disease) and it enhances the action of trastuzumab, a specific monoclonal antibody designed to work on this gene. The supplementation with fish oil, which is rich in Ω-3 PUFAs and extra virgin olive oil constitute the basis of an "anti her-2-neu cocktail", as was described by European researchers [24, 25].

Another usual treatment related to BC, the chemotherapy, is applied as an attempt to destroy cells which could have evaded the breast region and spread to the rest of the body. The features are rather similar to the previous described situation, but more intensely. With the aim of killing a presumably limited number of malignant cells, *the whole body* suffers the aggression of drugs and in particular those tissues which have a high turnover like epithelial ones are the ones who are more injured. The liver catches toxic substances from the circulation, in order to eliminate them through the bile system. The patient should take into account that her liver can be overwhelmed during the chemotherapy cycles: aside from doing what is mandatory to do (rebuilding carbohydrates, proteins and fats, i.e.), it is in charge of detoxification of the whole organism. The liver should be carefully handled. If the patient uses to eat plenty of fats like the one of cow or pork, from the skin of chicken, from dairy foods, from mayonnaise, or even that of vegetable sources like sunflower, soy or corn oils, – or even worse, trans-fatty acids which are present in margarines, snacks, fries, etc. –, she cannot expect that everything works well. The liver should be relieved from such overwork, for example, basing the diet on fruits *ad libitum* during a whole day after the chemotherapy cycle.

Aside from the liver, the impact that the bone marrow receives in its hemopoyetic role is high. Usually after chemotherapy the parameters in the blood cell count are modified in the sense of reduction, indicating anemia, leukopenia and perhaps trombocytopenia. Chemotherapy will temporally kill isolated tumoral cells, but the permanent responsibility concerns the immune system. This latter must be adequately active, hence, it should be maintained in good conditions, as much as possible. For example, the supplementation with squalene – derived from extra virgin olive oil or from shark liver oil [23] – might increase the activity of key elements such as Natural Killers and T-lymphocites.

When it is possible for the patient, some physical exercise will be worthy: the muscle provides an essential nutrient, glutamine, to lymphocytes. Physical exercise must be taken into account. Otherwise, the patient may be condemned to an excessive inactivity only for caution (unless there is anemia as a side effect of therapy). The point is that if the patient loses muscle mass, her immune system might be under the normal performance. Besides, tumour cells live better in anaerobic or low oxygenated environments and oxygen is harmful for them: this is well known by specialists. If the whole organism is better oxygenated, the cytotoxicity of chemotherapy and radiotherapy on malignant cells will be enhanced and it will contribute to protect healthy cells (which are a wide majority). Again, through the combination of dietary components like olive oil as well as fatty fishes (tuna, sardines, salmon, etc.) together with physical exercise there might be a better management of oxygen at the tissue level.

Let us make some considerations about hormones in the treatment of BC. Not all cancers have estrogen or progesterone receptors. Usually hormonal therapy has been more effective when it is administered for mammary tumours which have hormonal receptors than when tumours do not have them. The specialist will not prescribe hormonal therapy in this latter situation. What is hormonal therapy for? To prevent against or to block the action of hormones which would accelerate the growth and proliferation of tumour cells. Time ago, together with breast surgery an oophorectomy was done: the estrogenic action was surgically reduced. Theoretically this interruption could be also caused by radiotherapy.

Currently there are drugs which attempt to impact without being aggressive, although they are not completely harmless: there are the selective estrogen receptor modulators (SERMs), as tamoxifen, raloxifen, toremifen; there are also the aromatase inhibitors (anastrozol, letrozol) and other drugs which disrupt receptors making difficult their binding to hormone (fulvestran). As it can be seen, SERMs seek to trick the cells through intelligent ways. Only those hormones which have the adequate form bind the receptors, like pieces of a puzzle. The more receptors are bund with the proper hormones, the faster grow some type of cancers. But these drugs affect the amount of available estrogen to bind the receptor, or they bind it with something similar to avoid that the hormone binds it, or even they damage the receptor. Anti-estrogen therapy in women with BC can affect lipid profiles, cardiovascular risk, and liver function [26] and some data suggest that metabolic syndrome may be associated with a more aggressive tumour biology [27].The presence of a metabolic syndrome and the elevation of C-reactive protein are indicating that the chronic inflammation is active [28] and deserve to monitor the patient in order to prevent and reduce morbidity and mortality also unrelated to BC. **Now it is clear why it is not convenient to bear an excess of body fat and without changing the nutritional style, if this latter is excessive in Ω-6 PUFA: the patient has mainly disadvantages.**

If the histochemical study of the surgically removed piece indicates that it was moderately or strongly positive for estrogen receptors (RE+), we could add to the previous strategy something else: a higher contribution of soy products and legumes in order to profit from the usefulness of the phytoestrogens these foods have. In fact, if there are actually receptors, let's contribute with bind them to dietary low active estrogens. It does not seem to be convenient the intake of elaborated phytoestrogens without previous consultation: the effect could be inverted to the expected one, if doses are raised to a pharmacologic level. If on the contrary, the study indicates negative or weakly positive receptors, it could be recommended to put into practice everything that was indicated to produce "good" estrogens and to improve immunity: losing body fat and increase the muscle mass, supplementing Ω-3 PUFA, dramatically suppressing the intake of trans- and Ω-6 fatty acids, and having a high intake of cruciferous vegetables. In addition, including extra virgin olive oil, plenty of fruits especially citrus (orange, lemon, grapefruit, kiwi) and green tea with the aim of improving the antioxidant capabilities, will be always useful. These recommendations seem to be probably the core of a new dietary pattern for the patient, based on part of the evidence generated by epidemiologic and experimental research. We believe that this is a rationale for the patient to continue in better conditions.

Frequently, several patients who had normal menstrual cycles at the moment of their diagnosis, become postmenopausal after chemotherapy. The damage on the ovaries – theoretically necessary, sometimes – is, in other words, to provoke the menopause in an anticipated time. Together with this hormonal change determined by therapy, it is not unusual that women – young or middle-age ones – experience a body remodelling similar to the one that women who naturally cease their menses do. There is a reduction of their metabolic rate, expressed by an increase of body weight; the waist tends to increase its circumference; the adipose skinfolds in arms, trunk and lower limbs also increase their thickness. Obviously, such physical change is not only an aesthetic problem to be solved. The body composition has changed: whether the total weight has changed or not, the body fat will surely have increased, probably together with a simultaneous lose of muscle mass. We do not hear specialists speaking with worry concerning this point, and we assume that it could be not a minor issue. It seems as it is not perceived that if these events occur, the own hormonal and metabolic circumstances of the patient change towards a bad condition, as it was quoted above [28]. It cannot be reasonably expected to have the same therapeutic success in a woman who has added several kilograms of fat to her body. Changing the viewpoint: if losing fat excess improves survival, what do you think it could happen if the patient accumulates adipose excess? After doing certain changes regarding nutrition and physical activity, we are convinced that the time for having a consultation with the Endocrinologist has come, if the patient does not experience favourable modifications in her body.

The arrival of menopause does not imply only a body remodelling, but also an increase of cardiovascular pathologies. During some years, from the viewpoint of Cardiology, it was thought that the main responsible of cardiovascular diseases was the fall of oestrogen levels when the ovarian function failed. Some of the large studies with HRT (hormonal replacement therapy) have shown that there was no reduction of cardiovascular diseases in those who used this therapy compared to those women who had not received the hormonal substitution. At least initially, the problem is centered in the insulin synthesis, which changes as a consequence of hormonal changes. If HRT has not been able to reduce the cardiovascular changes, the putative protection is not fulfilled: **a HRT is not justified if the objective is reducing the probabilities of cardiovascular pathology.** Furthermore, leaving aside aspects such an eventual increase of risk of BC (something which is never negligible and mandatory to evaluate before prescribing hormones), the hormonal therapy does not reduce the insulin production. On the contrary, it could increase this latter. And the pro-inflammatory cytokines (such as tumor necrosis factor alpha, interleukin-1, epidermal growth factor, and insulin-like growth factor-1), produced in the adipose tissue tend to increase. The "bad" eicosanoids increase the insulin production and this latter increases the biosynthesis of the active Ω-6, which is the arachidonic acid. There is a real *circulus viciosus*. Hence, in natural or artificial menopause induced by medical treatments, the excess of Ω-6 fats are harmful. They play against the patient's objectives. How can such circulus viciosus be broken? Among other ways, contributing with plenty of Ω-3 PUFA in the diet, through fish intake or through nutritional supplements. Through competition with Ω-6 for the same receptors, the Ω-3 PUFA reduce the cytokines and insulin synthesis, by increasing the sensitivity of cells to this latter.

Also the antiangiogenic properties of foods, nutrients and bioactive substances are under study. Such capabilities are expected to be used in the prevention of certain cancer types and/or in the coadjuvance in conventional therapies. Foods which are rich in vitamin E (tocopherol), for example, can be very useful Vitamin E has not only antioxidant but also antiangiogenic capabilities [29]. There is a recently synthesized vitamin analog, the tocotrienol, which seems to be promising. The foods which contribute with vitamin E work by inhibition of the action of a substance located at the endothelium of blood vessels, the Vascular Endothelial Growth Factor (VEGF). Do you know who does usually stimulate the VEGF, which is a key factor in the regulation of angiogenesis? The pro-inflammatory cytokines do, which were aforementioned when we talked about their intense production in obesity (through an excess of adipose tissue). Do you realize? An excessive adipose mass in the body, enhances in addition the vascular neosynthesis, which facilitates the proliferation and development of tumour cells. These are the reasons why we insist that the patient should not have overweight if she was ever diagnosed with BC. It should not be allowed to prolong this situation, if it has ever occurred. Once again, we remember the reader that most studies have shown that survival of BC improves if a previously existing overweight is reduced [9–18].

It was already mentioned that not only vitamin E participates in the protection against angiogenesis, but also flavonoids do. These are cited as one of the protective agents of fruits. Among flavonoids, the subgroup called ANTOCYANINS has powerful antiangiogenic capabilities. They are present in strawberries, raspberries, blueberries, and cranberries. Their high content in antocyanins is beneficial for health due to their antioxidant capability, but also because they help with cell DNA reparing and protecting its completeness [30].

The intake of these "berries" fruits is proposed as an interesting help role in the strategy against BC for any patient. We are thinking specially of those patients dealing with a relatively disadvantageous situation, as for example, with negative hormonal receptors, but also when the axillary status has revealed the tumour extension beyond the breast gland. We can help the most orthodox oncologic strategy if we cut the nutritional nourishment of those possible remaining cells, when having an intake of functional antiangiogenic foods. Diet seems to provide protective elements which are better and thoroughly known, from which such protective potential should not be denied. Experimental research has given some evidence to be taken into account [31].

It seems unfair not recommending to patients the intake of plenty of fruits only based on "*It is not shown that the consumption of fruit A or fruit B is protective against cancer*" or even on the base that "*How many fruits must be eaten in order to reach the pharmacologic doses of drug X*? (perhaps thinking on bevacizumab, for example)" We think that these are insufficient arguments. Nobody, in fact, has established that emphasizing the intake of certain fruits the cure of BC is guaranteed, but that is not a reason to avoid indicating its consumption. We are not talking about the use of simultaneous medications. **It is a matter of favouring the organism with as much as possible, adding and not substracting.** We suggest you not to accept but neither generate by yourself a false opposition sometimes created between conventional treatments and nutritional support, because there is not an actual opposition. Nutrition is a complement.

A CANCER NEEDS GENERATING NEW BLOOD VESSELS TO GROW AND DEVELOP ITSELF. PUT YOURSELF IN ACTION CUTTING THE NUTRITIONAL SUPPLIES, RECOMMENDING THE INTAKE OF FOODS WITH ANTIANGIOGENIC PROPERTIES.

Since the hormonal environment occasionally does not seem to facilitate things, we should think in making difficult the neo-angiogenesis and at the same time, improving as much as possible the immune status. The immunity enhancement has several ways to be favoured. Let us take into account once again the intake of Ω-3 PUFAs. In addition, it is also feasible the increase of squalene intake, coming from olive oil, or even better from shark liver oil (from deep waters), several fold more concentrated than in olive oil. There is limited clinical evidence, but there is a good support of experimental and epidemiologic evidence to recommend a supplementation of this kind.

Additional comments deserve, to our knowledge, some products which in the last years were known through mass media: prebiotics and probiotics. A useful contribution for health has been recognized to them. A complete spectrum of "fermented milks" or similar ones, recommended because of their presence of lactobacillus (i.e., LGG or LCD) whose action on the intestinal transit and bacterial composition constitute a strong point. They have become a potential preventive factor against colon cancer and other serious pathologies of the bowel. A recent study which analyzed antioxidant supplements including vitamins C and E in the first 6 months after BC diagnosis [32] reported that this practice may be associated with reduced risk of mortality and recurrence. Another study found that activities of various antioxidant enzymes as superoxide dismutase, catalase, glutathione-S-transferase and glutathione reductase, and the levels of reduced glutathione were significantly increased ($P<0.01$) while, the levels of malondialdehyde and DNA damage were significantly ($P<0.01$) reduced in the vitamin C and E supplemented group relative to those of patients receiving chemotherapy alone [33].

We agree with their opinion: Such results do not support the recommendation that BC patients should avoid use of vitamin supplements. We also consider necessary to emphasize here, that the enhancement of the immune system, always recognized as convenient and necessary, could be – among other factors – potentially helpful against BC at any time, also after the diagnosis [34].

IF THE BREAST GLAND DEVELOPED A CANCER, THE IMMUNE SYSTEM HAS SOMEHOW FAILED. THE LATTER COULD BE RESTORED HELPING THE ORGANISM WITH APPROPRIATE FOODS.

References

1. Menke CH, Biazús JV, Cavalheiro JA et al (1999) Dieta e cancer de mama. In: Basegio DL (ed) cancer de mama. Revinter, Rio de Janeiro, pp 89–99
2. Salminen E, Bishop M, Poussa T et al (2004) Dietary attitudes and changes as well as use of supplements and complementary therapies by Australian and Finnish women following the diagnosis of breast cancer. Eur J Clin Nutr 58(1):137–144
3. McEligot AJ, Largent J, Ziogas A et al (2006) Dietary fat, fiber, vegetable, and micronutrients are associated with overall survival in postmenopausal women diagnosed with breast cancer. Nutr Cancer 55(2):132–140
4. Fink BN, Gaudet MM, Britton JA et al (2006) Fruits, vegetables, and micronutrient intake in relation to breast cancer survival. Breast Cancer Res Treat 98(2):199–208
5. Skeie G, Hjartaker A, Lund E (2006) Diet among breast cancer survivors and healthy women. The Norwegian Women and Cancer Study. Eur J Clin Nutr 60(9):1046–1054
6. Rock CL, Flatt SW, Natarajan L et al (2005) Plasma carotenoids and recurrence-free survival in women with a history of breast cancer. J Clin Oncol 23(27):6631–6638
7. Berrino F, Villarini A, De Petris M et al (2006) Adjuvant diet to improve hormonal and metabolic factors affecting breast cancer prognosis. Ann N Y Acad Sci 1089:110–118
8. Rock CL, Demark-Wahnefried W (2002) Nutrition and survival after the diagnosis of breast cancer: a review of the evidence. J Clin Oncol 20:3302–3316
9. Carmichael AR, Bates T (2004) Obesity and breast cancer: a review of the literature. Breast 13(2):85–92
10. Kroenke CH, Chen WY, Rosner B et al (2005) Weight, weight gain, and survival after breast cancer diagnosis. J Clin Oncol 23:1370–1378
11. Holmes MD, Chen WY, Feskanich D et al (2005) Physical activity and survival after breast cancer diagnosis. JAMA 293:2479–2486
12. Loi S, Milne RL, Friedlander ML et al (2005) Obesity and outcomes in premenopausal and postmenopausal breast cancer. Cancer Epidemiol Biomarkers Prev 14(7):1686–1691
13. Whiteman MK, Hillis SD, Curtis KM et al (2005) Body mass and mortality after breast cancer diagnosis. Cancer Epidemiol Biomarkers Prev 14(8):2009–2014
14. Tao MH, Shu XO, Ruan ZX et al (2006) Association of overweight with breast cancer survival. Am J Epidemiol 163(2):101–107
15. Abrahamson PE, Gammon MD, Lund MJ et al (2006) General and abdominal obesity and survival among young women with breast cancer. Cancer Epidemiol Biomarkers Prev 15(10):1871–1877

16. Kushi LH, Kwan ML, Lee MM et al (2007) Lifestyle factors and survival in women with breast cancer. J Nutr 137:236S–242S
17. Dal Maso L, Zucchetto A, Talamini R et al (2008) Effect of obesity and other lifestyle factors on mortality in women with breast cancer. Int J Cancer 123(9):2188–2194
18. Dawood S, Broglio K, Gonzalez-Angulo AM et al (2008) Prognostic value of body mass index in locally advanced breast cancer. Clin Cancer Res 14(6):1718–1725
19. Pierce JP, Faerber S, Wright FA et al (2002) A randomized trial of the effect of a plant-based dietary pattern on additional breast cancer events and survival: the Women's Healthy Eating and Living (WHEL) study. Control Clin Trials 23(6):728–756
20. Saxton JM, Daley A, Woodroofe N et al (2006) Study protocol to investigate the effect of a lifestyle intervention on body weight, psychological health status and risk factors associated with disease recurrence in women recovering from breast cancer treatment [ISRCTN08045231]. BMC Cancer 6:35
21. Newman VA, Thomson CA, Rock CL et al (2005) Achieving substantial changes in eating behavior among women previously treated for breast cancer -an overview of the intervention. J Am Diet Assoc 105(3):382–391
22. Ohkuma T, Otagiri K, Tanaka S et al (1983) Intensification of host's immunity by squalene in sarcoma 180 bearing ICR mice. J Pharmacobiodyn 6:148–151
23. Newmark HL (1999) Squalene, olive oil, and cancer risk. In: Bradlow HL, Fishman J, Osborne MP (eds) Cancer prevention: novel nutrients and pharmaceutical developments, vol 889. Annals of the New York Academy Science, New York, pp 193–203
24. Menendez JA, Vazquez-Martin A, Ropero S et al (2006) HER2 (erbB-2)-targeted effects of the omega-3 polyunsaturated. Fatty acid alpha-linolenic acid (ALA; 18:3n-3) in breast cancer cells: the<<fat features>>of the<<Mediterranean diet>>as an<<anti-HER2 cocktail>> Clin Transl Oncol 8(11):812–820
25. Sant M, Allemani C, Sieri S et al (2007) Salad vegetables dietary pattern protects against HER-2-positive breast cancer: a prospective Italian study. Int J Cancer 121(4):911–914
26. Redig AJ, Munshi HG (2010) Care of the cancer survivor: metabolic syndrome after hormone-modifying therapy. Am J Med 123(1):87.e1–6
27. Healy LA, Ryan AM, Carroll P et al (2010) Metabolic syndrome, central obesity and insulin resistance are associated with adverse pathological features in postmenopausal breast cancer. Clin Oncol (R Coll Radiol) 22(4):281–288
28. Thomson CA, Thompson PA, Wright-Bea J et al (2009) Metabolic syndrome and elevated C-reactive protein in breast cancer survivors on adjuvant hormone therapy. J Womens Health (Larchmt) 18(12):2041–2047
29. Miyazawa T, Tsuzuki T, Nakagawa K et al (2004) Antiangiogenic potency of vitamin E. Ann N Y Acad Sci 1031:401–404
30. Bagchi D, Roy S, Patel V et al (2006) Safety and whole-body antioxidant potential of a novel anthocyanin-rich formulation of edible berries. Mol Cell Biochem 281(1–2):197–209
31. Kang X, Jin S, Zhang Q (2009) Antitumor and antiangiogenic activity of soy phytoestrogen on 7, 12-dimethylbenz[alpha]anthracene-induced mammary tumors following ovariectomy in Sprague-Dawley rats. J Food Sci 74(7):H237–H242
32. Nechuta S, Lu W, Chen Z et al (2011) Vitamin supplement use during breast cancer treatment and survival: a prospective cohort study. Cancer Epidemiol Biomarkers Prev 20(2):262–271
33. Suhail N, Bilal N, Khan HY et al (2011) Effect of vitamins C and E on antioxidant status of breast-cancer patients undergoing chemotherapy. J Clin Pharm Ther. doi:10.1111/j.1365-2710.2010.01237.x
34. Yazdi MH, Soltan Dallal MM, Hassan ZM et al (2010) Oral administration of Lactobacillus acidophilus induces IL-12 production in spleen cell culture of BALB/c mice bearing transplanted breast tumour. Br J Nutr 104(2):227–232

Chapter 18
Nutritional Strategy: From Populations to Individuals

Several data, statements and discussions which were given herewith are giving some basis to put on action strategies. These are strategies at the individual level, at the family or the work level, in the best scenario. However, talking about strategies also is meaning to refer us to the idea of planning. Planning involves establishing goals and the definition of alternative strategies in order to achieve such goals. From a practical viewpoint, it is not possible to eliminate achieving goals by chance, but a good planning can increase the odds of success.

Nevertheless, it is not always possible to make a plan. In other words, there would be circumstances under which planning might be completely useless, especially when you do not have the power of doing things, of accomplishment, of putting theory in practice. Talking about the specific issue of diet, we are convinced that there is a need of a programmatic, systematic and massive activity to make feasible the spread of elemental concepts about the benefits of a prudent diet. In spite of a future refinement and improvement of certain concepts about the roles of given macronutrient and bioactive substances, about their mechanism of action, etc, we consider that there are so evident features that delays for their spreading would be nonsense.

Planning in the dietary area points to a primary prevention and the communication through the corresponding publicity plays a key role. The role of social communicators is pivotal: there is a need of knowing which people can be reached, how could be these people reached and what kind of messages should be transmitted to the target population. The intake of those dietary items which were mentioned in this book as potentially protective should be turned attractive and convincing at all ages, but with special emphasis in children and young people. The different economic capabilities of certain subgroups within a population should be also taken into account, in order to give them adequate and reasonable alternatives. On the other hand, and without excluding the latter phrase, we are also convinced that new risk populations or risk subgroups should be redefined – at least, an attempt is worthwhile – in order to propose more intense and better defined actions for them, compared to the general population. The physician can become a very useful information

A.L. Ronco and E. De Stéfani, *Nutritional Epidemiology of Breast Cancer*,
DOI 10.1007/978-94-007-2397-9_18, © Springer Science+Business Media B.V. 2012

vector, from the office as a center of knowledge spreading, recognizing the small scale that each patient and her family nucleus represent.

The strategies designed to minimize the cancer risks, besides, usually cover a wide population range. Occasionally it is recognized that the target group could be more limited and better defined. We have widely talked about this in the chapter of Secondary Prevention and it has been our research priority during some years we have worked on the area. The main idea was to have in the future superspecific preventive guidelines to be given to those persons who request them. In other words, the hope was – and it still is – to achieve a "tailored" prevention projected on the basis of an individual risk profile.

Around a decade ago, European proposed something similar in the issue of July/2001 of the European Journal of Cancer, through the Brussels Statement promoted by the European Coalition of Breast Cancer [1]. The 4th point stated that "The Conference encourages the researchers to identify a standardised risk assessment methodology suitable for European women", in order to facilitate the research in preventive measures such as, for example, innovative lifestyle modifications and others. In those years, at the end of the 90's (advancing at least two years the Europeans' initiative) and also at the beginning of the current century, our main objective was the preselection of possible patients with higher risk of having a BC, through a novel methodology that used artificial intelligence programs and whose results gave a good base – obviously needing to be improved and refined – for it practical application. What for the preselection? For example and as basic tasks, in order to make mammograms with more frequent periodicity than for general population, and to give preventive nutritional advice. A woman would receive information allowing her to reduce her risks and at the same time she could be recommended to have a different frequency of radiology exams. This latter would reduce the potential role of the "window period" between consecutive mammograms. This basic strategy led us to think that it was somehow advanced to its time and to its place.

Different studies on the supplementation of several substances have demonstrated that carcinogenesis can be inhibited through the intake of a variety of chemical products in the diet which are nutrient and non nutrients. An inhibition of tumorigenesis through the blockage of carcinogen activation was observed, as well as through antioxidant and antiproliferative activity, in order to mention common examples. Nevertheless, experimental studies in animals have helped us, on one hand, to understand the possible actions of dietary components in the modulation of carcinogenesis, but on the other hand we should be cautious about extrapolating to humans the information obtained from animal studies. Important differences have been seen between the metabolism of carcinogens in animals and humans. In addition, several experimental studies have used high doses of "preventive" products to be analyzed, and we do not always know whether the doses used in such products could be effective in humans (due to low levels), or if they could be toxic (due to high levels or a prolonged intake). Hence, the use of combinations of several preventive agents which are "softer" or tolerable would be a ***more practical*** approach for the prevention of cancer in general population. This is a reality when a more frequent intake of fruits and vegetables, for example, is proposed as a simple initial measure to reduce in the future the cancer rates.

We have already mentioned that some researchers of the developed World have demonstrated the efficacy of a multimodal approach of the problem, through telephone counsel, informative reunions, periodic bulletins and cooking classes [2], achieving some changes in the dietary habits of women who were previously treated because of having a BC diagnosed. It seems that a strategy should be developed following this path and not through isolated and uncoordinated impulses.

We are facing some paradigms which can be followed and developed and adapted to the own profile of each population and its culture and customs. It has been already demonstrated that an intervention with exercises and diet in patients with BC under chemotherapy ***is something feasible*** [3]. In particular, diet was able to improve quality of life in BC patients, mentally as well as physically [4]. Regarding all these facts, there is a change of mind that should be operating in us but as a society and not only in the patients.

Anyway, one must recognize that some of these points correspond to be managed by specialists in Public Health and authorities of the healthcare systems. They also are part of that society who needs to open its mind to the acquisition of new elements (and not always expensive ones) in order to improve the results, before and after the disease. Undoubtedly, the idea of health authorities promoting diet and exercise in institutions admitting patients afflicted with BC sounds somehow strange. The World has still not reached that and the underdeveloped societies even lesser. We think that it is not always a matter of extraordinary financial resources to account with in order to achieve certain goals. Sometimes, the will and coordination operating together are those who achieve them.

We want to emphasize, anyway, the positive role of spreading at a reduced scale that each woman can have beginning from her own family group. We have already mentioned the idea of ***transgenerational prevention***. It is of utmost importance. But we must consider the whole family core, including the husband or partner, together with children, also expanding the influence to siblings and their husbands and wives, when they are present. We can think about some features of the nutritional counseling: it is cheap, relatively easy and it could reach the 100% of women. In addition, from a practical viewpoint and also from the viewpoint of the health impact, it appears as more attractive the risk reduction in 1/3 in the 100% of women than a risk reduction of 2/3 in a selected high-risk group, perhaps a 10% of women. If secondary prevention is advancing one step before the disease, you Doctor, Nutritionist or health professional can advance another step with primary prevention.

Probably some time will be needed to have a consensus about a general dietary strategy for primary prevention of BC. In order to cover the largest fraction of population, we must restrict some aspects which at the individual level might be adequate, because variability among populations is high. Despite some exceptions (i.e. at a genetic level) we can manage a general concept that **physiology is similar among women from different continents and countries, but environmental factors are not**. In particular diet, the most important one, it is not. Some dietary patterns which are country-specific or even region-specific are being recognized, and this point has been analyzed in the corresponding chapter. It sounds as logic, besides, that there are not too much common features between some Spanish and Scandinavian populations, for example. We expect to find some similarities in the observations on the menstrual and reproductive history, which were performed in women of different parts of the World. However, we cannot expect such similarity for a possible role of diet, due to the important differences that currently exist between Western and Eastern societies, between South and North, between rich and poor populations, between literate and illiterate women. That is why migrants studies have been so useful and why so remarkable differences of incidence exist in the World.

When doing these considerations, it seems almost inevitable that a reflection arises: if environmental factors are the main ones which condition the genesis of BC, and if those identified environmental factors differ so much among populations, then, how can we imagine that any environmental factor be applied to any population at any place, in order to reduce the impact of the disease? Moreover, if diet is the most important of those environmental factors, how we will do in order to apply a dietary factor which is important within a given population in other very different population? There is a risk that its application might not be useful. The environmental factors are not all universal: this is a concept we should thoroughly think about. Some of them (i.e. a high intake of red meat exposed to direct heat) fulfil that requisite and the evidence collaborates in such sense. But on the contrary, since diets are complex because they are composed by several ingredients and in different proportions, it is not likely that the same occurs with all those ingredients. We should admit the possibility of varieties for each population.

The scientific literature generated in the last years, guides towards a reinforcement of the idea of risk and prevention individuality [5]. It makes nonsense to insist about proposing a simple low-fat diet. The absolute amount of dietary fat is not a major problem, but a qualitative one. There are some fats that increase the risk if their intake is excessive and there are other fats whose insufficient intake becomes a risk for the disease (i.e. the omega-3 PUFAs). It should be taken into account that an inadequate reduction of certain fats means a deprivation of liposoluble vitamins (A,D,E,K), which could represent health problems. Just as it usually happens in all scientific fields, along time we were obliged to accept that the facts probably were not such as the initial evidence suggested. Fat-rich diets were associated with a higher incidence of BC in animal experimental studies; the studies analyzing correlation between the fat disappearance in the market and the incidence rates of the disease showed that those populations who were more exposed to fat intake displayed more BC; nevertheless, the cohort studies did not evidence a higher risk for total fat intake.

Besides, it is not either convenient to simplify reducing the fat intake, just as a magic solution. If fat percentage falls from a 50% to a 25%, the respective carbohydrate and protein percentages increase automatically. For example, we cannot considerably raise the carbohydrate proportion without leading to an excess which probably derive into a hyperinsulinism. The energy cannot be given mainly based on fruits and vegetables. We should moderate the proportions of carbohydrates and proteins, in order to slow down their absorption without producing insulin peaks, which would be potentially harmful if they are systematically repeated. In this sense, we consider a very good choice that proposed by B. Sears [6], who talks about moderate proportions in carbohydrates, proteins and fats. Aside from these similar proportions, eating proteinic foods (i.e. meats, dairy) together with carbohydrates would be recommendable, since the latter can have a slower absorption and determine a slower insulin release by the pancreas, together with glucagon release by this organ. With that aim, the recommendation of eating every 4–5 h if possible before having the appetite sensation (such as diabetic people), is excellent and well supported.

It was necessary to refine the epidemiologic research to begin finding what was beyond total fat: some of the fat subtypes have influence in one sense and some other subtypes in the opposite sense. We remark that although physiology is essentially similar among persons, biology shows individual differences: there are people who respond with differences of intensity but in the same sense, when they are exposed to a given agent. In other words, there will be women in whom a given exposure to certain fats will be harmful and others in whom completely neutral. In the same way, it is already known how there are women who process faster and women who process slower the heterocyclic amines produced in the cooking process of fried or barbecued meat. These differences, depending on certain gene polymorphisms, increase the probability that some of them be afflicted by mammary carcinogenesis and others will not, because their organisms achieve sooner or later the detoxification of the quoted substances [7].

This does not mean that we are obliged to manage only a limited group of general recommendations. Regarding that nutrition has an important local and regional value, if risk and protective factors are identified at a local or regional level, we can count on a wider spectrum for recommendations to general population. We need to emphasize again that: since physiology is universal, recommendations on a physiological basis have universal application. But on the contrary, ***since diet is local or regional, nutrition-based recommendations might have potential application at a local or regional level***. They could be restricted concerning their universality, but increase their useful value at a national or regional scale.

What kind of potential usefulness would have in Scandinavian women the intake of a "stew" – a potentially protective way of cooking meat among Uruguayan population –, being prepared just as in Uruguay or Argentina? Perhaps they could manage a new and different choice of meat preparation, but, what about the meat types, the vegetables features, for example? In the Scandinavian geographic and socio-demographic context, with extreme cold weather, lower vitamin D synthesis, low birth rates, etc, what is to be expected? We do not have answers to these questions, especially when several years of exposure are needed. The modality of stewed meat could be protective within the Rio de la Plata way of life, but we do not have certainty that its apparently protective association could be extrapolated to places located so far in the World.

We ignore the hormonal receptors level of each woman (assumed as normal) and there is still lack of evidence that may lead us towards the nutritional style for a woman with very positive estrogen receptors or for a woman with negative receptors.

We are based only on data from those who have been surgically operated and their information was obtained from the pathologist who analyzed the corresponding tissues. When mentioning the hormonal receptors, recommendations are supported mainly on a logic criterium and the biologic plausibility. If for example, no protective effect from fruit intake is found in a studied population (some studies on BC reported this fact), enhancing the fruit consumption with the expectation of reducing the risk of the disease does not seem much reasonable. Obviously, the positive contributions of fruits cannot be denied, and one cannot avoid recommending their intake, since it is feasible that they actually are protective against several other possible diseases. On the contrary, we have already confirmed again and again that the intake of citrus fruits is relevant concerning their protective role against BC among the Uruguayan women. After this confirmation, we recommend a high intake of those fruits, despite large international studies have not found the same results. Citrus fruits are worthy for the Uruguayan woman within their dietary frame, and that is enough for us. We repeat again the concept to the reader: from now on, we should be accepting the local or regional value of foods, looking for a good health.

The reader might have wondered once or more, what will be the right concept when one report communicates that a given food reduces the chances to develop the disease and other paper says that such food does not reduce nor increases the chance of developing a disease. Those who are accustomed to epidemiologic words and to investigate in this field, will not feel strange. It is convenient to express it in other words. All this has to do with evidence: the concepts in scientific research are perfectible and the evidence accumulates in one or in other sense. Since there are no final questions, there are neither definite answers. While evidence is getting bigger in one sense more than in the other, we begin to accept that an event is more likely to occur the higher is the exposure to a factor. This fact, which is true in groups, does not occur always in individuals.

References

1. Piccart M, Cataliotti L, Buchanan M et al (2001) Brussels Statement document. Eur J Cancer 37(11):1335–1337
2. Newman VA, Thomson CA, Rock CL et al (2005) Achieving substantial changes in eating behavior among women previously treated for breast cancer – an overview of the intervention. J Am Diet Assoc 105(3):382–391
3. Demark-Wahnefried W, Kenyon AJ, Eberle P et al (2002) Preventing sarcopenic obesity among breast cancer patients who receive adjuvant chemotherapy: results of a feasibility study. Clin Exerc Physiol 4(1):44–49
4. Wayne SJ, Baumgartner K, Baumgartner RN et al (2006) Diet quality is directly associated with quality of life in breast cancer survivors. Breast Cancer Res Treat 96(3):227–232
5. Hanf V, Gonder U (2005) Nutrition and primary prevention of breast cancer: foods, nutrients and breast cancer risk. Eur J Obstet Gynecol Reprod Biol 123:139–149
6. Sears B (2005) En la zona con omega 3 Rx. Ediciones Urano, Barcelona
7. Ambrosone CB, Freudenheim JL, Sinha R et al (1998) Breast cancer risk, meat consumption and N-acetyltransferase (NAT2) genetic polymorphisms. Int J Cancer 75(6):825–830

Chapter 19
Development of an Individual Prevention Tool: The Breast Cancer Risk Profile

Summary

In order to give personalized preventive recommendations, on a basis of country-specific research findings and putative risk and protective factors which are mostly modifiable, we developed an individual risk profile report oriented to lower the woman's risk level of breast cancer as much as possible. The available data are requested through a thorough questionnaire on sociodemographics, family history of cancers, reproductive history, diet, lifestyle and occupation, completed with a detailed anthropometric assessment, which allows calculation of body composition and somatotype. Additional information is obtained from non-clinical tests as mammography and selected laboratory results. A series of 20 items – which includes family history of cancer; reproductive factors; intake of: red meat, white meat, dairy foods, oils and fats, high glycemic load foods, vegetables and fruits; alcohol consumption; physical activity; psychosocial stressors; metabolic disturbances; other medical factors; fat-to-muscle ratio; serum vitamin D level; urine 2:16 α-OH estrogens ratio; serum triglycerides/HDL ratio; fasting insulinemia, and mammographic density – is taken into account to compose a tailored risk profile, which enables us to give the patient a number of useful guidelines. Patients should undergo a follow-up during a minimum time of 1 year, with the aim of checking whether the expected changes are having place or not. Although generalizability of the proposal is limited in the case by populational features of Uruguayan women, it is feasible from a practical viewpoint, taking into account the necessary resources for its application.

Background

Along the last decades, scientific literature on BC has consistently stated the convenience and need of more personalized preventive strategies. Concerning secondary prevention, the low benefit/cost ratio of mass screenings led to some

A.L. Ronco and E. De Stéfani, *Nutritional Epidemiology of Breast Cancer*,
DOI 10.1007/978-94-007-2397-9_19,

researchers to test selective screenings [1–9], with the aim of improving such ratio, but those strategies usually failed at the same point: many "false negatives", which preclude any strong impact on public health. When such attempts are analyzed in detail, it can be appreciated that only a few variables had been used as classificators.

In this sense, the Gail-Constantino method [10, 11] was an interesting proposal for risk prediction, but it can be argued that non-white and non-American women as well others with different environmental or ethnical factors could not receive the benefit of its classification capabilities.

Other proposals like the one of Djordjevic [12, 13], using an arithmetic score based on 27 variables, and ours [14–17], using artificial neural networks models working with 30–55 variables – related to socio-demographics, family history of cancer, reproductive history, dietary history and lifestyle –, led us to think that whereas with few classificatory variables we were able to work at a population level, we could operate at an individual level only working with a large number of them [18]. Nevertheless, its practical application was difficult due to its own complexity and length.

Instead of assessing complex individual risks for further classification to be used in secondary prevention, a multifactorial disease as BC gives the chance to design a simple but complete report based on the main risk factors destined to preventive guidelines. After having identified the principal risk and protective factors for BC among Uruguayan women [19], we developed such type of report, which is currently in a pilot phase, and one of the objectives of this chapter is to communicate is to present its background and features. The first communication about the Breast Cancer Risk Profile (BCRP) was done within a recent international congress [20].

2/16 α-OH Estrogens Ratio

Although there is still controversy about it, the 2 α-OH estrogens have been considered as "good" ones and the 16α-OH estrogens as "bad" [21]. Experimental and clinical evidence suggests that 16 α-OH estrogen metabolites, biologically strong estrogens, are associated with BC risk, while 2 α-OH metabolites, with lower estrogenic activity, are weakly related to this disease [22–26]. So, Women who metabolize a large proportion of their estrogen via the 16 α-hydroxylation pathway could be at a higher risk of BC [27]. Body composition was associated with 2 α-OHE1 and 16 α-OHE1 levels: while thicker skinfolds were associated with higher 16-α OH levels [28], an increase in lean body mass was associated with an improvement in 2/16 α -OHE1 ratio [29]. It has been suggested that women at higher risk for developing BC because of low 2/16 ratio may reduce their risk by participating in lifestyle interventions such as exercise/calorie restriction [30].

Vitamin D

Currently, substantial epidemiologic and experimental data support a role for vitamin D in cancer prevention, despite of some inconclusive evidence [31, 32]. On the basis of ecologic correlations of BC incidence rates [33] or BC mortality rates and solar radiation exposure levels [34, 35] it has been suggested that a lack of sun exposure, which would mean a deficiency of vitamin D, could be a risk factor for BC. According to a recent pooled analysis, intake of 2000 IU/day of Vitamin D3 and a very moderate exposure to sunlight, could raise serum 25(OH)D to 52 ng/ml, a level associated with reduction by 50% in incidence of BC [36]. The original study of Thomas et al. [37] reported a large proportion of hypovitaminosis D found in an American general hospital in population. Besides, preliminary results of a pilot study on measurement of serum vitamin D in healthy young adults performed some years ago in Uruguay [38] revealed a high frequency of hypovitaminosis D in the studied sample. Also, a recent study on postmenopausal women reported a seasonal variation of plasmatic vitamin D levels, with maximal values in summer and minimal ones in winter [39]. Also, considering that human breast cells have vitamin D receptors, there is a biologically plausible basis for the hypothesis that vitamin D can contribute to protect against BC [40].

Triglycerides/HDL Ratio Hypertension, Diabetes, Insulin Resistance

The incidence of BC in the Western world runs parallel to that of the major components of the insulin resistance syndrome: hyperinsulinemia, dyslipidemia, hypertension, obesity and atherosclerosis. The literature has already recognized possible roles for hypertension, obesity, increased levels of insulin and Insulin-like Growth Factor I in the risk of BC [41–43], mainly among postmenopausal women. Women with abdominal obesity exhibit evidence of insulin resistance and hyperinsulinemia [44]. The metabolic syndrome, which is characterized by visceral obesity, glucose intolerance, hypertension, and dyslipidemia (low serum high-density lipoprotein cholesterol HDL-C and high serum triglycerides), has a high and increasing prevalence in parallel with increasing BC incidence worldwide [45]. There is evidence that the growth of BC is favoured by specific dietary fatty acids, visceral fat accumulation and inadequate physical exercise, all of which are thought to interact in favouring the development of the insulin resistance syndrome [41]. Obesity increases the risk of vitamin D deficiency [46]. Once vitamin D is synthesized in the skin or ingested, it is deposited in body fat stores, making it less bioavailable to subjects having large of such fat stores.

Psychosocial Stress

Stress, mood, emotions, social support are among the main psychological variables whose relationships with BC have been studied [47, 48] Among psychological variables that can influence on the course of cancer are grief, desperation, depression and abandonment. But for other factors, literature still remains inconsistent [49–52]. Psychological stress, generated by desperate circumstances, very demanding tasks or the lack of social support is possible to be harmful for health [53]. The hypothesis on which this is based states that both chronic and acute stressing factors alter the susceptibility of the host or even they become directly pathogenic as they affect neuroendocrine functions [54]. Animal experimentation had shown that psychosocial factors can influence on tumor evolution [55]. Furthermore, psychological factors were even postulated as promoters of cancer development [56]. We have recently published some results that support the existence of certain associations of different psychosocial aspects and the risk of BC. Significant increases in risk were associated with dissatisfaction from social status, from friends' relationships, from job/profession and also from received education [57]. A borderline two-fold increase in risk was also observed for the occurrence of a first traumatic episode since age 50. Other sources of dissatisfaction or stressful events have tended to display non significant increases in risk or lack of association. No potential stressor was found negatively associated, in the sense of a protective effect.

Anthropometric Assessments

A positive association of central adiposity with postmenopausal BC risk and also a weaker association for pre-menopausal women were found in some studies [58–65]. Our results show that certain body measurements are associated with BC risk in the analyzed population, despite of menopausal status and BMI level [66–68]. In our studies on body composition and somatotype, the highest quartiles of the fat amount, the fat percentage and the endomorphism showed significant risk increases of BC, whereas the ectomorphism was borderline associated. On the other hand, muscle weight and fraction were always inversely associated to the risk of BC. After having found an increase of risk with high adipose amount and fraction, as well as with a slender or round body type, strong linear trends, and biological plausibility for the associations, we proposed that the body fat through its 3 components (amount, fraction and distribution) might be independent risk factors for the studied population.

Methodology Features

A review of updated specialized literature on BC risk factors and an analysis of the Uruguayan epidemiologic studies on BC [18, 19, 69] were performed. The questionnaire that has been used for the local studies has been tested for reproducibility with good results [70] and is the base for requesting information to patients. It includes a food frequency questionnaire (FFQ) with 120 items; a complete history of tobacco, alcohol and *mate* consumption; a complete menstrual and reproductive history; a detailed family history of cancers; some selected items on metabolic disturbances (history of hypertension, diabetes, hypercholesterolemia, hypertriglyceridemia, gall bladder lithiasis and hyperuricemia); a socio-demographic section. We added queries on psychosocial stressors from an adapted questionnaire used a few years ago [57] and also a complete series of anthropometric measures involved in recent studies, which enables us to calculate body composition and somatotype [66, 67].

Anthropometry equipment includes a height scale and headboard. For body measurements a plastic centimeter at intervals of 0.5 cm (circumferences), a vernier caliper (diameters) and a skinfold caliper (skinfolds) are used. Subjects are weighed wearing minimal clothing. If two consecutive measurements are similar, the obtained value is registered as valid. If both are different (± 1 mm for skinfolds and diameters, ± 0,5 cm for circumferences), a third one is taken and the median value is then registered. Measurements are performed according to Carter's Instruction Manual [71].

The questionnaire is administered to each patient in person by a trained nurse. Questions and anthropometric measurements require around 1 hour of time and are performed at the medical office.

The 20 items that were used to build the BCRP – including their categories of high-risk- were the following:

1. Menstrual-reproductive factors (menarche < age 12, nulliparity, first delivery after age 30, no breastfeeding, menopause > age 55)
2. Family history of cancer (sister with BC at age < 48; mother with BC at age < 55; mother + sister with BC and/or ovary cancer (any age)); >1 sister with BC (any age); father with BC; mother + aunt with BC and/or ovary cancer (any age); sister + aunt with BC (any age); sister or mother with ovary cancer; grandmother + mother with BC and/or ovary cancer (any age)
3. Red meat intake (beef, barbecue, fried meat >3 times/week)
4. White meat intake (not fried fish <1 time/week; fried fish; chicken with skin/fried)
5. Fruit intake (orange, tangerine, orange juice <3 units/week; non citrus fruits < 3 units/week)
6. Vegetable intake (tomato <2 units/week; lentils, beans <1 time/week; cauliflower, broccoli, cabbage <1time /week; green leaf vegetables <2 times/week)
7. Dairy foods (whole milk, fatty cheeses >4 times/week; cream, caramel > 1 time/week; yoghurt, ricotta cheese < 2)
8. Oils and fats (sunflower or soy oil >4 times/week; eggs, mayonnaise >3 times/week; snacks like French fries >2 times/week; no olive oil intake)
9. High glycemic load foods (white sugar, custard, dessert, marmalade > 1 time/day; pasta >3 times/week; white bread, cakes, other bakery products >1 time/day; soft drinks with sugar > 1 small bottle/day)
10. Anthropometric features (fat >27%; muscle <38%; fat/muscle ratio >1.7; body mass index >30 kg/m2)

Table 19.1 Selected cutoff points used for classification in the risk profile report

Variable	Low risk	Medium risk	High risk
2/16 αOH-estrogen ratio	>2	1.7–2	<1.7
Triglycerides/HDL ratio	<2	2–4	>4
Serum vitamin D level (ng/ml)	>40	30–40	<30
Fasting insulinemia (μU/ml)	<10	10–15	>15
Anthropometry (fat/muscle ratio)	<1.2	1.2–1.8	>1.8

11. Physical activity for leisure (<2 times/week)
12. Other medical items (thyroid diseases, polycystic ovary syndrome, hypertension, benign breast diseases)
13. Triglycerides/HDL ratio (according to Table)
14. 2/16 α-OH estrogens ratio (according to Table)
15. Serum vitamin D level (according to Table)
16. Fasting insulinemia (according to Table)
17. Metabolic disturbances (dislypidemia, hyperuricemia, diabetes)
18. Psychosocial stress (dissatisfaction from social status, friends relationships, job/profession and received education; traumatic episode that changed life for >2 weeks)
19. Alcohol consumption (beer, hard liquor >2 times/week)
20. Mammographic density (according to Table)

In order to classify each item, we established the following criterium: Variables were divided into tertiles, according to the controls' distribution, that means, the reference is the normal population. The assignment of a low, medium and high risk value was done depending on the variable nature and its association to the risk of BC. Some variables (dietary, anthropometric) were divided according to such criterium. Therefore, a low value of red meat consumption leads to classify this item as "low risk" but if it describes the intake of citrical fruits, it would classify this latter as "high risk". Other variables (laboratory tests, mammographic density, family history of cancer) allow a classification based on known cutoff points. Table 19.1 summarizes the cutoff points used for classification in this latter group. A third group of variables (menstrual-reproductive, psychosocial stress, other medical factors) requires a subjective and thorough procedure for combining several items, based on the knowledge of them.

The report consists of an initial sheet including the 20 selected areas (Fig. 19.1), each one of which has an established risk classification level that is fulfilled according the previously described criteria. The right cell of each item is completed with a cross or tick. Then, additional sheets including recommendations according to each analyzed item complete the report. A detailed anthropometric description is displayed, which can be compared with future assessments.

Patient: Date:

		LOW	MED	HIGH
Classic factors	Menstrual-reproductive			
	Family history of cancer			
Dietary factors	Red meat intake			
	White meat intake			
	Fruit intake			
	Vegetable intake			
	Dairy foods			
	Oils and fats			
	High glycemic load foods			
Medical factors	Anthropometric features			
	Physical activity			
	Other medical items			
	Triglycerides/HDL ratio			
	2/16 α-OH estrogens ratio			
	Serum vitamin D level			
	Fasting insulinemia			
Other factors	Psychosocial stress			
	Tobacco smoking			
	Alcohol drinking			
	Mammographic density			

Fig. 19.1 Sheet features of the risk profile

Breast Cancer Risk Profile

The proposed strategy does not imply to consider or discard well-known intervention measures like prophylactic mastectomy or chemoprevention, but it is actually focused on modifying several modifiable factors – mainly related to nutrition and lifestyle – in a tailored way. A high-risk category could be assigned based mainly on nutritional, metabolic or anthropometric features, even in the absence of classic risk factors. We have already recognized some years ago [17] that the nutritional profile might be considered as a potential risk profile of populations and individual subjects.

Currently, scientific evidence coming from basic experimental, epidemiologic or clinical research enables us to consider BC as a complex hormonal, metabolic and also immune problem. Although hormones have been recognized for long time as the core of the problem, recently the 2:16 α-OH estrogens ratio has been suggested as an independent risk factor [72], which is particularly influenced by diet, anthropometric features, lifestyle and genetics.

For pure primary prevention and also for prevention of BC recurrence, we think that there is a great potential of impact on the cancer risk through the management of the levels of "good" (2 α-OH) and "bad" (16 α-OH) estrogens. This can be achieved by correcting the current levels of some selected items. Even though it is not acceptable the idea of an only cure or preventive measure for BC, the fact that several measures have convergence on the control of amount and quality of estrogens, is something we can take profit of.

Besides, periodically monitoring markers like the 2/16 α-OH estrogen ratio, the serum vitamin D level, the triglycerides/HDL cholesterol ratio and the fasting insulinemia, allows us to know about the background metabolic-hormonal condition of the woman's body. If the patient is a cancer patient, we are offering her complementary surveillance to that performed by the Oncologist or the Mastologist. These specialists usually perform a follow-up mainly based on tomography, scintigraphy and cancer biomarkers together with a clinical examination. While they are looking for any cancer signals, we are looking for certain signals which can reflect a physical conditioning favourable or not to cancer. Hormonal and metabolic profiles suggest a potential role for the Endocrinologist in the management of patients, perhaps in such a way it might has not been thought previously.

Years ago, an ELISA method was available for direct measurement of the sum of 2-OHE1 and 2-OHE2 metabolites and of 16α-OHE1 [73]. It was accepted that the value of the 2/16α ratio in a single urine sample reflects reasonably well an individual's level of the biomarker over a 2 month period [74]. For urine specimens a reference limit of>2.0 is generally used for the 2α-OHE1/16α-OHE1 ratio measured by the ELISA method, and this can derive into the concept that people with 2/16α ratio values below 2.0 should be advised of measures that can stimulate 2-hydroxylation [72].

It is important to remark that the recommendations derived from the BCRP are aligned with the established therapies. There is no potential conflict. Furthermore, the scientific evidence brings us support in the sense that one of the main objectives to reach through the BCRP is the quantitative and qualitative change of endogenous estrogens – mainly the achievement and maintenance of an adequate 2/16 α-OH estrogens ratio-. To our knowledge, this is a core zone of the BC problem, to which there is a convergence of several lines (e.g. reproductive, dietary, anthropometric, environmental).

Some limitations of the method are to be recognized. First, the collected information takes into account local or regional data, which were thoroughly obtained through case-control studies. This fact limits generalizability of the procedure, since some items that are country-specific (diet, anthropometry) cannot be extrapolated elsewhere. Each country or region should construct its own reference values. Second, also related to this latter, appropriate cut-off points could be assigned only for some laboratory results, but neither for dietary intakes nor for anthropometric results or for psychosocial stressors, provided they all might represent population-specific features. Third, the risk category assignment of certain items is arbitrarily performed, albeit it is done on a basis of knowledge derived from the specific studies.

Whereas values obtained from laboratory tests lead to a quantitative classification, nutritional and other items allow us to perform mostly qualitative estimations.

Additional questions arise from the proposed strategy. One of them is referred to the opportunity for the recommended changes derived from the BCRP. In asymptomatic women, we are not able to express a risk reduction in terms of time requirements for such reduction. Albeit it is reasonable to accept that every woman can benefit herself from major nutritional and lifestyle changes, it is also easy to suppose that the potential impact on BC risk would be stronger, the earlier those changes take place. We could move backward in time, recognizing that during childhood it would be good and during life in utero perhaps it would be the best period for a new style.

Other question refers to the individual degree of proposed guidelines. We should recognize that the knowledge basis was achieved on epidemiologic studies involving certain population groups. So, each subject who is interviewed and measured through the BCRP shares some features with other different subjects, but an assumption of a given risk or protective level is still merely speculative. In a future, the results of nutrigenetics and nutrigenomics perhaps will clarify these points, but in the meantime, we must deal with some degree of uncertainty.

In conclusion, we described the background and features of the so-called BCRP report, which intends to become an individual preventive tool and is still in a pilot phase of development. The report is based on 20 items, most of which were selected from relevant data coming from local case-control studies. Although generalizability is limited by this local value of certain variables, methodology seems to be feasible elsewhere from a practical viewpoint.

References

1. Dunn JE (1969) Epidemiology and possible identification of high-risk groups that could develop cancer of the breast. Cancer 23:775–780
2. Fournier D, Kuttig H, Müller A et al (1977) Brustkrebsfrüherkennung: Kontrolle von Risikogruppen oder Massescreening – wer soll geröntgt werden? Med Welt 28:359–363
3. Soini I, Hakama M (1978) Failure of selective screening for breast cancer by combining risk factors. Int J Cancer 22:275–281
4. Toti A, Piffanelli A, Pavanelli CN et al (1980) Possible indication of breast cancer risk through discriminant functions. Cancer 46(5):1280–1285
5. Seidman H, Stellman SD, Mushinski MH (1982) A different perspective on breast cancer risk factors: some implications of the nonattributable risk. CA Cancer J Clin 32(5):301–313
6. Schechter MT, Miller AB, Baines CJ et al (1986) Selection of women at high risk of breast cancer for initial screening. J Chron Dis 39(4):253–260
7. Mettlin C (1994) The relationship of breast cancer epidemiology to screening recommendations. Cancer 74:228–230
8. Torner J, Fernández Martínez I, Granell J et al (1996) Screening masivo versus screening selectivo. Rev Senologia y Patol Mam 10(1):31–43
9. Chart PL, Franssen E (1997) Management of women at increased risk for breast cancer: preliminary results from a new program. CMAJ 157(9):1235–1242

10. Gail MH, Brinton LA, Byar DP et al (1989) Projecting individualized probabilities of developing breast cancer for white females who are being examined annually. J Natl Cancer Inst 81:1879–1886
11. Costantino JP, Gail MH, Pee D et al (1999) Validation studies for models projecting the risk of invasive and total breast cancer incidence. J Natl Cancer Inst 91:1541–1548
12. Djordjevic M, Vuletic L, Jovicevic-Bekic A et al (1994) Follow-up of risk groups for breast cancer 1990–2000. In: Sankaranarayanan R, Wahrendorf J, Demaret E (eds) Directory of on-going research in cancer epidemiology 1994, IARC Scientific Public. N° 130. International Agency for Research on Cancer, Lyon, p 510 (abstract 1242)
13. Djordjevic M, Babic M, Drecun V et al (1999) Results of the questionnaired selective screening for the breast cancer. In: Proceedings of the I conference on screening and early detection of cancer, Development of a European Strategy, Vienna, Abstract 9006, p 39
14. Ronco AL (1998) Evaluation of classificatory capabilities of an artificial neural network in search of breast cancer risk populations: a pilot study, X International congress of breast diseases, Oporto, 31/V–4/VI, 1998, The Breast J 4(Suppl 1):S22. Abstract No 120
15. Ronco AL (1999) Discriminating breast cancer high-risk individuals with artificial neural networks: a novel approach to selective screenings. In: Proceedings of the I conference on screening and early detection of cancer, Development of a European Strategy, Vienna, 18–19 Nov 1999, Abstract 9030, p 51
16. Ronco AL (1999) Use of artificial neural networks in modeling associations of discriminant factors: towards an intelligent selective breast cancer screening. Artif Intell Med 16(3):299–309
17. Ronco AL, De Stéfani E (1999) Role of classical and dietary discriminant factors for classification of breast cancer high-risk populations: a study with neural networks. Cancer Strategy 1:203–209
18. Ronco AL, De Stéfani E, Deneo-Pellegrini H (eds) (2008) Epidemiología Nutricional del Cáncer de Mama. Ed.de la Plaza, Montevideo
19. Ronco AL, De Stéfani E, Stoll M (2010) Hormonal and metabolic modulation through nutrition: towards a primary prevention of breast cancer. Breast 19:322–332
20. Ronco AL, Maisonneuve J, Stoll M, et al (2010) The breast cancer risk profile report: development of a personalized preventive tool. XVI World congress on breast diseases, Valencia, 20–22 Oct 2010
21. Bradlow HL, Telang NT, Sepkovic DW et al (1996) 2-hydroxyestrone: the "good" estrogen. J Endocrinol 150(Suppl):S259–S265
22. Kabat GC, Jen Chang C, Sparano JA et al (1997) Urinary estrogen metabolites and breast cancer: a case-control study. Cancer Epidemiol Biomarkers Prev 6:505–509
23. Ho GH, Luo XW, Ji CY et al (1998) Urinary 2/16α-hydroxyestrone ratio: correlation with serum insulin-like growth factor binding protein-3 and a potential biomarker of breast cancer risk. Ann Acad Med Singapore 27:294–299
24. Coker AL, Crane MM, Sticca RP et al (1997) Re: ethnic differences in estrogen metabolism in healthy women. J Natl Cancer Inst 89:89
25. Meilahn EN, De Stavola B, Allen DS et al (1998) Do urinary oestrogen metabolites predict breast cancer? Guernsey III cohort follow-up. Br J Cancer 78:1250–1255
26. Muti P, Bradlow HL, Micheli A et al (2000) Estrogen metabolism and risk of breast cancer: a prospective study of the 2:16alpha-hydroxyestrone ratio in premenopausal and postmenopausal women. Epidemiology 11(6):635–640
27. Cauley JA, Zmuda JM, Danielson ME et al (2003) Estrogen metabolites and the risk of breast cancer in older women. Epidemiology 14(6):740–744
28. Campbell KL, Westerlind KC, Harber VJ et al (2005) Associations between aerobic fitness and estrogen metabolites in premenopausal women. Med Sci Sports Exerc 37(4):585–592
29. Campbell KL, Westerlind KC, Harber VJ et al (2007) Effects of aerobic exercise training on estrogen metabolism in premenopausal women: a randomized controlled trial. Cancer Epidemiol Biomarkers Prev 16(4):731–739

30. Westerlind KC, Williams NI (2007) Effect of energy deficiency on estrogen metabolism in premenopausal women. Med Sci Sports Exerc 39(7):1090–1097
31. Garland CF, Garland FC, Gorham ED et al (2006) The role of vitamin D in cancer prevention. Am J Public Health 96(2):252–261
32. Cui Y, Rohan TE (2006) Vitamin D, calcium, and breast cancer risk: a review. Cancer Epidemiol Biomarkers Prev 15(8):1427–1437
33. Gorham ED, Garland FC, Garland CF (1990) Sunlight and breast cancer incidence in the USSR. Int J Epidemiol 19(4):820–824
34. Gorham ED, Garland CF, Garland FC (1989) Acid haze air pollution and breast and colon cancer mortality in 20 Canadian cities. Can Public Health 80:96–100
35. Garland FC, Garland CF, Gorham ED et al (1990) Geographic variation in breast cancer mortality in the United States: a hypothesis involving exposure to solar radiation. Prev Med 19:614–622
36. Garland CF, Gorham ED, Mohr SB et al (2007) Vitamin D and prevention of breast cancer: pooled analysis. J Steroid Biochem Mol Biol 103(3–5):708–711
37. Thomas MK, Lloyd-Jones DM, Thadhani RI et al (1998) Hypovitaminosis D in medical inpatients. N Engl J Med 338(12):777–783
38. Mendoza B, Ronco AL (2001) Importancia de los niveles séricos de vitamina D-3. Tendencias 9(18):97–101
39. Mendoza B, Ronco AL, Mintegui G et al (2006) Serum vitamin D status among postmenopausal Uruguayan women. In: Proceedings of the international osteoporosis foundation world congress, Toronto, 2–6th June 2006, Abstract p704su, p S208
40. Mendoza BA, Ronco AL (2007) Vitamin D and breast cancer: a short review. Biomedicina 2(3):139–148
41. Stoll BA (1999) Western nutrition and the insulin resistance syndrome: a link to breast cancer. Eur J Clin Nutr 53(2):83–87
42. Furberg AS, Veierod MB, Wilsgaard T (2004) Serum high-density lipoprotein cholesterol, metabolic profile, and breast cancer risk. J Natl Cancer Inst 96:1152–1160
43. Sinagra D, Amato C, Scarpilta AM (2002) Metabolic syndrome and breast cancer risk. Eur Rev Med Pharmacol Sci 6:55–59
44. Kissebah AH, Vydelingum N, Murray R et al (1982) Relation of body fat distribution to metabolic complications of obesity. J Clin Endocrinol Metab 54:254–260
45. International Agency for Research on Cancer (2002) Cancer preventive effects. In: Vainio H, Bianchini F (eds) Weight control and physical activity IARC. Handbooks of cancer prevention, vol 6. IARC Press, Lyon, pp 83–206
46. Arunabh S, Pollack S, Yeh J et al (2003) Body fat content and 25-hydroxyvitamin D levels in healthy women. J Clin Endocrinol Metab 88(1):157–161
47. LeShan L (1966) An emotional life history pattern associated with neoplastic disease. Ann NY Acad Sci 125:780–793
48. Hagnell O (1966) The premorbid personality of persons who develop cancer in a total population investigated in 1947 and 1957. Ann NY Acad Sci 125:846–855
49. Fox BH (1995) The role of psychological factors in cancer incidence and prognosis. Oncology (Huntingt) 9(3):245–253
50. Protheroe D, Turvey K, Horgan K et al (1999) Stressful life events and difficulties and onset of breast cancer: case-control study. BMJ 319(7216):1015–1016
51. Price MA, Tennant CC, Smith RC et al (2001) The role of psychosocial factors in the development of breast carcinoma: part I. The cancer prone personality. Cancer 91(4):679–685
52. Price MA, Tennant CC, Butow PN et al (2001) The role of psychosocial factors in the development of breast carcinoma: part II. Life event stressors, social support, defense style, and emotional control and their interactions. Cancer 91(4):686–697
53. Elstad JI (1998) The psycho-social perspective on social inequalities in health. In: Bartley M, Blane D, Davey Smith G (eds) The sociology of health inequalities. Blackwell, Oxford, pp 39–58

54. Krieger N (2001) Glossary of social epidemiology. J Epidemiol Community Health 55:693–700
55. Schell LM, Liebermann LS (1981) Noise stress and cancer. In: Bammer K, Newberry BH (eds) Stress and cancer. C.J.Hogrefe, Toronto
56. Greer S, Watson M (1985) Towards a psychobiological model of cancer: psychological considerations. Soc Sci Med 20(8):773–777
57. Ronco AL, Silveira S, De Stéfani E et al (2007) Sociocultural and psychologic factors and breast cancer: a case-control study in Montevideo, Uruguay. Biomedicina 1(3):6–17 (in Spanish)
58. Hall IJ, Newman B, Millikan RC et al (2000) Body size and breast cancer risk in black women and white women. The Carolina Breast Cancer Study. Am J Epidemiol 151:754–764
59. Shu XO, Jin F, Dai Q et al (2001) Association of body size and fat distribution with risk of breast cancer among Chinese women. Int J Cancer 94:449–455
60. Macinnis RJ, English DR, Gertig DM et al (2004) Body size and composition and risk of postmenopausal breast cancer. Cancer Epidemiol Biomarkers Prev 13:2117–2125
61. Lahmann PH, Hoffmann K, Allen N et al (2004) Body size and breast cancer risk: findings from the European Prospective Investigation into Cancer and Nutrition (EPIC). Int J Cancer 111:762–771
62. Chow LW, Lui KL, Chan JC et al (2005) Association between body mass index and risk of formation of breast cancer in Chinese women. Asian J Surg 28:179–184
63. Krebs EE, Taylor BC, Cauley JA et al (2006) Measures of adiposity and risk of breast cancer in older postmenopausal women. J Am Geriatr Soc 54:63–69
64. Okobia MN, Bunker CH, Zmuda JM et al (2006) Anthropometry and breast cancer risk in Nigerian women. Breast J 12:462–466
65. Wu AH, Yu MC, Tseng CC et al (2007) Body size, hormone therapy and risk of breast cancer in Asian-American women. Int J Cancer 120:844–852
66. Ronco AL, Mendoza B, Varas X et al (2008) Somatotype and risk of breast cancer: a case-control study in Uruguay. Braz J Epidemiol 11(2):215–227
67. Ronco AL, Boeing H, De Stéfani E et al (2009) A case-control study on fat to muscle ratio and risk of breast cancer. Nutr Cancer 61(4):466–474
68. Ronco AL, De Stéfani E (2010) Interrelationships between body composition and somatotype and the risk of breast cancer. XVI World congress on breast diseases, Valencia, 20–22 Oct 2010
69. World Cancer Research Fund/American Institute for Cancer Research (2007) Food, nutrition, physical activity, and the prevention of cancer: a global perspective. American Institute for Cancer Research, Washington, DC
70. Ronco AL, De Stefani E, Boffetta P et al (2006) Food patterns and risk of breast cancer: a factor analysis study in Uruguay. Int J Cancer 19:1672–1678
71. Carter JEL (2002) The Heath-Carter anthropometric somatotype – instruction manual. TeP and Rosscraft, Surrey
72. Lord RS, Bongiovanni B, Bralley JA (2002) Estrogen metabolism and the diet-cancer connection: rationale for assessing the ratio of urinary hydroxylated estrogen metabolites. Altern Med Rev 7(2):112–129
73. Klug I, Dressendorfer R, Strasburger C et al (2000) Cortisol and 17-hydroxyprogesterone levels in saliva of healthy neonates. normative data and relation to body mass index, arterial cord blood pH and time of sampling after birth. Biol Neonate 78:22–26
74. Chen Z, Zheng W, Dunning LM et al (1999) Within person variability of the ratios of urinary 2-hydroxyestrone to 16alpha-hydroxyestrone in Caucasian women. Steroids 64:856–859

Index

A.L. Ronco and E. De Stéfani, *Nutritional Epidemiology of Breast Cancer*,
DOI 10.1007/978-94-007-2397-9, © Springer Science+Business Media B.V. 2012